Training the Body to Cure Itself

Training the Body to Cure Itself

HOW TO USE EXERCISE TO HEAL

Edited by Alice Feinstein

By the Editors of **PREVENTION** Magazine Health Books

Doug Dollemore ❏ Sara J. Henry ❏ Marcia Holman ❏ Sid Kirchheimer
Gale Maleskey ❏ Hollis Paschen ❏ Joseph Wargo ❏ Pat Wittig

 Rodale Press, Emmaus, Pennsylvania

If you have any questions or comments concerning this book, please write:

>Rodale Press
>Book Readers' Service
>33 East Minor Street
>Emmaus, PA 18098

The illustration on page 9 was adapted from "Exercise and Nutrition in the Elderly," by William J. Evans, Ph.D., and Carol N. Meredith, *Nutrition, Aging and the Elderly,* edited by H. N. Munro and D. E. Danford (Plenum Publishing Corporation, 1989).

The illustration on page 162 was adapted from "Angiographically Demonstrated Arterial Spasm in a Case of Benign Sexual Headache and Benign Exertional Headache," by P. L. Silbert and associates, *Australian and New Zealand Journal of Medicine,* vol. 19, no. 5, 1989.

The box on jet lag on page 190 is reprinted from *Twirling & Jet Lag,* with permission from The Dawn Horse Press.

The exercises on page 483 were adapted from *Back Care Basics: A Doctor's Gentle Yoga Program for Back and Neck Pain Relief,* by Mary P. Schatz, M.D. (Rodmell Press, 1992).

Library of Congress Cataloging-in-Publication Data

Traning the body to cure itself : how to use exercise to heal / edited by Alice
    Feinstein ; by the editors of Prevention Magazine Health Books.
        p.   cm.
    Includes index.
    ISBN 0-87596-131-2   hardcover
    1. Exercise therapy.   I. Feinstein, Alice.   II. Prevention Magazine
Health Books.
RM725.T73   1992
615.8'2—dc20   92-13615
                                                CIP

Distributed in the book trade by St. Martin's Press

    4   6   8   10   9   7   5   hardcover

Notice

This book is intended as a reference volume only, not as a medical guide or manual for self-treatment. If you suspect that you have a medical problem, please seek competent medical care. The information here is designed to help you make informed decisions about your health. It is not intended as a substitute for any treatment prescribed by your doctor. Before beginning any exercise program, check with your doctor, who can help you design a program to meet your personal health needs.

Training the Body to Cure Itself

Managing Editor: Alice Feinstein

Editors of *Prevention* Magazine Health Books: Doug Dollemore, Sara J. Henry, Marcia Holman, Sid Kirchheimer, Gale Maleskey, Ellen Michaud, Hollis Paschen, Joseph Wargo, Pat Wittig

Other Contributors: Joe Barks, Paris Mihely-Muchanic, E. J. Muller, Jane Sherman, Porter Shimer

Research Chief: Ann Gossy

Illustration Coordinator: Paris Mihely-Muchanic

Research Staff: Christine Dreisbach, Melissa J. Dunford, Jewel Flegal, Anne Remondi Imhoff, Karen Lombardi, Cemela London, Melissa Meyers, Paris Mihely-Muchanic, Deborah J. Pedron, Bernadette M. Sukley, Michele Toth

Production Editor: Jane Sherman

Copy Editor: Barbara M. Webb

Indexer: Ed Yeager

Book and Cover Designer: Lynn N. Gano

Illustrator: Narda Lebo

Office Manager: Roberta Mulliner

Secretarial Staff: Julie Kehs, Mary Lou Stephen

Contents

Part II Exercise Therapies

Introduction: Get Moving for Better Health

Imagine before you a golden vial containing a miraculous elixir. A daily drop of this vital fluid confers upon you a more youthful appearance, while boosting your energy and enhancing your creative powers. Imagine that this precious substance alleviates pain, prevents disease, grants you euphoric waves of pleasure, and, used over time, can actually add years to your life.

Sounds like an exclusive new designer drug, right? Like maybe people would do anything to get their hands on it . . . travel to distant lands, spend fabulous sums of money, plead to be admitted to the select circle that has access to those golden drops.

Would you walk a mile for it? Every day?

Okay, you've seen the cover of this book. You know *Training the Body to Cure Itself* is about exercise—walking, running, bending, stretching, lifting weights, and so on. The "miraculous elixir" that I'm talking about is actually exercise in its various forms. And rather than "golden drops," the only liquid substance involved is sweat. The spectacular results promised are real, though. And, while they're free, you *will* have to work for them.

Ah, there's the rub . . . work. If you still think of exercise in terms of loud-mouthed, whistle-blowing gym teachers or arrogant athletes strutting their superior stuff, you may have a few surprises in store for you in the pages of this unique book. These days the work involved in exercising for health offers so many rewards that it's more than worth it. But what type of exercise should you do? How do you get started safely if you're out of shape? Exactly how hard will you have to work and what will it feel like? What kinds of results can you expect? You'll find the answers to these questions within these pages.

To create *Training the Body to Cure Itself,* the editors of *Prevention* Magazine Health Books talked to hundreds of doctors, medical researchers, and exercise experts throughout the nation about how the body benefits from the right kind of movement—the positive effects on each and every cell, the healing that takes place, the chemical and structural alterations in the body that enhance the ability to resist disease. These experts say that *everyone* can benefit from exercise. And they provide specific instructions on how to do so . . . and why.

Medical science finds out more amazing things about exercise every day. Just recently, for example, a study conducted at the University of Colorado at Boulder looked at 11 men and women aged 70 to 92. These elderly people—average age 80—spent six months in an exercise program that involved pumping iron. Under close supervision they lifted weights that for them were fairly heavy. By the end of the study all the participants showed considerable gains in balance and strength— some of the women more than doubled their strength in certain areas.

Think about what that means. We're not talking about building muscles that are going to make a person look better in a bathing suit (although exercise can certainly do that). In an older individual, strength and balance are the kinds of things that allow for continued independence—the physical attributes that make it possible to pick up a bag of groceries, get in and out of the car and up and down the stairs.

Doctors and researchers interviewed for this book said that among other things, exercise can help prevent heart disease, build strong bones, rev up your sex life, dispel arthritis pain, prevent back pain, preserve your memory, chase away the blues, and enhance your creativity. Written in a list like this, these kinds of claims sound almost unbelieveable, but these experts also came through with the kind of information that can help you reap these benefits for yourself. Part 1, Exercise Prescriptions, details the specific kinds of exercise to do for more than 50 common health problems. In many cases there are actual routines to follow, complete with illustrations and detailed instructions.

In almost every case, the experts also said, "Go for a walk." Perhaps that's not so surprising, considering what a perfectly natural exercise walking is. This is what they advised: Go for a regular walk, and if getting out in the fresh air and pumping your legs and swinging your arms doesn't quite satisfy you or hold your interest, find some other vigorous, repetitive activity, such as swimming or dancing or riding a bicycle. And do it often. And stick with it.

So many medical experts recommended this practice, for so many different conditions, that we created part 2, Exercise Therapies. This section is designed to help you get started on an appropriate exercise program, stay motivated, and make it a part of your life.

Training the Body to Cure Itself is all about one of nature's best medicines— movement. You were meant to move. Put your body in harmony with what it was created to do and you're on the road to a lifetime of good health. This book tells you how.

Alice Feinstein
Managing Editor
Prevention Magazine Health Books

Part I
Exercise Prescriptions

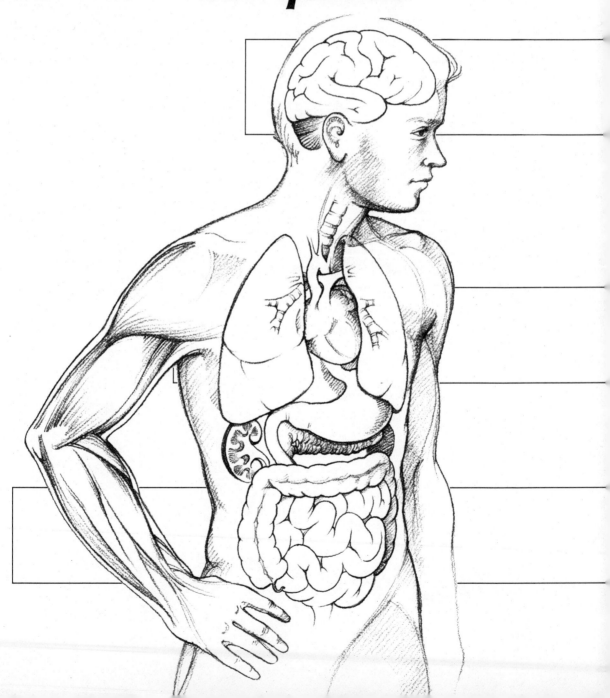

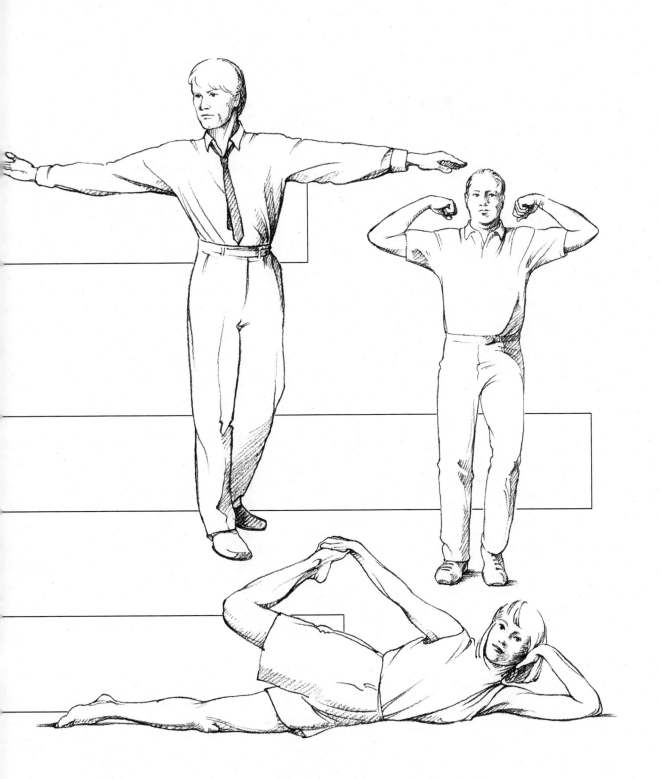

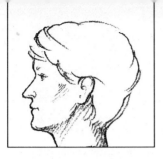

Aging

*T*he day she decided to stop acting her age, Alverta Hettinger made one of the best choices of her long life.

It happened 13 years ago when she joined the Sun City (Arizona) Poms, a group of 19 women aged 60 to 84 who do dance routines that include tumbling, leg splits, and human pyramids. They perform at least 50 times a year at conventions and trade shows in the Phoenix area.

"You really have to stay active with a physical program to be able to do this. I play golf, I walk 2 or 3 miles a day, I swim, and I'm learning to play tennis," says Alverta, who is still going strong at age 70. "I truly feel better now than I did when I was 50 and didn't exercise at all."

Discover Your Own Fountain of Youth

Hettinger's story wouldn't surprise many experts on aging who say that exercise may be the closest thing we have to a fountain of youth.

"By taking yourself from a sedentary state to a physically trained state, you can, in effect, reduce your biological age by 10 or 20 years," says Roy Shepard, M.D., Ph.D., a professor of applied physiology in the School of Physical and Health Education and the Department of Preventive Medicine and Biostatistics at the University of Toronto.

Others say the effects are even more dramatic than that.

It is often said that exercise, if it could be bottled, would be the most potent prescription we have for a healthy existence, says Elizabeth McNeely, R.N., Ph.D., who is a nurse gerontologist at Emory University School of Nursing in Atlanta.

How potent? Well, researchers say that some of the physical limitations that Americans accept as a natural consequence of aging—including heart disease, reduced vigor, and waning muscle strength—can be prevented with regular exercise.

"If we stay active, many of the things that supposedly decline with age really don't decline," says William Simpson, M.D., professor of family medicine at the Medical University of South Carolina in Charleston.

Study after study bears this out. For example, researchers measured the effects of aging on 756 athletes aged 35 to 94, who participated in events such as rowing, swimming, and track and field during the 1985 World Masters Games in Toronto. "We found some people in their late sixties and seventies who had about the same cardiopulmonary fitness as you would expect from sedentary 25-year-olds," says Terence Kavanagh, M.D., director of the Toronto Rehabilitation Centre and princi-

EXERCISE: YOU'RE NEVER TOO OLD TO START

It is never too late in life to begin an exercise program. Just ask Joan Rowland, who was diagnosed with angina at age 60.

To combat the condition, her cardiologist prescribed walking. It wasn't long before she entered her first racewalking competition. Within five years she set a world record and nearly 15 national ones.

"It seems I was born to racewalk," she says. "Many racers plan a strategy, but not me. I just empty my head, put a smile on my face, and start moving. It's exhilarating."

Aging experts wish more older people would share Joan's go-get-'em attitude.

"A lot of people have a fatalistic attitude and think, 'Oh well, I'm 60, I can't do that anymore,' " says Michael Kaplan, Ph.D., program coordinator for physical performance and functioning at the National Institute on Aging. "Well, older people can have the same strength and the same endurance as young people if they work at it. People can do a lot more than they think they can." He advises, however, that they seek the supervision of their doctor before beginning an exercise program.

Too Few Do

Unfortunately, only 31 percent of Americans between the ages 45 and 64, and 27 percent of people 65 and over, exercise regularly. Possibly as a consequence of that, 40 percent of Americans older than 75 are unable to walk two blocks, according to the National Institute on Aging. Nearly 32 percent are unable to climb stairs, and 22 percent can't lift 10 pounds.

Older Americans may exercise less because they believe that the need for it diminishes with age, says Sara Harris, executive director of the Center for the Study of Aging in Albany, New York. She recalls when representatives of her organization tried to discuss the importance of exercise at senior centers.

"Some of the people at those centers would get furious with us," she says. "They'd say, 'We've worked all our lives. We don't have to do that. We just want to enjoy ourselves.' They didn't seem to realize that exercise would help them enjoy their life more."

But experts say those seniors are missing a vital point: Light to moderate exercise can combat aging and make their life more rewarding.

"I think several things keep people away from exercise. In particular is the notion that they have to go out and jog for 20 minutes three times a week to do themselves any good. That's just not true, particularly for older people," says David Corbin, Ph.D., professor of health education at the University of Nebraska in Omaha and author

pal author of the study. When compared to sedentary people their own age, they averaged twice the cardiovascular fitness. Plus, they had more lean body mass and a stronger cardiovascular system.

But what is most astounding is the amount of effort that went into getting them in such good shape, says Dr. Kavanagh.

Most trained less than 7 hours a week in preparation for the games. "These were people who were interested in having a good time and weren't fanatical trainers in any sense," he says. "They were more typical of the average recreational sports person rather than the elite athlete. Yet the results of their exercise habits were marked.

of *Reach for It,* an exercise handbook for older adults.

Fun-and-Games Exercises

The value of moderate exercise for senior citizens was demonstrated in a Japanese study of 12 elderly people who had played gate-ball (a game similar to croquet) six days a week for at least 3 years. After evaluations, the researchers determined that the men, whose chronological age averaged 76 years, physically were at least 4½ years younger.

Elderly people who play tennis and other racquet sports benefit from enhanced muscle strength, according to researchers at McGill University in Montreal. In the study, 20 male and female tennis players aged 65 and older demonstrated significantly more strength and endurance than 20 sedentary men and women of the same age.

And t'ai chi, a form of Chinese martial arts that emphasizes slow body movement, can help elderly people improve their balance. Initial results of an ongoing study in Atlanta of 215 elderly people, 50 of whom practice t'ai chi, are encouraging.

"The improvement in how people move is, to say the least, dramatic," says Steven Wolf, Ph.D., physical therapist at Emory University School of Medicine and the study's principal investigator.

One man who, before practicing t'ai chi, fell often and needed to sit down to remove his shoes was able to do that task standing in a hallway without support after 15 weeks of participation in the martial art.

Juggling is another activity that older people can do to help increase movement, Dr. Corbin says.

"It helps with coordination, and it's just a fun thing to do," he says. To learn juggling, Dr. Corbin recommends that you start with chiffon scarves.

"The scarves float, so you have more time to catch them and learn the technique," he says.

The senior citizens in his program became so proficient at the task that they actually did better than some of the younger people tested.

In fact, Dr. Corbin suggests that exercising with younger people is a good way for seniors to gain confidence in their physical abilities and keep motivated.

"I have university students work out right along with older people so they can see what the older people can do, and in some cases, they find the older people are better than they are," Dr. Corbin says. "The older people get a chance to see that younger people aren't all they're cracked up to be."

It seems that even modest exercise can push functional aging back 20 years."

Fighting Father Time

If you think looking and feeling in shape is a great incentive to get out and exercise, consider this: Exercise can even help you live *longer.*

In one study, Dutch researchers followed the death rate among 2,259 participants in a 120-mile ice skating race in 1956. The skaters included highly trained athletes as well as weekend warriors. Over the next 32 years, their death rate was 24 percent lower than that of the general population. Based on their findings, the researchers concluded that vigorous physical exercise contributes to longevity.

In a similar study of 636 middle-aged Finnish men conducted over a 20-year period, researchers found that physically active men lived an average of 2.1 years longer than their peers who were sedentary.

Then there's the classic study of 16,936 Harvard alumni aged 35 to 74, who were followed by Stanford University researchers for 12 to 16 years. Death rates were 25 to 33 percent lower among those alumni who burned off more than 2,000 calories exercising each week. For an average-sized man, that's equivalent to running or walking 3 miles a day, or climbing 38 flights of steps every day.

You don't have to be a lifelong athlete to get a lease on longer life. The Stanford researchers concluded that people who start exercising between the ages of 35 and 55 can probably add two years to their life expectancy. Even if you start exercising in your seventies, you can add an extra six months to your life.

Formula for a Longer Life

If you mix exercise with other healthful living practices, your prospects for a longer life get even greater, says Kenneth Manton, Ph.D., professor and assistant director of Duke University's Center for Demographic Studies. What does it take? In addition to exercising, you should maintain your ideal weight, not smoke, keep your cholesterol low, and follow a low-fat diet, says Dr. Manton.

Dr. Manton came to this conclusion after using an innovative computer program to reanalyze data from several major studies, including the famed 20-year Framingham Heart Study. He concluded that a healthful lifestyle that includes regular physical exercise, begun at age 30, has the potential to extend the average life expectancy in this country by as much as 15 years.

"Many of the debilitating conditions we often assume to be natural to the aging process are, in fact, consequences of lifestyle, which can be controlled," Dr. Manton says. "Our study showed that proper nutrition and exercise, for example, can do a great deal to reduce risks of early death due to cardiovascular disease or cancer."

But it's exercise itself that many doctors believe will help make *all* your years—no matter how many there are—productive and disease-free.

"Many people become disabled at 65 and die at 85. Wouldn't it be better to be able to spend those 20 years as an active person, get disabled at 85, and die at 85?" says Paul Rousseau, M.D., chief of the Department of Geriatrics at Carl T. Hayden Veterans Administration Medical Center in Phoenix. "That's what exercise can do for the body. It's better to compress all that illness into a short period of time and let the other years be quality years."

Stop the Signs of Aging

Some physical decline is part of the natural aging process. As we age, reaction time slows (one of the reasons older people fall 40 percent more often than younger folks), we accumulate more body fat, and we have a tendency toward high cholesterol and high blood pressure.

The heart's ability to pump blood drops an average of 58 percent between the ages of 25 and 85, experts say. By age 70, lung capacity can decrease by 40 to 50 percent and muscle strength by 20 percent. Bone loss of 1 percent per year usually begins in women by age 35 and in men by age 55.

The body also gradually becomes less efficient at processing the sugar in the bloodstream. As blood sugar levels rise with age, the chances of developing diabetes increase.

With exercise, however, many of these telltale signs of aging can be much less profound. In a study of 30 men at San Diego State University, researchers monitored the effects of aging on two groups—15 men aged 45 to 68 who had been exercising regularly for 23 years, and 15 formerly active men who hadn't exercised in 18 years.

Although maximum aerobic power among the exercisers decreased 13 percent over the years, researchers found the decline was three times greater in the sedentary men. The exercisers averaged about 15 percent body fat, while the nonexercisers had at least 25 percent body fat. In addition, resting blood pressure was unchanged in the exercisers, but it rose significantly among the nonexercisers. In fact, 60 percent of the sedentary men suffered from high blood pressure at the conclusion of the study.

"Study after study shows that the signs that we traditionally link with aging—increased body fat, weak muscles, a shrinking skeleton—all are simply a result of being less active as we grow older," says William Evans, Ph.D., chief of the physiology laboratory at Tufts University in Boston and coauthor of *Biomarkers*, a book about aging.

Now consider what can happen to the body when it *stops* exercising. A Swedish physiologist asked five young men to remain bedridden 24 hours a day for three weeks to study their body's physiological response. All of the men experienced a drop in their aerobic capacity equivalent to almost 20 years of aging!

"A lot of the effects of aging are self-inflicted," Dr. Kavanagh says. "The less you do, the easier you fatigue. And the more you fatigue, the less you are able to do. It's a vicious cycle."

Breaking that cycle is critical to aging well, experts say.

"I think it's just common sense," Dr. Kavanagh says. "Just look around you and you'll see that the people who are physically active work harder, tire less, and enjoy themselves a lot more."

"Regular physical activity is excellent for everyone," Dr. Kavanagh says. "But it has to be regular; it can't be inconsistent. It needs to be something that you do at least three times a week."

Which brings us to the question: What kind of exercise is best to hold back the aging process?

Make It Aerobic

Aerobic exercise—such as swimming, running, dancing, cycling, and walking—is the most powerful weapon we have to combat many of the effects of aging, according to the results of several studies.

In one study, 32 men aged 47 to 84 participated in an eight-year study of aerobic fitness at Washington University School of Medicine in St. Louis. Eighteen of the men were athletes who had been in training for about ten years. The other 14 participants were sedentary. Researchers found that the aerobic capacity in the active men decreased about 4 percent during the eight years, but it decreased nearly 10 percent in the sedentary men.

At the same institution, men and women aged 60 to 69 who participated in a study of the effects of moderately intense walking and jogging increased their maximum exercise capacity by 30 percent in 12 months.

At Duke University, 75 elderly veterans aged 65 to 74 exercised three days a week for two years. The 90-minute workouts included 15 minutes of stationary bicycling, 20 minutes of lower back and abdominal exercises, and 30 minutes of walking. As a result, the veterans' flexibility increased, their resting heart rate decreased, and their blood pressure dipped.

Aerobic exercise also can significantly affect other conditions, such as high cholesterol. For example, in a study of 34 healthy women aged 61 to 81 at Florida Atlantic University in Boca Raton, investigators found that those who walked three times a week at a speed that elevated their heart rate to 70 or 80 percent of their maximum pumping capability reduced their blood cholesterol levels and their risk of heart disease.

And researchers at California State University, Fullerton, followed the progress of 21 women aged 57 to 85, who did 20 to 25 minutes of low-impact aerobics followed by another 20 to 25 minutes of calisthenics three times a week for three years. The researchers concluded that the exercisers significantly improved their flexibility, balance, and reaction times in comparison to a similar group of women who participated in arts and crafts workshops.

Aerobic exercise may even improve your love life. In a study of 160 swimmers aged 40 to 60, researchers at Harvard University found that swimmers in their forties were as sexually active as 20- or 30-year-olds. In addition, they reported that the 60-year-old swimmers were nearly as passionate as those in their forties.

"People in their forties, fifties, and sixties can be just as active as people in their twenties. It's not that these people are going to live forever or that aging isn't going on. But they do prove that you can be strong, agile, and sexy well into your life," says Phillip Whitten, Ph.D., an anthropologist and sociologist who teaches human behavioral biology at Harvard.

Aerobic workouts are important because without adequate oxygen, the body doesn't perform at its best, Dr. Kavanagh says. "If you let your muscles go to pot, you're artificially reducing your oxygen uptake. If you do that, you really can't function well. You think slower, you move slower. You're just less capable of taking advantage of this world," he says.

So how do you take advantage of this high-octane energy booster? What do you do if you've already slumped into a sedentary lifestyle?

Brisk walking is an excellent aerobic exercise for beginners, doctors say, because it's easy and can give you all the health-enhancing and age-resisting benefits of more strenuous aerobic activities, such as jogging and stair climbing. Walking will also get you in condition for more rigorous activities such as running, biking, and

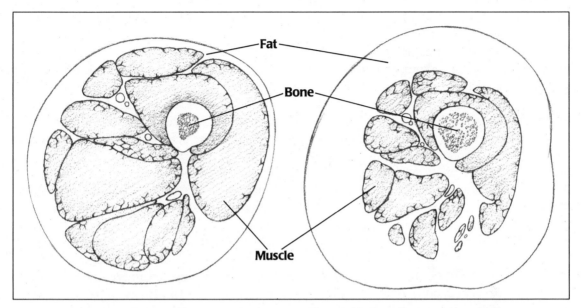

Fat

Bone

Muscle

As we age, the body tends to put on fat and lose muscle—but you can fight back with exercise. The thigh of a 20-year-old female athlete (left) is backed with firm muscle.

The thigh of a sedentary 64-year-old woman (right) is mostly fat. The key to changing the proportion of muscle and fat in the older woman is regular exercise.

swimming. (To learn how to begin a walking program, see "Walking" on page 458.)

Make the Most of Your Muscles

Aerobic exercise is just one component of an antiaging package. You should also consider some form of weight training, experts say.

Researchers at Tufts University found that weight training significantly improved the muscle strength of 12 previously sedentary men aged 60 to 72. During the 12 weeks of weight lifting, the muscle strength increases ranged from 107 percent to 226 percent. Overall, their total muscle mass increased by an average of 10 percent.

More important, these gains were similar to those reported by healthy younger men undergoing a similar training regimen.

In another study, the Tufts researchers studied the effects of resistance training on ten frail 90-year-old residents of the Hebrew Rehabilitation Center in Boston. The men and women who participated in the study did weight-training exercises with their legs three times a week for eight weeks. At the end of the study, researchers found that muscle strength increased 174 percent. Two people no longer needed to use canes to walk, and one person who initially couldn't rise unaided from a chair was able to do so when the study concluded.

"Because muscle strength decreases 30 to 40 percent during the course of the adult life span, it is likely that at the end of the training these subjects were stronger than they had been in many years previously," according to the Tufts researchers. "Our findings suggest that a portion of muscle weakness attributed to aging may be modifiable through exercise."

These findings are significant, note the researchers, because retaining muscle strength and flexibility could help prevent falls, a major cause of disability and death in the elderly.

At-Home Toning

If joining a health club to work out is about as appealing to you as going to Daytona Beach at Easter time, listen to this: Experts say there are a number of clever (and inexpensive) ways to flex your muscle without setting foot in a gym. All you need to do is find yourself a bicycle inner tube.

"It is an excellent exercise apparatus," says David Corbin, Ph.D., author of *Reach for It,* an exercise guidebook for older adults. "The resistance offered by the inner tube can be varied from exercise to exercise, from person to person, and from one part of the body to another by varying how or where the tube is held."

Inner tubes have several advantages, Dr. Corbin says. Used tubes usually can be obtained free at most bicycle shops. The tubes can be used by all ages and by people with a range of disabilities. The tube exercises also can be done sitting or standing.

To do a rowing exercise, for example, sit in a chair and hook one end of the tube under both feet. Grab the other end of the tube in a overhand grip with both hands. Pull the tube toward your chin in a rowing motion. Repeat five to eight times.

To strengthen your legs, try tube jogging. Sit in a sturdy chair and loop one end of the tube over both feet. Hold the other end of the tube with both hands about 18 inches apart. Move your feet in a jogging motion. Make sure that you sit on the front portion of the chair and lean heavily on the chair back. Continue jogging for about 1 minute. Gradually increase your time, up to 5 minutes. This exercise also can be a good warm-up for a long, brisk walk, Dr. Corbin says.

If you're intimidated by the thought of exercising with a group, ask a friend or your spouse to join you, Dr. Simpson suggests.

"Exercising with a partner certainly helps, particularly if that someone is willing to get out there with you at 6:00 in the morning to encourage you," he says.

And on those days when you need even more incentive, remember that exercising not only will help you feel younger, it'll make you look younger, too.

"Everyone thinks I've been to a spa," says Sunny Griffin, of Playa del Rey, California, who took up downhill skiing at 30 and classical ballet at 40, and now spends her time mountain climbing.

"It sometimes startles me when I remember that I'm over 50," she says. "The concept of old just doesn't relate to my life. People say, 'Gee, you look good for 50,' and I always think, 'This is what 50 is supposed to look like!' "

MUSIC, MAESTRO, PLEASE

Ever find yourself "conducting" your favorite orchestra? As music swells from the stereo, your spirits rise, and your arms lift of their own accord and begin beating time . . .

If so, have we got an exercise for you! All it takes is music, a baton, and a healthy imagination.

Vigorously conducting a recorded orchestra can be great aerobic exercise, says William Simpson, M.D., professor of family medicine at the Medical University of South Carolina in Charleston. And it's a fun way to replace your walking or jogging routine on those days when the weather is bad. He cautions, however, that individuals with high blood pressure or angina should consult a physician before engaging in upper body exercises.

"Anything that encourages range of motion is positive," Dr. Simpson says. "The nice thing about conducting is that the music gives you a beat so you have a pace to maintain. The music is pleasant to listen to, and it turns something that may seem like exercise into something that seems like fun."

William McGlaughlin, music director of the Kansas City Symphony, is one conductor who is intrigued by the idea. He recalls when two Kansas City Chiefs football players tried to help him conduct. "It was a 10- or 12-minute piece, and they couldn't make it through it," he says. "That's how difficult it can be. It really is a good upper body exercise."

So what orchestral works might provide you with a suitable challenge? McGlaughlin suggests the final movement from Tchaikovsky's Fourth Symphony. "It's fun, and it's not hard to learn how to follow it. It's fast and loud, which means you can flail your arms around to your heart's content," McGlaughlin says.

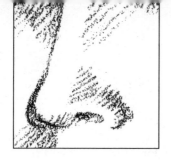

Allergies

Y ou wake up feeling like the sandman left a few sandbags in your nose. And your eyes are so watery, anybody looking at you would think your best friend just died. Well, maybe you are in mourning—for your good health. Because it's allergy season again.

But instead of rolling out of bed and heading for the medicine cabinet, try another form of instant and effective relief—a short session of vigorous exercise.

"Vigorous exercise is one of the body's most efficient ways to control nasal congestion," according to Robert S. Zeiger, M.D., chief of allergy at Kaiser Permanente Medical Center in San Diego.

It's unclear exactly how exercise helps unclog the nasal passages. One theory is that it helps redistribute nasal blood flow. This redirected blood flow may reduce the amount of water circulating through the nasal mucus.

Exercising seems to clear congestion rapidly, and the effects last up to a half hour. "Engaging in some exercise upon rising in the morning and before retiring can be beneficial if you have chronic nasal problems," says Dr. Zeiger.

Making Exercise Easier

Allergy sufferers can have special problems when it comes to exercise, however.

For one thing, they can't breathe! Also, they might suck in more of what caused their symptoms in the first place. Here are a few tips for allergic folks who want to enjoy the allergy-beating (and health-enhancing) benefits of exercise.

Start with a squirt. Dr. Zeiger suggests that if you suffer from chronic nasal problems, squirting some commercial saline solution in your nose *before* beginning your routine may be quite helpful. He says that this procedure may help to thin and drain mucus both during regular activity and during exercise.

Get your allergies under control. If you seem to be sensitive to airborne irritants, work with your doctor to treat the allergy, advises Ellen Garibaldi, M.D., director of the Adult Asthma Exercise Program at St. Louis University Medical Center. Rather than having to work at avoiding irritants, you may be able to reduce or even eliminate your allergic reaction to them, she says.

Don't jog in the smog. When you exercise you can get a double dose of air pollutants such as ozone and sulfur dioxide. These gases can irritate the airways and may increase your sensitivity to anything in the air that you're allergic to.

Check prevailing winds. Even a little exercise can carry a lot of pollen into the airways. On windy days, when the pollen is whipping about, you're better off exercising indoors, says Gerald Klein, M.D., director of the Allergy and Immunology Medical Group in Vista, California. If you must exercise outdoors, take an antihistamine 30 minutes before going out. Also, try wearing the type of cotton mask used by industrial workers to filter out air particles.

Become an afternoon exerciser. Pollen counts tend to peak at dawn and again at dusk, says Dr. Klein. If you want to exercise outdoors, wait until 2:00 to 5:00 P.M., when pollen is at its lowest.

Avoid dry environments. Don't work out on overheated or ice-cold air-conditioned racquetball courts, for example. If you're exercising outside in frigid weather, wear a scarf over your mouth to warm and humidify inhaled air.

Breathe through your nose. The sinuses and nose are built-in humidifiers, says Dr. Klein.

If stuffiness makes nose-breathing impossible, take a decongestant before exercising.

WHAT TO DO IF YOU'RE ALLERGIC TO EXERCISE

The exercise allergy we're talking about isn't an acute attack of laziness every time you think about putting on walking shoes. It's a *serious* (even life-threatening) condition called "exercise-induced anaphylaxis."

In some people, exercise triggers extremely high levels of histamine, a body chemical that, among other effects, causes airways to swell—and perhaps shut completely. "It's a relatively rare condition, but severe enough that you should know what to do if you have it," says Albert L. Sheffer, M.D., clinical professor of medicine at Harvard Medical School.

If you have an itchy rash (another symptom of histamine release) or feel faint after exercising, see an allergist. He can discover if you have the condition. If you do,

he'll probably advise you to carry a kit that enables you to inject yourself with adrenaline if you have anaphylaxis during exercise. (These kits are the same as those carried by people who have anaphylactic reactions to bee stings.) He may also advise you to try the mildest form of exercise: easy-does-it walking. It's also a good idea to exercise with a friend; you could be in the midst of an anaphylactic episode before you know it, and you might not be able to inject yourself.

Finally, if you have an exercise allergy, don't eat for at least 4 hours before exercising. Certain foods (celery and seafood are the worst) may trigger anaphylaxis. Aspirin and ibuprofen are other potential triggers.

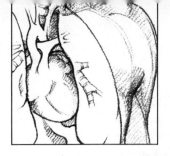

Angina

*I*t may happen as you tee off on the golf course, when you're walking around the block, or when you're just taking out the garbage. But wherever you are when angina first strikes, it scares the heck out of you.

And it should—the suffocating tightness you feel across your chest is a warning sign of coronary artery disease. But just because you have angina doesn't mean you should cancel your country club membership, throw your walking shoes into the closet, and spend the rest of your life nestled in a lounge chair.

In truth, that may be the worst thing you can do, because regular exercise done with a physician's approval can relieve certain types of angina and help you live a more fulfilling life.

"There is simply no doubt that some people with angina can benefit remarkably from exercise," says Paul Thompson, M.D., medical director of cardiac rehabilitation at Miriam Hospital in Providence, Rhode Island. "Exercise can control and lessen the frequency of angina. I have a couple of angina patients who have gotten to the point where they can jog a couple of miles a day."

Just make sure you don't dash out to the local running trail until *after* you've seen a physician. Coronary artery disease is a serious condition that requires medical attention. An inappropriate exercise program could induce a heart attack. Get your doctor's approval before beginning any regular physical activity.

But in general, the type of angina you have will determine whether exercise is a good treatment for you. Unstable angina, for example, may be triggered by minimal activity such as light housework, or it can even occur when you're resting. If you have this type of angina, exercise probably isn't a good idea. Instead, other treatment such as surgery may be necessary.

However, if you have stable angina, meaning that your chest pains occur *only* when you're exerting yourself, then exercise might help you immensely, says C. Noel Bairey, M.D., medical director of the Preventive and Cardiac Rehabilitation Center at Cedars-Sinai Medical Center in Los Angeles.

"Exercise really can have a *tremendous* impact on a person who has stable angina," Dr. Bairey says. "If a person is willing to stick with an exercise program, they can dramatically reduce their symptoms, reduce their use of medication, and feel better."

On the other hand, being sedentary will only make stable angina worse, Dr. Thompson says.

"Doing less is self-defeating because you're going to get angina more and more often," he says.

A Roadblock to Your Heart

The pain of angina is caused by a temporary, partial obstruction of your arteries. As you work or exercise, your heart needs more blood. But your body can't meet that demand because arteries that have been narrowed by a spasm or a buildup of fatty deposits restrict blood flow to your heart. When the heart can't get enough blood, it hurts. People who suffer from it describe that dull ache as "feeling like a weight," "squeezing," and "pressure."

An angina episode generally lasts less than 5 minutes. It usually can be relieved with rest or by drugs such as nitroglycerin that dilate arteries so more blood reaches the heart, says Renae Guiterrez, Ph.D., a patient education specialist at the Mayo Clinic Scottsdale in Arizona.

Putting the Squeeze on Angina

Exercise does at least four things that help relieve angina. Regular physical activity dilates vessels, increasing blood flow, and it improves your body's ability to extract oxygen from the bloodstream, Dr. Bairey says.

But a long-term program of regular exercise ultimately lowers your heart rate and increases its pumping ability, so it takes less effort to circulate blood through your body, Dr. Thompson says.

"If you slow the heart rate down, the heart needs less blood. What exercise training does is lower the heart rate it takes to do certain activities," he says. "For example, a fellow who gets angina while taking out the trash may have a heart rate of 120 beats a minute. But if he gets in shape, he may only get a heart rate of 105 doing the same task, so he doesn't get angina anymore."

Walking is a good exercise that conditions the heart and combats angina, Dr. Thompson says.

"It varies from patient to patient, but I like to have them start out with 5 or 10 minutes of walking a day, then add 5 minutes a week until they're walking 40 to 60 minutes a day," he says. "Pretty soon, we find they can exercise longer and longer with less and less pain."

Others favor a diverse approach. Dr. Bairey, for example, has her patients do a variety of activities. A typical workout to combat angina might include 10 minutes of warm-up and stretching exercises, 20 minutes of treadmill walking, 20 minutes of stationary rowing or bicycling, and finally 10 more minutes of stretching to cool down.

But how can you exercise safely and comfortably without pain? Dr. Bairey and Dr. Thompson recommend that you take a nitroglycerin pill right before you begin your workout.

"Taking nitroglycerin is always best before you exercise because it dilates coronary arteries and increases blood flow to the heart," Dr. Thompson says.

But if you do get angina when you're working out, don't ignore it, Dr. Bairey says.

"When you get angina, it's a warning sign that your heart isn't getting enough blood," she says. "It's *not* something that if you just bear through it, it will get better. You may not need to stop, but you always want to slow down when you get it until it goes away."

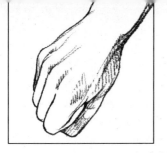

Anxiety

The young man felt confident the morning he took the entrance exam to Harrow, a prestigious British prep school. After all, he had mastered French, history, grammar, and geography—the topics he expected to see on the test. But to his astonishment, he was asked to translate passages of Latin and Greek. Despite having studied those two languages for more than a year, he panicked and couldn't understand a single word of either text.

In despair, he wrote his name at the top of the page. Then he sat grimly staring at the barren page until the test ended.

Winston Churchill, the man who would later symbolize Great Britain's resolute fighting spirit during World War II, had been beaten—by his own anxiety.

"I think all of us can relate to test anxiety. I think everyone gets symptoms of it at one time or another in their lives. If you're put in a situation where you're being evaluated and the pressure is on you, I think anxiety is a natural response," says Robert Topp, R.N., Ph.D., assistant professor of nursing at Indiana University in Bloomington.

While anxiety may be a natural response to life's pressures, that isn't much of a comfort to a teenage boy nervously asking a girl to the prom or to a corporate executive making her first presentation to the company board of directors.

But fortunately, anxiety has a natural cure—exercise.

Turning On Your Own Tranquilizers

Exercise frequently works better than quiet rest and other relaxation techniques at reducing anxiety. Just why that is still mystifies scientists.

One popular theory suggests that exercise triggers the release of mood-altering chemicals, such as endorphins and serotonin, in the brain. Another possibility is that simply taking a break from your daily routine can reduce anxiety. Other researchers are investigating the possibility that exercise subdues anxiety by improving a person's self-image.

Surprisingly, scientists say that anxiety isn't all bad. Many therapists believe that personality development is impossible without *some* anxiety. Others think it sparks innovative thinking.

"I suspect if we didn't have a bit of anxiety in our lives, we wouldn't accomplish much," says Robert S. Brown, Sr., M.D., Ph.D., clinical professor of behavioral medicine and psychiatry at the University of Virginia.

"Anxiety is a warning signal much like the smoke alarm in your house. If the smoke alarm went off, you would certainly get up and try to find out where the fire is or get out of the house," he says.

Put simply, the body is conditioned to experience anxiety in a threatening situation, real or imagined—it's a primitive reflex. But the constant pace of stress in modern life doesn't allow us to expend the energy generated from that reflex.

"My simple prescription is exercise," says Dr. Brown. "The fitter you are, the better prepared you'll be to handle your stresses, including anxiety."

Scientific research supports the notion that exercise may help reduce anxiety to a more tolerable level in many circumstances.

In one study of 45 students at the University of Pennsylvania, for example, Dr. Topp found that students who participated in aerobic dance classes three times a week significantly lowered their test anxiety levels in less than two months. (They improved their fitness, too.)

In another study, researchers in Kansas concluded that people who jogged 20 minutes a day three times a week were less anxious and expressed less anger, hostility, and aggression than nonexercisers.

Walk Your Way to Calmness

Does all this research mean that you have to lace up your aerobic shoes or hit the jogging trail to banish anxiety? Not on your life.

Even if you're not a regular exerciser, you may be able to reduce your anxiety by simply taking a brisk walk, says David Roth, Ph.D., associate professor of psychology at the University of Alabama in Birmingham.

"The one-shot exercise session does appear to have antianxiety effects," he says. "The effects are temporary; we really don't know how long they last. But I would guess the effects would last for at least 1 hour afterward."

The effects of regular exercise may last even longer than that, according to John Raglin, Ph.D., assistant professor of kinesiology at Indiana University.

In his two-part study, 15 men aged 25 to 60 were randomly assigned to sit quietly in a room or participate in an aerobic exercise of their choice—jogging, racquetball, basketball, swimming, or cycling. During the next session, the groups switched roles.

After each session ended, blood pressure and anxiety levels were monitored for several hours.

While Dr. Raglin concluded that quiet rest does reduce anxiety, he found that exercise had a longer-lasting impact. In some cases, exercise relieved the men's anxiety for up to 3 hours.

Go Ahead, Try Something New

"Any moderate exercise is beneficial if it makes people feel good about themselves and is likely to lead to physical health improvements," says Dr. Roth. "Whether it's aerobic exercise or some other type may be of lesser importance."

Research supports Dr. Roth's claim. In a study of patients suffering from severe mental disorders, including panic attacks, Norwegian researchers found that both aerobic and nonaerobic exercise effectively reduced people's anxiety.

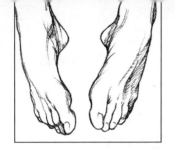

Arthritis

I had never done what you would call exercise," says Emmet Fulkerson, a 73-year-old Cincinnati man with long-term rheumatoid arthritis. "When my arthritis was better, I'd be more active, and when it was bad, I'd cut back."

Then, a flare-up and a winter of inactivity melted 15 pounds, mostly muscle, off him shortly before he was due to leave for a trip to Paris. "I told the doctor I wasn't sure I had the strength to carry my luggage," Emmet explains. The doctor suggested he try a new arthritis exercise center nearby. Two months later, with six weeks of gentle, light weight lifting under his belt, he made the trip to Paris.

"I carried my hand luggage without pain," he says. "And I also was able to handle my suitcase for a short distance. That was something I hadn't been able to do for about three years. I could also walk longer and wasn't nearly as tired as I used to be."

Emmet is so pleased with his progress that he's continuing the weight-lifting program on his own at his company's fitness center. "I used to have pain in my shoulders in bed at night, just from the weight of my body pressing on them. Now I have none of that," he says. His doctor has been so impressed he plans to suggest exercise to more of his patients.

Doctors used to advise people with arthritis to get plenty of rest—up to 12 hours a day. And they'd recommend even *more* down time if a patient complained of being weak or tired or if arthritis symptoms flared up.

Doctors Say: Get Moving

While this laid-back prescription might delight afternoon game-show fans, doctors now know that too much rest ultimately makes arthritis symptoms *worse*, not better. It makes joints stiffen up and become even more painful. It weakens muscles and depletes stamina, which turns climbing stairs or shopping into exhausting chores. It erodes people's ability to do simple, everyday things for themselves, which can lead to dependence, fear, and depression. And it turns fun things like travel into frustrating misadventures if someone lacks the strength or nimbleness to climb the steps into a bus or pick up a suitcase.

That's where exercise comes in. Studies done during the last ten years or so consistently show that low-impact exercise such as swimming, biking, or walking is nothing but good for people with arthritis. It improves muscle strength, builds stamina, and allows joints to move better, with less pain and swelling. It allows some people to cut back on anti-inflammatory drugs. Plus, exercise can replace feelings of fatigue and depression with new energy and a sense of hope and control.

"I've seen a remarkable aura of optimism develop in our exercise groups," says C. William Castor, M.D., professor of internal medicine in the Rheumatology Division and Rackham Arthritis Research Unit at the University of Michigan Medical Center in Ann Arbor. "Even people who initially had to be coaxed into the program soon see how much more they can do, with energy to spare. Many say they intend to continue exercising after a study is over."

Those attending arthritis exercise classes can tell you exactly what benefits they have reaped.

"My chiropractor told me if I didn't start exercising I would become a cripple," says Violet Adams, a Perkasie, Pennsylvania, woman who's had rheumatoid arthritis for years. She signed up for an Arthritis Foundation–sponsored water exercise class at the YMCA after her feet and ankles became so painful she couldn't walk, even with support. Six months later, she says proudly, "Now I don't need a walker. And the classes, and the people in them, are wonderful."

Use It or Lose It

Studies—and real-life experiences—show that exercise provides this wide array of benefits without harming joints. Not only that, it helps *most* people with rheumatoid arthritis or osteoarthritis, the two most common forms. (It may also improve symptoms in people with related conditions such as ankylosing spondylitis, a form of spinal arthritis.)

While most research focuses on people with mild or moderate arthritis, experience shows that people whose arthritis is so bad they can't walk or use their hands can regain some use with proper exercise, doctors say.

People who've had arthritis for years, or those who are quite old, can improve. "Age doesn't seem to have a bearing on it," says Donald Kay, M.D., of the Boone Clinic in Columbia, Missouri. "Even people in their mid-eighties have improved with exercise." So have people with artificial hip, shoulder, or knee joints.

Give Your Joints a Lube Job

Just how does exercise help relieve the symptoms of arthritis?

"Moving the joints is now known to be essential to joint health," explains Mary P. Schatz, M.D., of Nashville, Tennessee. Dr. Schatz is a pathologist at the Centennial Medical Center, an instructor of yoga, and author of *Back Care Basics: A Doctor's Gentle Yoga Program for Back and Neck Pain Relief.*

A normal joint consists of the ends of two bones, both covered with glistening, smooth cartilage and surrounded by a fibrous capsule of tissue, called the synovium. Inside this capsule is a thick, slippery fluid that lubricates the joint, nourishes the cartilage, and helps to keep it clean. Around the outside of this capsule are the muscles, ligaments (which connect bone to bone), and tendons (which connect muscle to bone).

In rheumatoid arthritis, the lining of the synovial capsule becomes inflamed. The inflammation causes the breakdown

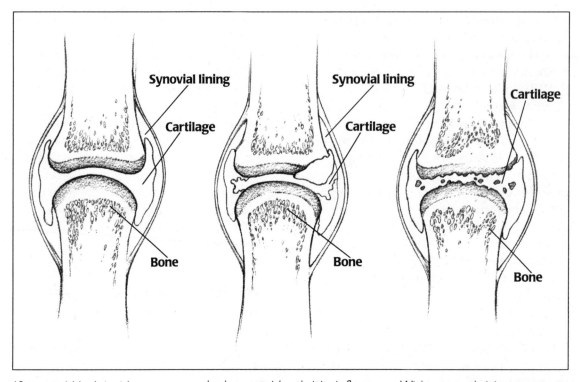

If you could look inside a normal joint, you would see an orderly arrangement of bone and cartilage that works smoothly and keeps you moving effortlessly.

In rheumatoid arthritis, inflammation causes thickening of the synovial lining—a thin tissue that surrounds the joint capsule—and an increase in synovial fluid, which serves as a lubricant. The joint swells and becomes stiff and painful.

With osteoarthritis, overuse or injury may hasten the natural degeneration of cartilage. When new bone grows to repair the damage, the growth may occur as painful spurs or projections.

of synovial tissue and swelling that stretches and weakens the tendons, ligaments, and joint capsule. The synovial lining overgrows into the joint capsule in an attempt to heal. The synovial fluid declines in quality as a result of inflammation, and its ability to nourish, cleanse, and lubricate is diminished. Unless the process can be reversed, the whole joint slowly weakens and stiffens.

Moving the joint, as you would with exercise, induces the manufacture of synovial fluid and helps to distribute it over the cartilage and circulate it throughout the entire joint space, Dr. Schatz explains. Movement increases the circulation of blood and lymph into and out of the joint structures and adjacent soft tissues, reducing swelling, removing waste products, and increasing delivery of nutrients and oxygen to help heal joint tissues.

In osteoarthritis, the cartilage and the bone beneath it start to break down. Instead of being replaced in a smooth, even layer, new cartilage and bone are formed as projections or spurs. The cartilage grows thinner and thinner and may eventually erode away entirely, allowing bone to grate painfully on bone.

In people with osteoarthritis, exercise helps to maintain the cartilage by the same mechanism described for rheumatoid arthritis. It may also help the underlying bone to stay stronger by coaxing it to hold on to its calcium, Dr. Schatz says.

Exercise also strengthens shock-absorbing muscles and ligaments around joints, and thus takes some of the pressure off joints, Dr. Kay adds. This is a plus for people with either kind of arthritis.

Of course, it's important to have your type of arthritis diagnosed and to make exercise part of a total program that includes both medical care and self-help.

Okay, all this research has convinced you that you want to get those joints moving once again. The big question now is: What kind of exercise should you do?

The magic formula in any arthritis exercise program is to increase joint flexibility, muscle strength, and stamina—*without* stressing your joints. Pounding, high-impact activities or those that call for quick twisting movements—such as traditional aerobics or basketball—are out. Smooth, rhythmic movements are in.

These days, arthritis exercises usually fall into one of three categories: range-of-motion exercises, strengthening exercises, and aerobics. Often, all three kinds of exercise are recommended in one form or another. And some activities, such as swimming, biking, and walking, can fit into more than one category.

Take It to the Limit

Shoulder shrugs, leg and arm circles, waist bends, heel-toe taps, and some yoga poses qualify as range-of-motion exercises. Designed to take any joint in the body slowly and safely through its full, natural range, these exercises help to maintain and restore stiff, constricted joints. They can be done on land or in the water. Many people find them easiest to do in a pool of warm water, where heat and buoyancy ease movement.

"People may not realize how important range of motion is until they lose it," Dr. Castor explains. Try feeding yourself with a fork when you can't bend your elbow, or walking when your knee or hip won't bend or straighten. It takes much more effort. And if a major joint freezes up—a shoulder, hip, or knee, let's say—your entire balance can be thrown off, Dr. Castor says.

That's one reason doctors recommend that range-of-motion exercises be done every day. And there is no substitute for them, doctors and exercise therapists agree. "Normal daily activities do not provide full range of motion for all joints," says Dr. Castor. And while swimming, biking, or walking moves some joints, it's seldom full-range, or full-body.

"We exercise them all, even the joints we don't know we have," explains one Arthritis Foundation aquatics exerciser. "And we feel it when we don't," chimes in another. Those classes, and other land-

FENDING OFF FLARE-UPS

Rest, and more rest, used to be the Rx for an arthritis flare-up. A doctor would immobilize the swollen, painful joint—or your whole body, if necessary.

Even today, rest *may* be what's needed, especially if your flare-up is severe.

Now, though, in many cases, doctors encourage you to continue moving your joints; they provide medical guidance and have you cut back or modify your exercise program as needed.

Why do doctors these days recommend that you continue exercising? Because the alternative—resting the joint, even for a few days—leads to stiffness. "And if the joint becomes stiff and painful enough, people tend to drop out of an exercise program altogether," says Donald Kay, M.D., of the Boone Clinic in Columbia, Missouri. "It can be real hard to get them going again."

Even people who exercise will have flare-ups, he admits, "but no more than those who don't." Your exercise program should not be causing you additional joint pain or require that you take additional medications before, or after, your workout. If it does, you're overdoing it.

---

based ones offered by the Arthritis Foundation, include up to 70 different range-of-motion exercises that move you from head to toe. (See the illustrations on pages 28 and 38 for instructions on how to do some range-of-motion and flexibility exercises.)

Pump It Up

You don't need to look like Superman or Hulk Hogan to benefit from a muscle-strengthening program. Most people with arthritis are much weaker than people the same age without arthritis. Simply getting back to normal strength, or close to it, can make all the difference in the world, doctors say.

"Being able to get up and down the stairs, out of bed, and off the toilet by yourself may not seem like much to most people, but to someone with arthritis, it could mean the difference between being able to stay at home or having to go into a nursing home," says Larry Houk, M.D., a Cincinnati rheumatologist and director of the Arthritis Fitness Center.

Traditionally, muscle-building exercises for people with arthritis have included leg or arm lifts, water exercises, and biking or walking, usually without additional weight. The Arthritis Foundation's PACE (People with Arthritis Can Exercise) videotapes include some of these strengthening exercises, as do most arthritis exercise classes. These exercises do provide some muscle building. And most people can do them.

In the past few years, though, some doctors have taken advantage of sophisticated weight-training equipment, which allows some of their arthritis patients to pump iron in a modified version of the routine used by professional bodybuilders. The advantages: more muscle in less time, and the ability to build up certain specific muscles.

That's what Dr. Houk is doing. One of

his patients is Emmet Fulkerson, the man who was able to haul his luggage around Paris, thanks to weight training.

Dr. Houk has his patients use a variety of Nautilus and Hammar machines to exercise the major muscles around the joints most likely to be affected by arthritis—the hips, shoulders, and knees. He does not have them attempt to work the smaller joints with weights or use free weights. "They are too hard for people with arthritis to grip, and it's too easy to lose control of them," he says. He's worked with both men and women with osteoarthritis or rheumatoid arthritis.

His patients start out with very small amounts of weight—sometimes just the weight of the bar. And they are instructed to pump very slowly—5 seconds going up, 5 seconds coming down, at a weight that has them feeling some muscle fatigue at the ninth and final repetition in a set.

But don't head out to the local gym just yet.

"An initial evaluation and training are very important," Dr. Houk says. "Every individual needs to learn what he can and can't do, and that may change over time."

One of the first things people need to learn is to distinguish between the slightly burning pain of muscle fatigue and the dull ache, or even sharp pain, of joint stress.

Most people work for eight to ten weeks with Dr. Houk, then find a local gym or health club with similar equipment. They return for periodic evaluations and to modify their program if needed.

Right now, most doctors are taking a wait-and-see attitude toward weight training in arthritis patients.

"Until more research has been done and published, it's hard to know the risks and benefits this kind of exercise might have for someone with arthritis," Dr. Kay says.

If you're interested, your rheumatologist may be able to refer you to an appropriate training center where you can learn weight training. Or try contacting the nearest university hospital with a rheumatology division.

Huff and Puff

Aerobic exercise is any kind of activity that increases your body's ability to use oxygen. It's activity that increases your heart rate and breathing rate. It can be a heavy-breathing, sweat-producing performance or a fairly gentle sustained exercise that tones you only slightly. People with arthritis who become aerobically fit, over time, are usually able to exert themselves longer without feeling fatigue, which translates into more energy throughout the day for all kinds of activities, Dr. Castor explains.

Studies show that for most people, it's easy to get an aerobic workout without stressing fragile joints. Your choices are plentiful: water exercises such as "marching" across a pool in chest-deep water, rowing machines, cross-country skiing machines, bicycling on a stationary bike or outdoors, walking, swimming, and low-impact dance classes.

Go Jump in a Warm Pool

In a world where doctors often disagree about treatments, pool exercises are universally recommended for arthritis. The reason? "Nearly everyone can do them, and without hurting themselves," says Jo Ann Millet, who helped develop the Arthritis Foundation YMCA Aquatic Program on the East Coast and who now trains its instructors around the United States.

In the pool, movements are done against the resistance of the water, which is similar in effect to doing them on land with weights. In chest-deep water, the stress of impact is virtually eliminated because you weigh only about 10 percent of your on-land weight.

Water exercises include as many fancy moves as you'd find in an Esther Williams routine—walking across the pool, leg swings, lifts, circles, pedaling, and arm swings and circles. (See page 53 for examples of some of these exercises.) An additional portion of the class for encouraging endurance generally lasts 10 minutes in the regular "aquacise" class and 20 minutes in the advanced.

Some class participants also swim laps before or after class. But this requires more strength and endurance, Millet explains.

Even people in wheelchairs or those who use walkers can get into a pool with some help, Millet says. Most YMCAs have a lift or special steps that let you enter the pool without climbing down a ladder. To be certified by the Arthritis Foundation, the water temperature must be balmy— between 84° and 90°F—and the instructor must take the foundation's training. People who have trouble peeling off a wet bathing suit or negotiating a tiled floor may need to bring a family member to lend a hand; however, some Y's may have volunteers to assist.

"People are surprised to find out how much they can really do once they get into the water," Millet says.

Hop on a Bike

Cycling, especially stationary biking, is a favorite of arthritis specialists. One reason is that it's easy to measure how well people are doing on these bikes, and they can be set up just about anywhere.

Because the body's weight is on the seat, not on the legs, biking is considered a non-weight-bearing activity. It's especially helpful for people with arthritis who are overweight, says Thomas C. Namey, M.D., chief of the divisions of rheumatology and sports medicine at the University of Tennessee Graduate School of Medicine in Knoxville. "It allows them to get a good aerobic workout without pounding their knees, hips, ankles, and feet," he says.

Biking also helps strengthen the quadriceps, the muscles on the front of the thighs that help stabilize knees, and the gluteal, or buttock, muscles. This additionally takes some of the strain off the hip and knee joints, Dr. Namey says.

Who's a good candidate for cycling? "If you can stand and walk comfortably, you can probably cycle," Dr. Namey says. If you have a condition in the hips or ankles that prevents full range of motion, you may have trouble pedaling.

Some bike seats can hurt hips, so get one with a wide-cushioned, adjustable seat or a gel-based seat. Handlebars should be padded and easy to reach from a seated position. If you have back problems, be sure you can sit upright and don't have to bend forward to reach the handlebars, Dr. Namey says.

Warm up first by pedaling with low resistance for 5 minutes. Cool down the same way.

Make sure your seat is at the right height. When the pedal is at the bottom of its range, your leg should still be just slightly flexed, not perfectly straight. Try to achieve a cadence of at least 60 to 80 rpm (revolutions per minute).

Exercise cycles with handles that require back-and-forth arm movement in addition to pedaling are relatively new and may offer advantages. "They are excellent for people with arthritis," Dr. Namey says. "They help to spread the aerobic work to the upper extremities." (See "Stationary Bicycling" on page 434.)

Take a Stroll

If you can walk, and you find that it relieves your pain, many doctors recommend you make walking a part of your arthritis exercise. Start out slowly, going only as far as you can without feeling more pain than before you started. Walk three to four times a week, increasing your distance by no more than 10 percent every two weeks, Dr. Kay recommends.

Researchers at the University of Missouri who offered either water exercises or walking to arthritis patients found that people in both groups could work up to an aerobic rate. (Some doctors contend that it is hard for people with arthritis to walk fast enough to reap aerobic benefits.)

JUMP-STARTING YOUR RUSTY JOINTS

When the Tin Man in the *Wizard of Oz* wanted to get moving again, all he needed was a squirt of oil. When pain and stiffness have you immobilized, the challenge can be a little greater. What to do?

A phone call to your local chapter of the Arthritis Foundation may be your best first step. They'll send you brochures on a variety of exercise classes and at-home exercise videotapes, for range-of-motion, strengthening (without weights), and low-impact aerobic conditioning.

It's also wise to consult with the doctor who is treating your arthritis, experts agree. Your doctor may be able to evaluate your joints and muscles before you start and guide you toward the forms of exercises appropriate for your condition.

Your doctor will also know whether you are at risk for heart disease. If you are, you'll have to have a few additional tests to check your heart before you begin a more strenuous exercise program.

Experts also agree that getting special assistance in setting up your program can pay off big—by preventing "start-up" injuries. Special training should come from an expert in rehabilitative medicine and injury prevention. Several kinds of health professionals might fit that bill: physical therapist, sports medicine specialist, orthopedist, or physiatrist.

Do you want to go solo or join a group? Attending a class could mean the difference between sticking with a program and dropping out after a few fitful weeks. "The compliance rate for medically prescribed solitary exercise is terrible—fewer than 25 percent actually do it," says Donald Kay, M.D., of the Boone Clinic in Columbia, Missouri. "But when you put people together in a class, and make it a social event, the compliance rate goes up to about 85 percent."

EXERCISE CAN CAUSE ARTHRITIS: PROTECT YOURSELF

Ballet dancers get it in their toes, gymnasts in their elbows, swimmers in their shoulders, and soccer players in their feet. Even racehorses may develop osteoarthritis, usually in their much-abused forelegs.

It's not that exercise alone—even high-impact exercise like running—always causes osteoarthritis. Studies of long-time runners show they are *less* likely to have osteoarthritis than the general public.

But those findings don't mean *everyone* can pound the pavement with impunity, says Robert P. Nirschl, M.D., assistant professor of orthopedic surgery at Georgetown University School of Medicine in Washington, D.C., and medical director of the Virginia Sportsmedicine and Rehabilitation Institute in Arlington, Virginia.

"Those studies look at self-selected guinea pigs—people who were able to run for many years without injury. They don't consider all the people sidelined because of injuries," he says.

Who's most likely to be retired with early osteoarthritis? At highest risk are people who have inherited joint instabilities or misalignments, such as "loose" joints, knock-knees, or flat feet; people who are overweight; people who've had an injury to a joint or bone, such as a ligament tear or fracture, which may throw off the angle of a joint; and people who have chronic inflammation of joints for any reason.

If people at risk participate in fitness activities inappropriate for them, they may develop osteoarthritis long before they reach old age, Dr. Nirschl says.

To lower your risk of developing early osteoarthritis, he advises:

Make sure the exercise fits. Choose an activity that fits your body type. If you're overweight, out of shape, and have wobbly knees, then biking, swimming, or walking will be kinder and gentler to your flabby body than running, soccer, or football.

Easy does it. Start out slowly in any activity, no matter what your age. If your goal is fitness, beware of competitive streaks. "I've seen 80-year-old tennis players determined to beat the pants off their opponent," Dr. Nirschl says. "Competitiveness doesn't fade just because you're older, but it can always lead to injuries that set you up for osteoarthritis."

Know when to stop. Treat inflamed joints promptly and properly, with ice, rest, anti-inflammatory drugs, and a doctor's evaluation if necessary. Continue to gently move the joint only with a doctor's okay.

Cross-train. Alternate walking with biking or swimming. If possible, include light weight lifting to strengthen muscles around joints.

Do it right. Make sure you've moving with proper form when swimming, biking, and even walking. Find an expert to watch, evaluate, and correct you.

Protect yourself. Wear and use the proper equipment. Wear supportive, well-padded shoes. If you cycle, make sure your bike fits your body, and wear a helmet and gloves when you're outdoors. Proper clothes and equipment not only protect your body, they lift your spirits, contends Knoxville, Tennessee, rheumatologist Thomas C. Namey, M.D., who encourages his arthritis patients to enjoy the athletic look.

"We thought the pool group would do better, but we were surprised," says Dr. Kay. Both groups improved about equally in aerobic fitness and muscle strength. And in neither group were tender joints aggravated. "We found no evidence that weight-bearing walking exercise was detrimental," Dr. Kay says. "And we did have our share of chubbies."

The real test came when the study was over, though. Many people in the study *continued* to walk, even those initially in the water exercise group. And they were still walking a year later, and continuing to improve their fitness level, Dr. Kay says.

"Pools just aren't convenient for a lot of people, especially those in rural areas," he says. "Walking is convenient. A lot of our patients faithfully walk the malls, and they have no more flare-ups than those who don't walk." (See "Walking" on page 458.)

Motion Promotion

After pain, stiffness is one of the most common complaints of people with arthritis. These exercises are designed to improve or maintain the range of motion in your joints. They can help you to fully straighten or bend joints like your knees and elbows, circle your arms and legs, turn your head, twist your back, clench your fists, and wiggle your toes. They also help to keep joints healthy by improving blood flow and internal lubrication.

Most people with arthritis do range-of-motion exercises every day, often in a swimming pool. Although some other forms of exercise, like yoga, also move some joints through their full range of motion, there's no good substitute for these movements. Even if you have a flare-up, you may still be able to perform some movements to prevent joints from freezing up. Ask your doctor.

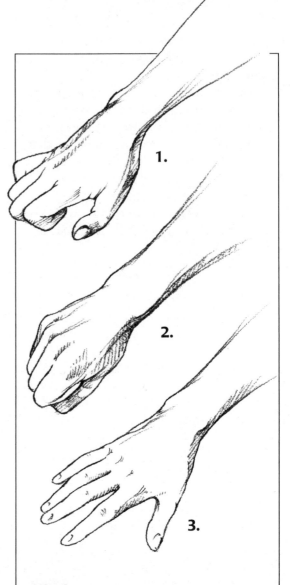

Hands

(1) Curl your fingers tightly, keeping the base knuckles straight, (2) then bend the knuckles to make a complete fist. (3) Open your hand wide, as if you were holding a large ball. Repeat several times. You can do this exercise either with both hands at once or one hand at a time.

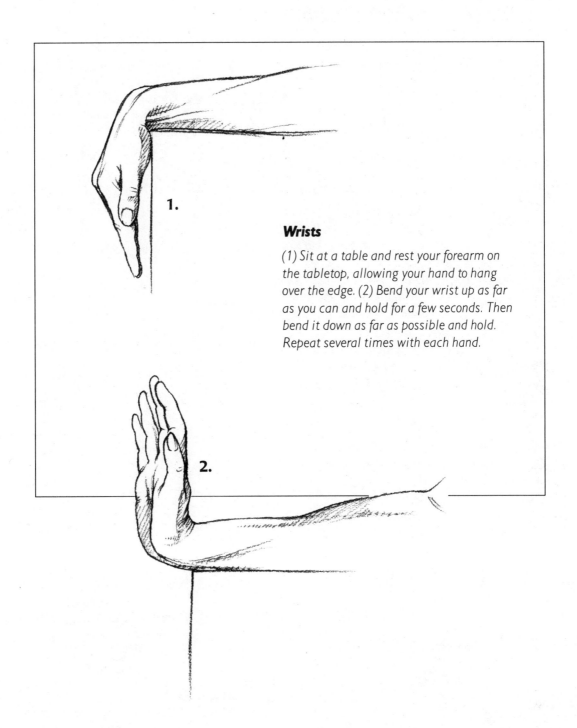

Wrists

(1) Sit at a table and rest your forearm on the tabletop, allowing your hand to hang over the edge. (2) Bend your wrist up as far as you can and hold for a few seconds. Then bend it down as far as possible and hold. Repeat several times with each hand.

Motion Promotion—Continued

Shoulders

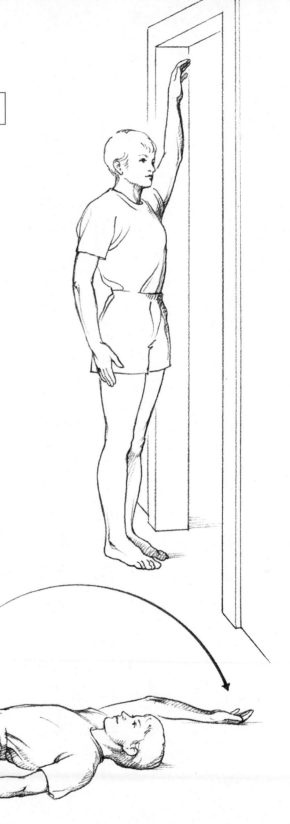

It's easy to test range of motion in your shoulder. Stand facing a wall or door frame, then reach up and mark the highest point you can touch with your fingertips. Keep your feet flat on the floor. Once a day, try to touch the mark, alternating arms. As long as you can touch it, you are maintaining your normal range of motion. (If you find that you can reach higher, mark that spot as your new self-test checkpoint.)

Lie on your back with your arms down at your sides. Slowly raise one arm over your head in a sweeping motion, keeping your elbow straight and your arm close to your head. Slowly bring your arm back down to your side. Repeat with the other arm, then repeat again, alternating arms.

Shoulders

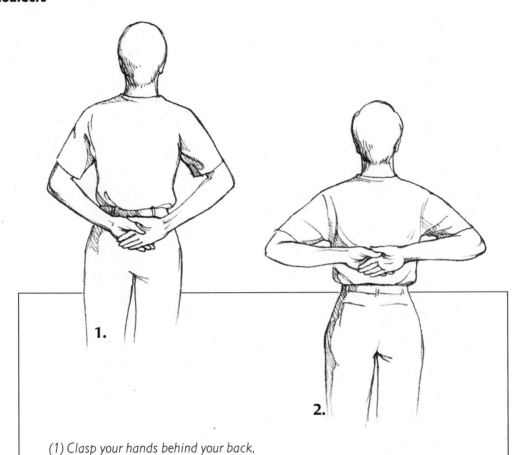

1.

2.

(1) Clasp your hands behind your back, about level with the end of your spine.
(2) Keeping your head erect and your back straight, bring your hands up as high as you can. Hold for a few seconds, then move them back down. Repeat.

Motion Promotion—Continued

Shoulders and Elbows

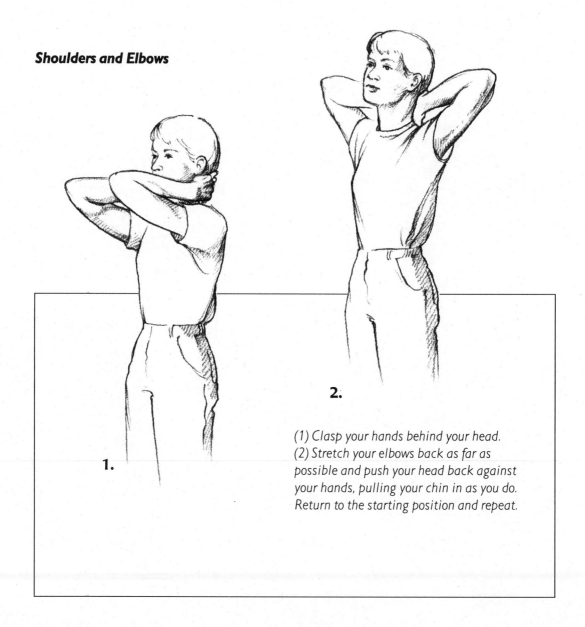

1.

2.

(1) Clasp your hands behind your head.
(2) Stretch your elbows back as far as
possible and push your head back against
your hands, pulling your chin in as you do.
Return to the starting position and repeat.

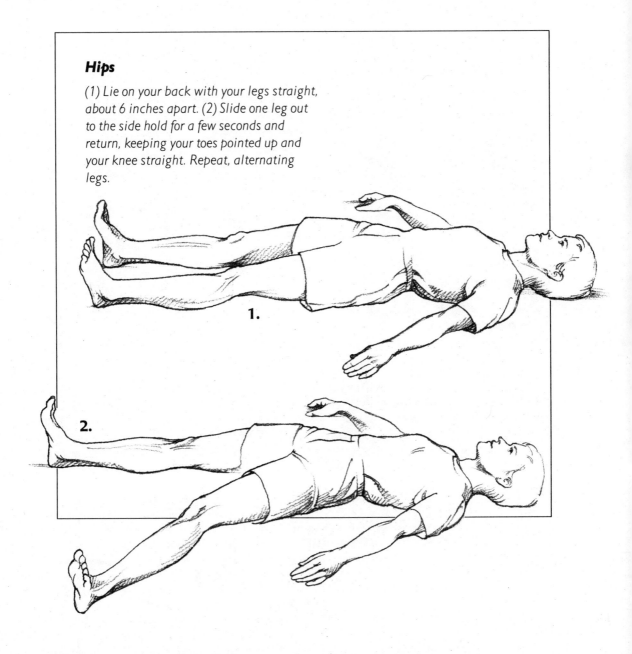

Hips

(1) Lie on your back with your legs straight, about 6 inches apart. (2) Slide one leg out to the side hold for a few seconds and return, keeping your toes pointed up and your knee straight. Repeat, alternating legs.

1.

2.

Motion Promotion—Continued

Hips

Lie in the same position as for the previous exercise, with your legs straight. Rotate one leg from the hip so your knee and foot point inward. Don't bend your knee. Then rotate your leg outward. Repeat with the other leg. Then do the entire series again, alternating legs.

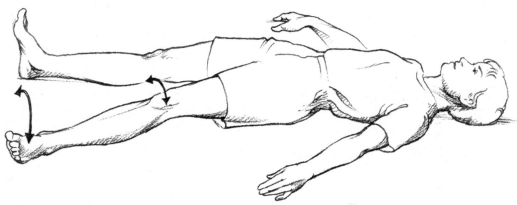

Hips and Knees

Lying on your back, bend your knee and bring it as close toward your chest as you can. Slowly straighten your leg as you return it to the floor. Repeat with the other leg, then repeat again, alternating legs.

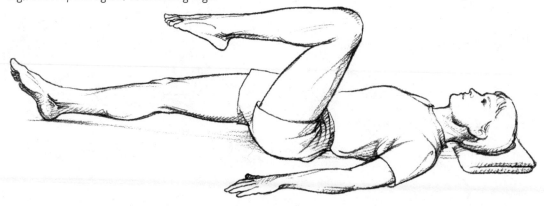

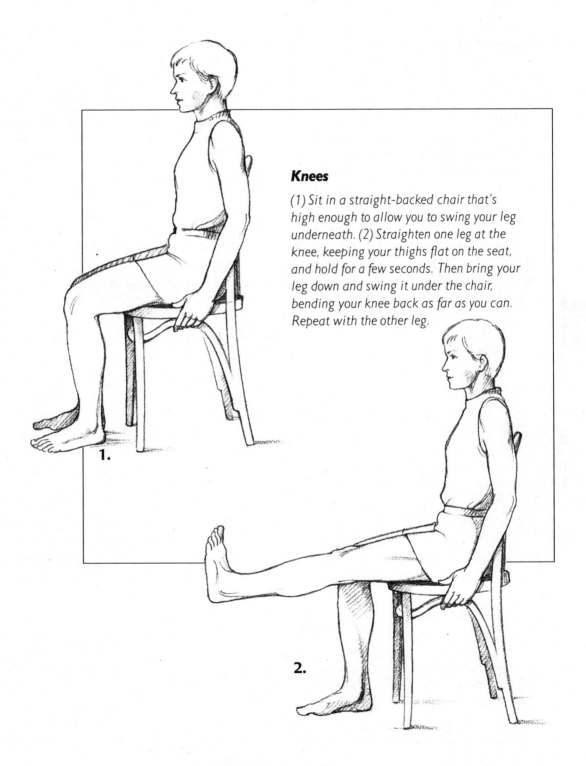

Knees

(1) Sit in a straight-backed chair that's high enough to allow you to swing your leg underneath. (2) Straighten one leg at the knee, keeping your thighs flat on the seat, and hold for a few seconds. Then bring your leg down and swing it under the chair, bending your knee back as far as you can. Repeat with the other leg.

1.

2.

Motion Promotion—Continued

Ankles

Sit comfortably with your bare feet flat on the floor. (1) Keep your heels on the floor and lift the toes and the front part of both feet as high as you can. (2) Return your feet to the floor, then raise your heels as high as possible. (3) Rotate your feet so that the soles face each other, (4) then rotate them away from each other. Hold each position for a few seconds, then repeat the entire series.

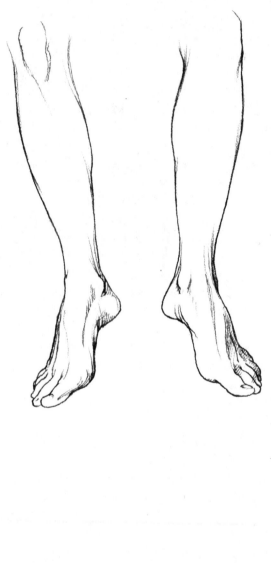

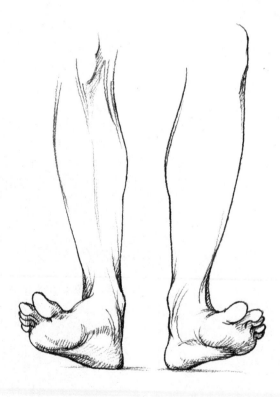

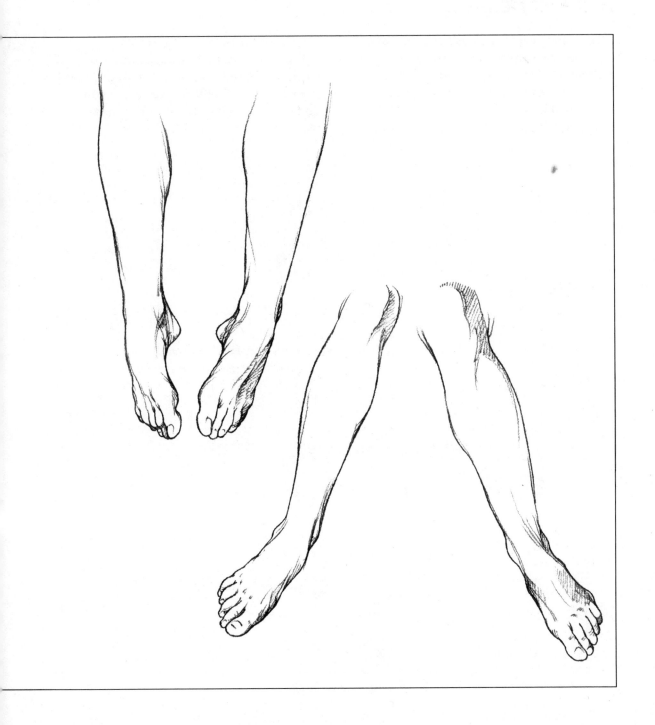

Focus on Flexibility

For some people, arthritis can lead to contracture, painful shortening of the muscles that leads to gnarled hands and a bent-over, shuffling walk. The exercises illustrated here gently work and stretch muscles to help prevent contractures and keep hands nimble and limbs useful.

If you're very stiff, you may have to work with a therapist to get started limbering up. Work slowly and gently, so you don't tear muscles. Be patient. It may take weeks to see improvement.

Hands

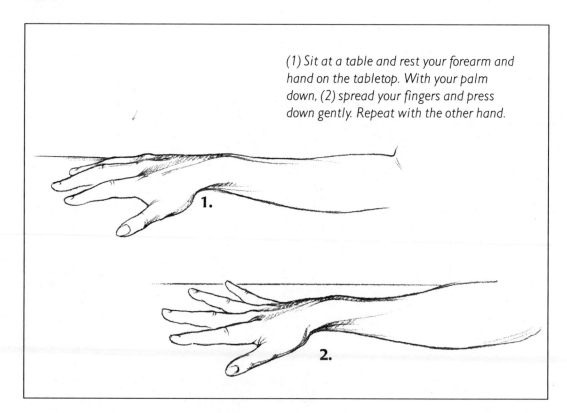

(1) Sit at a table and rest your forearm and hand on the tabletop. With your palm down, (2) spread your fingers and press down gently. Repeat with the other hand.

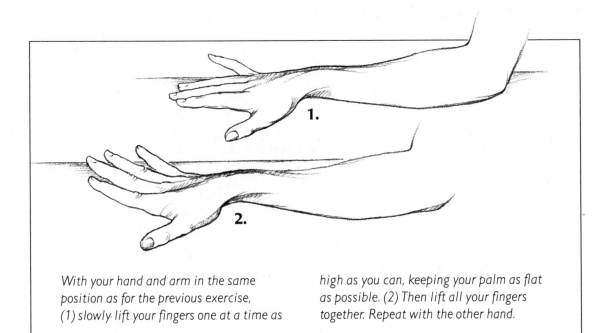

With your hand and arm in the same position as for the previous exercise, (1) slowly lift your fingers one at a time as high as you can, keeping your palm as flat as possible. (2) Then lift all your fingers together. Repeat with the other hand.

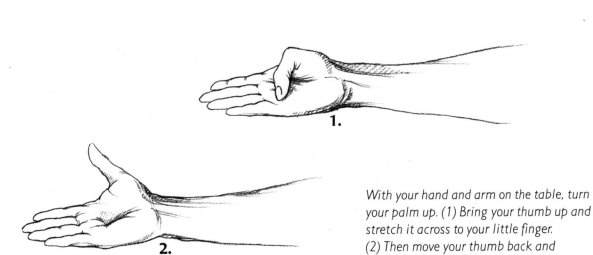

With your hand and arm on the table, turn your palm up. (1) Bring your thumb up and stretch it across to your little finger. (2) Then move your thumb back and stretch it out at almost a right angle to your hand. Repeat with the other hand.

Focus on Flexibility—Continued

Fingers

Hold your hand up and spread your fingers. Then touch each finger in turn to the tip of your thumb, as if making an "OK" sign. Repeat with the other hand.

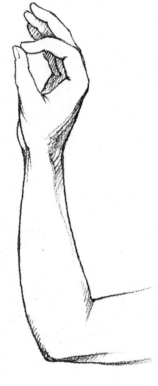

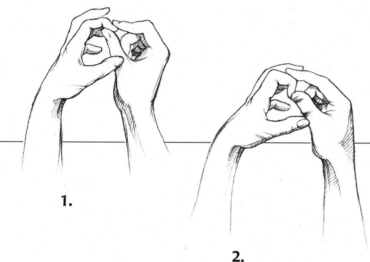

1.

2.

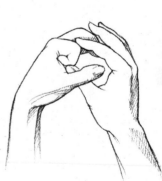

3.

You can do this exercise with one finger at a time or all together; the object is to touch your fingertips to your palm. (1) Bend the joint at the top of your finger, then (2) bend the middle joint. (3) Finally, bend the knuckle joint so that the finger is somewhat curled and touching the palm. If your fingers are very stiff, you can use the other hand to help the movement. Apply gentle pressure; don't force it.

To help keep your fingers from getting out
of alignment, try this sliding exercise.
Place your hand flat on a table, with your
fingers together and your thumb extended.
Slide your index finger out toward your
thumb, then slide each of the other fingers
over in turn. Repeat with the other hand.
You can use your other hand to help control
the movement if you have to.

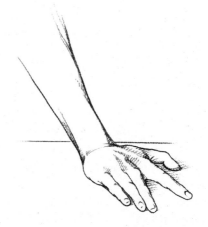

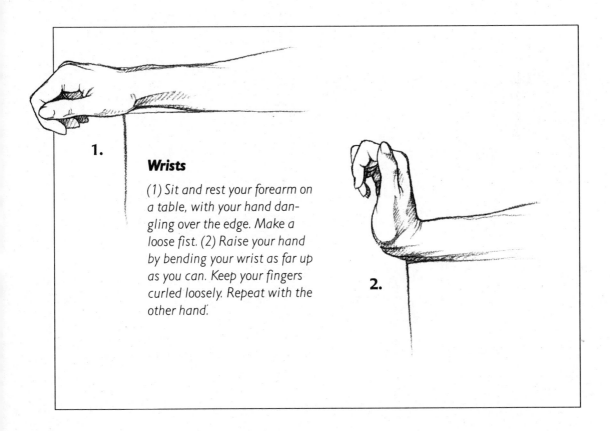

1.

Wrists

*(1) Sit and rest your forearm on
a table, with your hand dangling over the edge. Make a
loose fist. (2) Raise your hand
by bending your wrist as far up
as you can. Keep your fingers
curled loosely. Repeat with the
other hand.*

2.

Focus on Flexibility—Continued

Wrists

(1) Still sitting, rest your elbows on the table and place your palms together with your fingers slightly intertwined. (2) Press one hand back with the other, exerting pressure with the palm, not the fingers. The arm of the hand that is doing the pressing will have to come up from the table somewhat. Then reverse and press the other hand back. Press until the position is just slightly uncomfortable, but not to the point of pain. Repeat.

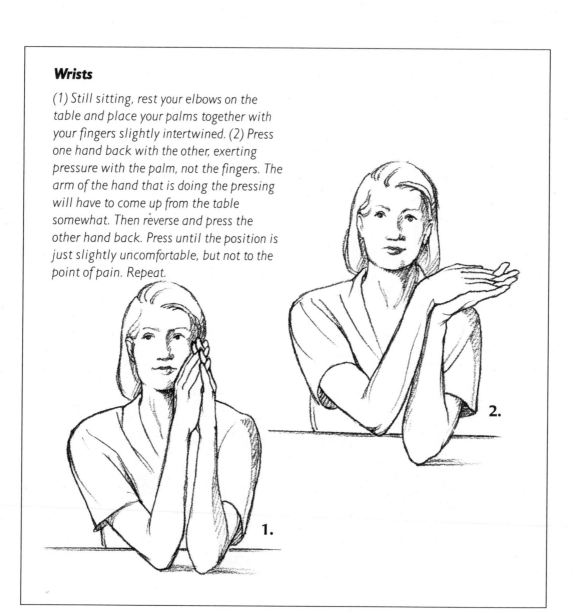

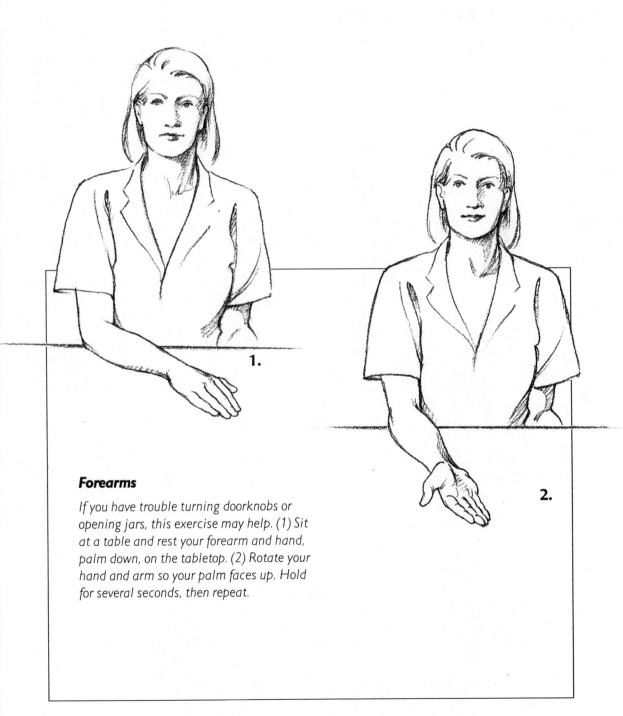

1.

2.

Forearms

If you have trouble turning doorknobs or opening jars, this exercise may help. (1) Sit at a table and rest your forearm and hand, palm down, on the tabletop. (2) Rotate your hand and arm so your palm faces up. Hold for several seconds, then repeat.

Focus on Flexibility—Continued

Elbows

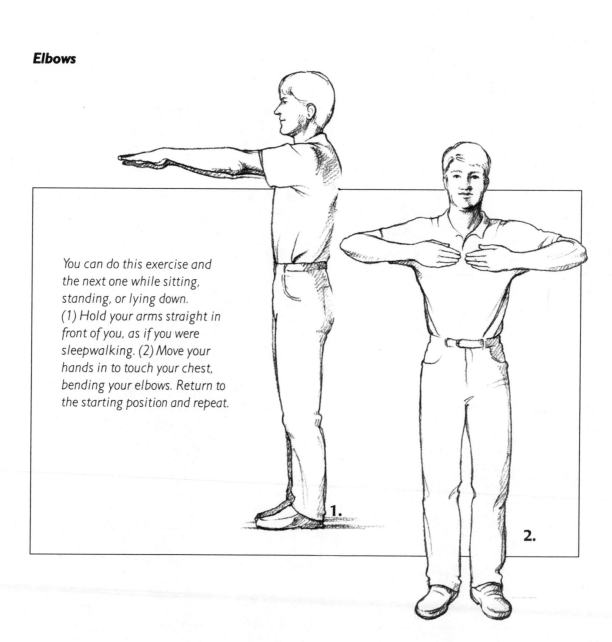

You can do this exercise and the next one while sitting, standing, or lying down. (1) Hold your arms straight in front of you, as if you were sleepwalking. (2) Move your hands in to touch your chest, bending your elbows. Return to the starting position and repeat.

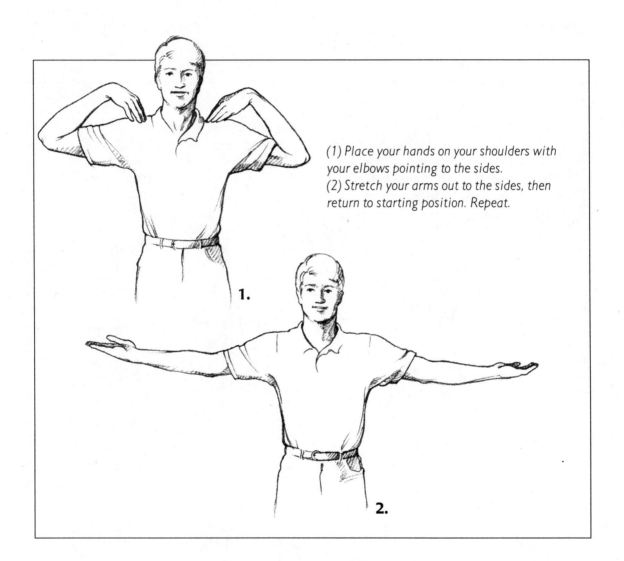

(1) Place your hands on your shoulders with your elbows pointing to the sides.
(2) Stretch your arms out to the sides, then return to starting position. Repeat.

1.

2.

Focus on Flexibility—Continued

Shoulders

This exercise may help if you have trouble reaching behind your head. (1) Lie on your back and rest your left elbow on the floor. Bend that arm up, with the palm of your hand facing inward. Reach across your body with the right arm and grasp the left arm just above the elbow, to support it. (2) Now extend your left arm as far as you can toward the floor, with the palm up. Hold for several seconds. Repeat on the other side.

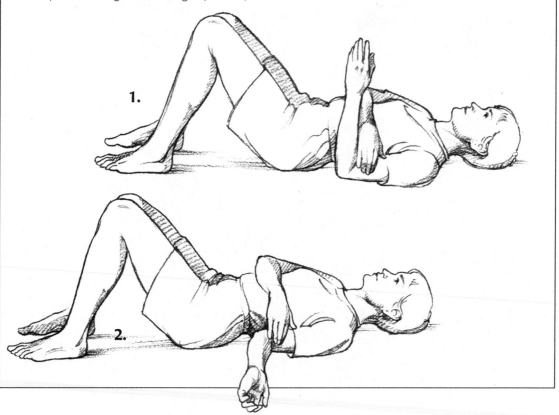

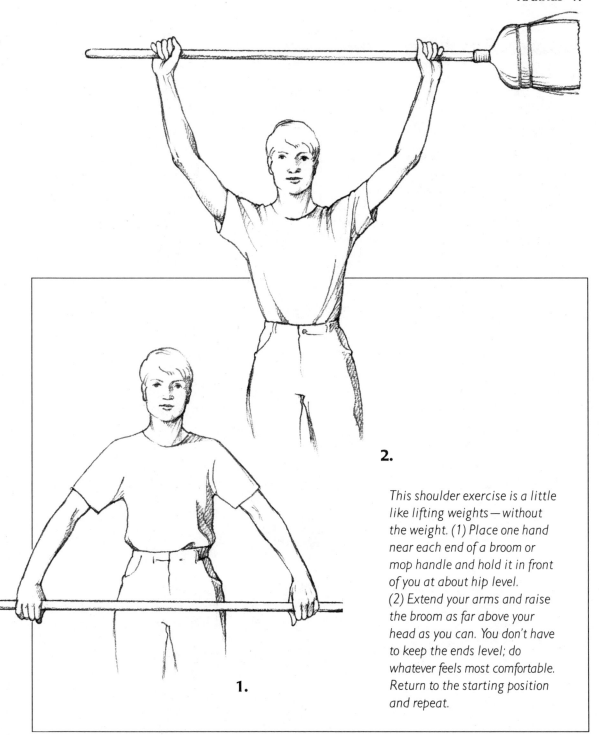

2.

This shoulder exercise is a little like lifting weights—without the weight. (1) Place one hand near each end of a broom or mop handle and hold it in front of you at about hip level. (2) Extend your arms and raise the broom as far above your head as you can. You don't have to keep the ends level; do whatever feels most comfortable. Return to the starting position and repeat.

1.

Focus on Flexibility—Continued

Shoulders

You'll need a piece of rope for this exercise. Place the rope over an open door so that one end hangs down on each side. Sit or stand with your back to the door and grasp one end in each hand, then pull down on one side, raising the other arm as you pull. Go just to the point of discomfort, hold for a moment, then reverse the motion and pull down on the other side. Repeat.

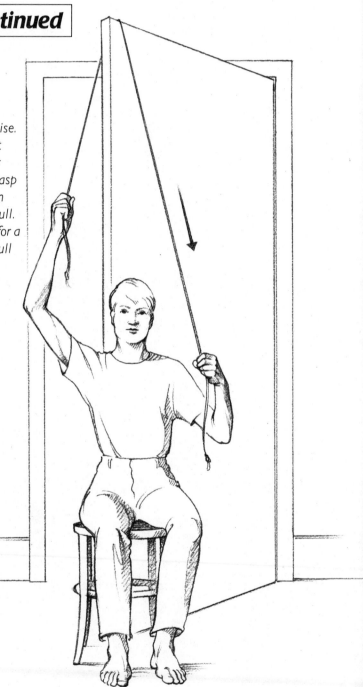

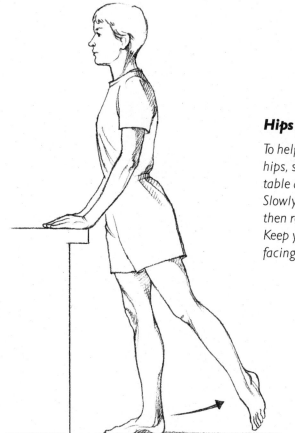

Hips

To help ease backward movement in the hips, stand erect facing a counter or sturdy table and support yourself with your hands. Slowly swing one leg back from the hip, then return. Repeat with the other leg. Keep your knees straight and your hips facing forward.

(1) Lie on your back with your arms extended to the sides, or place your hands behind your head. Bend your knees and put your feet flat on the floor, then cross one leg over the other knee, keeping both knees bent. (2) Rotating from the hips and keeping your upper body flat on the floor, turn your legs to one side and drop your knees toward the floor. Return to the starting position and repeat to the other side. Now cross your leg the other way and repeat.

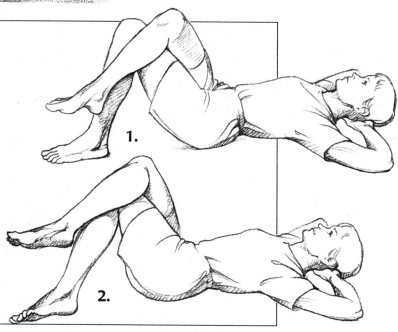

Focus on Flexibility—Continued

Ankles

Sit in a chair and place your bare feet flat on the floor. (1) Raise the front of your feet as high as possible while keeping your heels on the floor. (2) With your heels in the same position and toes up, keep your feet together and move them to the right. (3) Relax, then raise up on your toes as high as possible and move your heels to the left. Repeat in the opposite directions.

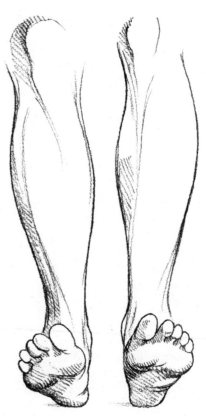

1.

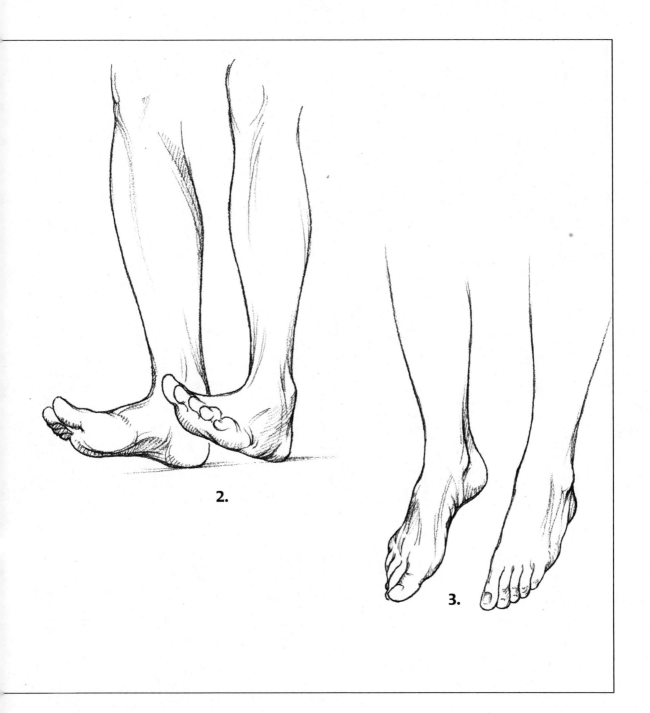

2.

3.

Focus on Flexibility—Continued

Feet

You can do this exercise while sitting or standing. (1) Put your right foot flat on the floor. (2) Now lift your arch only, not your toes, and try to slide your toes back toward your heel, as if you were trying to relieve an itchy foot without removing your shoe. (3) Then stretch your toes as far apart as you can. Repeat with the left foot.

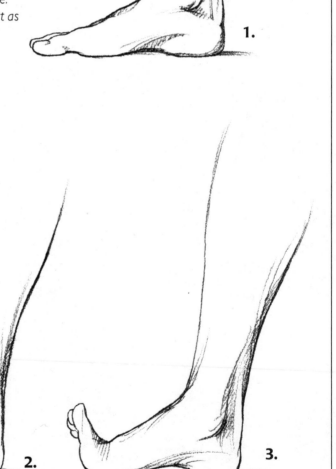

1.

2.

3.

Warm Water Works Wonders

In a pool, it's possible for people with arthritis to get an aerobic workout without pounding tender knees, to build muscles without lifting weights, and to move joints in a gravity-free environment. In general, start with three or four repetitions of any range-of-motion exercise, and work up to ten.

Some of these pool exercises are part of the Arthritis Foundation's YMCA Aquatic Program. They should be done in water that's about chest-deep. If you are having a flare-up, or have not exercised previously, move joints slowly and through fewer repetitions. Move an inflamed joint through its range of motion *gently*. If you've had joint replacement surgery, check with your doctor before you begin any exercise program about which movements you can safely do.

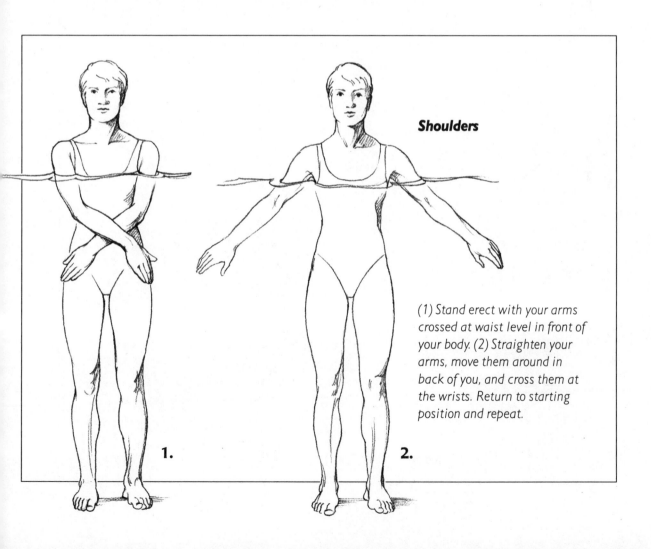

Shoulders

(1) Stand erect with your arms crossed at waist level in front of your body. (2) Straighten your arms, move them around in back of you, and cross them at the wrists. Return to starting position and repeat.

1.

2.

Warm Water Works Wonders—Continued

Shoulders

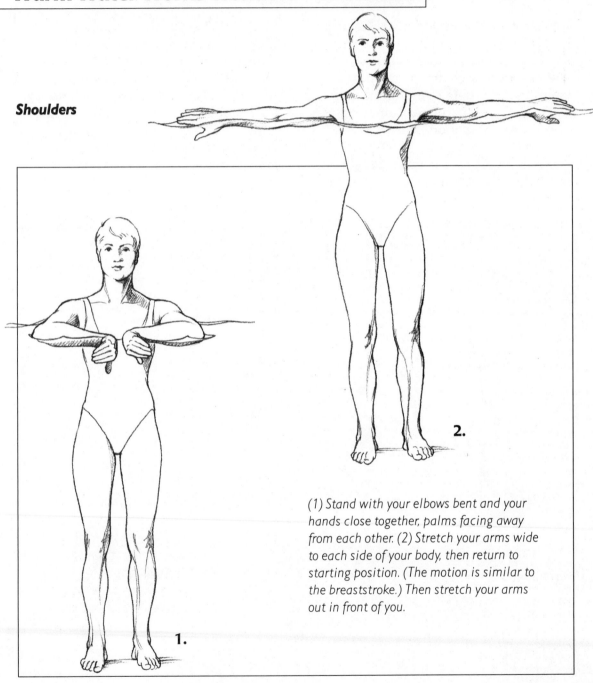

(1) Stand with your elbows bent and your hands close together, palms facing away from each other. (2) Stretch your arms wide to each side of your body, then return to starting position. (The motion is similar to the breaststroke.) Then stretch your arms out in front of you.

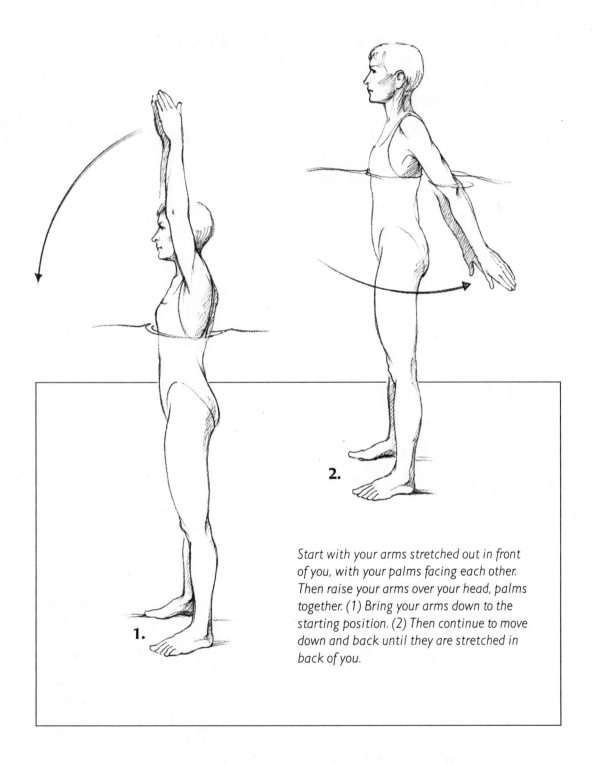

1.

2.

Start with your arms stretched out in front of you, with your palms facing each other. Then raise your arms over your head, palms together. (1) Bring your arms down to the starting position. (2) Then continue to move down and back until they are stretched in back of you.

Warm Water Works Wonders—Continued

Shoulders and Wrists

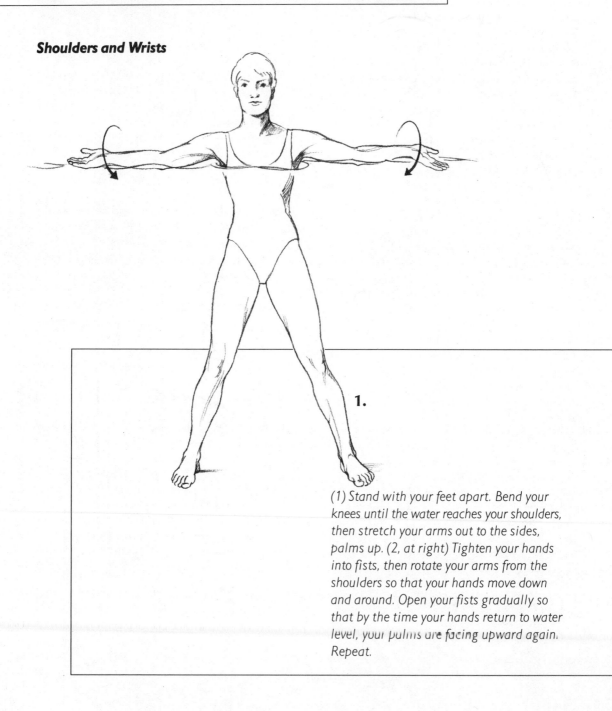

1.

(1) Stand with your feet apart. Bend your knees until the water reaches your shoulders, then stretch your arms out to the sides, palms up. (2, at right) Tighten your hands into fists, then rotate your arms from the shoulders so that your hands move down and around. Open your fists gradually so that by the time your hands return to water level, your palms are facing upward again. Repeat.

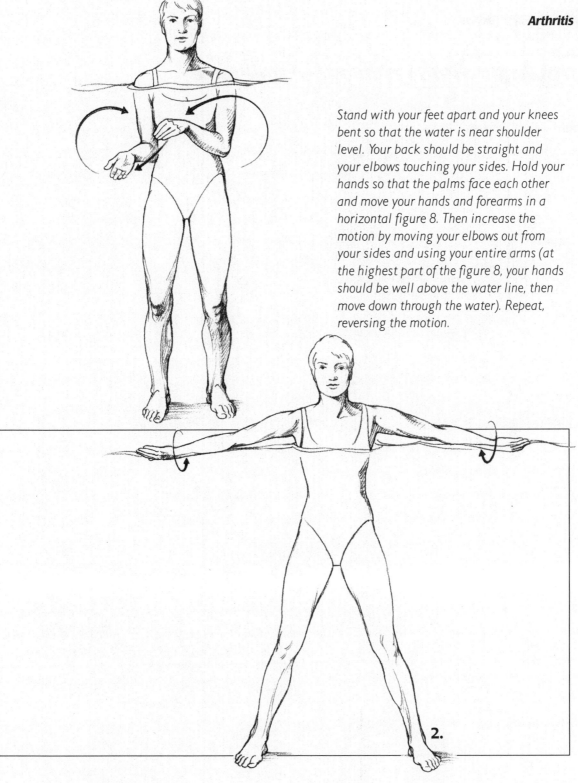

Stand with your feet apart and your knees bent so that the water is near shoulder level. Your back should be straight and your elbows touching your sides. Hold your hands so that the palms face each other and move your hands and forearms in a horizontal figure 8. Then increase the motion by moving your elbows out from your sides and using your entire arms (at the highest part of the figure 8, your hands should be well above the water line, then move down through the water). Repeat, reversing the motion.

2.

Warm Water Works Wonders—Continued

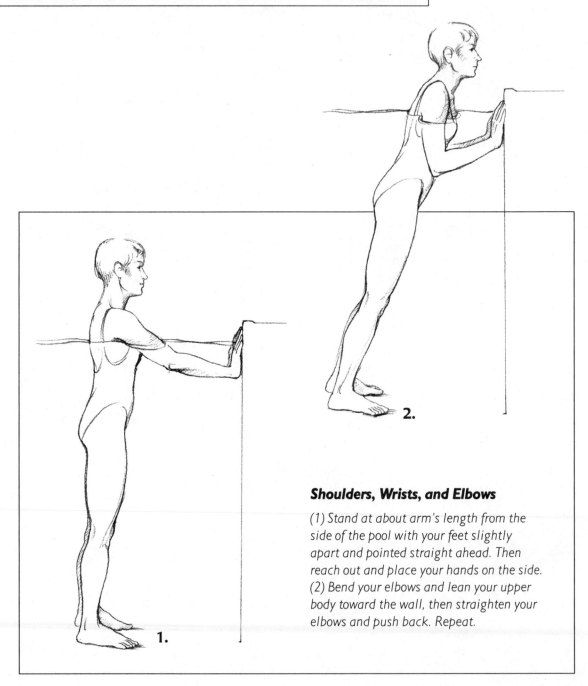

2.

1.

Shoulders, Wrists, and Elbows

(1) Stand at about arm's length from the side of the pool with your feet slightly apart and pointed straight ahead. Then reach out and place your hands on the side. (2) Bend your elbows and lean your upper body toward the wall, then straighten your elbows and push back. Repeat.

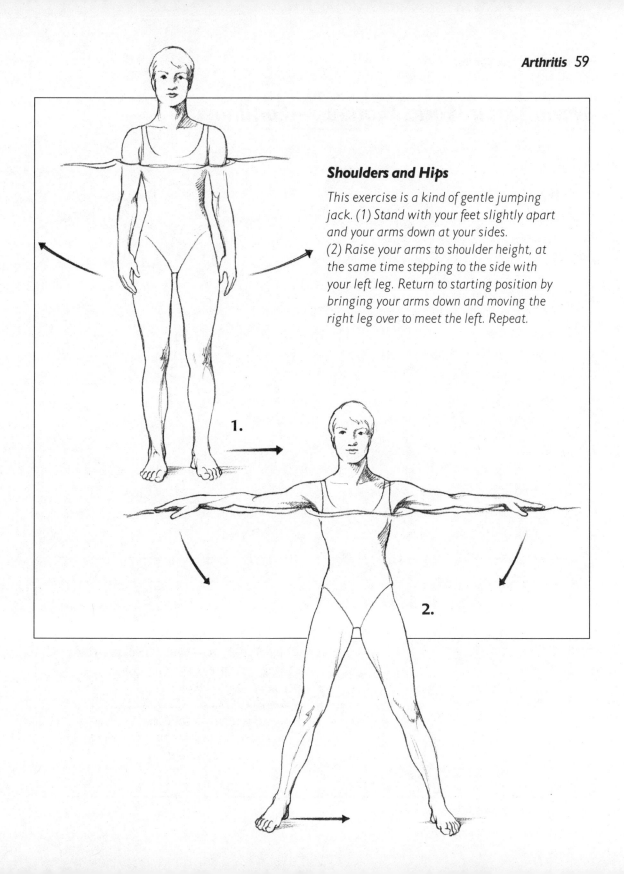

Shoulders and Hips

This exercise is a kind of gentle jumping jack. (1) Stand with your feet slightly apart and your arms down at your sides.
(2) Raise your arms to shoulder height, at the same time stepping to the side with your left leg. Return to starting position by bringing your arms down and moving the right leg over to meet the left. Repeat.

1.

2.

Warm Water Works Wonders—Continued

Legs

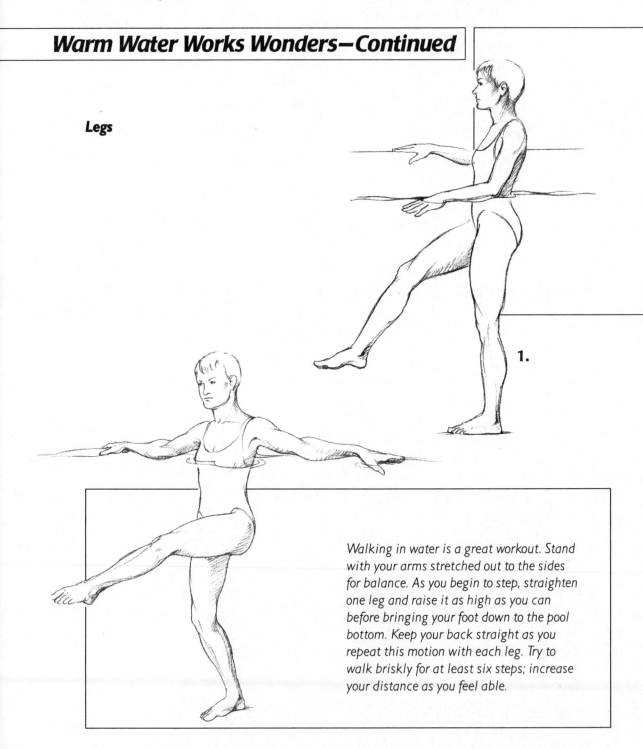

1.

Walking in water is a great workout. Stand with your arms stretched out to the sides for balance. As you begin to step, straighten one leg and raise it as high as you can before bringing your foot down to the pool bottom. Keep your back straight as you repeat this motion with each leg. Try to walk briskly for at least six steps; increase your distance as you feel able.

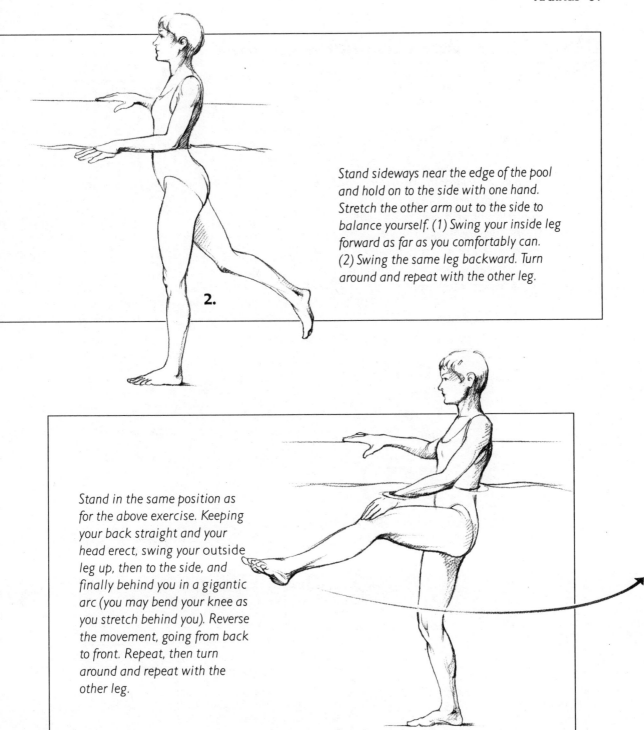

Stand sideways near the edge of the pool and hold on to the side with one hand. Stretch the other arm out to the side to balance yourself. (1) Swing your inside leg forward as far as you comfortably can. (2) Swing the same leg backward. Turn around and repeat with the other leg.

2.

Stand in the same position as for the above exercise. Keeping your back straight and your head erect, swing your outside leg up, then to the side, and finally behind you in a gigantic arc (you may bend your knee as you stretch behind you). Reverse the movement, going from back to front. Repeat, then turn around and repeat with the other leg.

Warm Water Works Wonders—Continued

Hips and Knees

*Stand sideways near the edge of the pool
and hold on to the side with one hand.
Extend your other arm for balance, if
necessary. Keeping your knee as straight as
possible, raise your outside leg and swing
it in a wide vertical circle, rotating from
the hip. Reverse the movement, then turn
around and repeat with the other leg.*

*Support yourself on the side of the pool
with your hands and elbows. Keeping your
back and buttocks pressed against the pool
wall, raise both legs parallel to the pool
bottom. Point your toes toward the ceiling
and spread your legs as far apart as you
can, then bring them together quickly as
you stretch your toes forward.*

1.

Stand with your back to the side of the pool
and place one hand on the edge to steady
yourself. (1) Lift one leg to the side.
(2) Then swing it back across in front of the
other leg. Repeat with the other leg.

2.

Warm Water Works Wonders—Continued

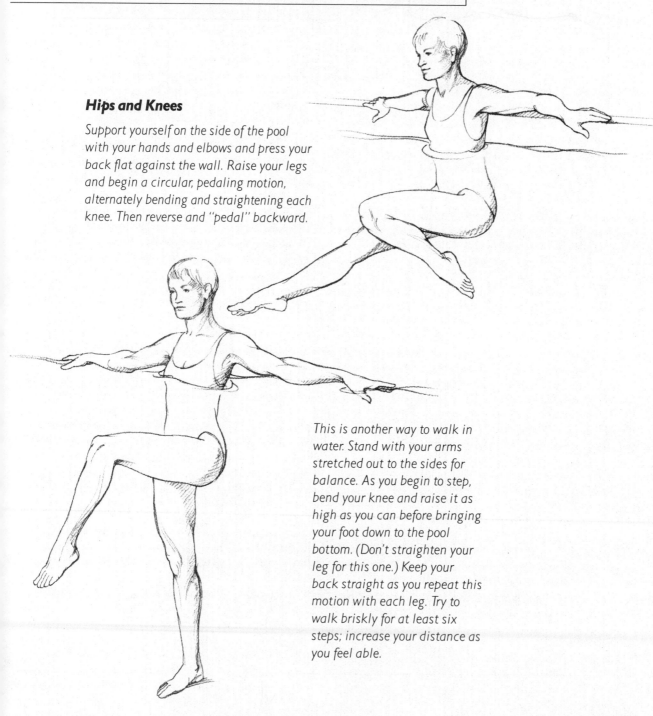

Hips and Knees

Support yourself on the side of the pool with your hands and elbows and press your back flat against the wall. Raise your legs and begin a circular, pedaling motion, alternately bending and straightening each knee. Then reverse and "pedal" backward.

This is another way to walk in water. Stand with your arms stretched out to the sides for balance. As you begin to step, bend your knee and raise it as high as you can before bringing your foot down to the pool bottom. (Don't straighten your leg for this one.) Keep your back straight as you repeat this motion with each leg. Try to walk briskly for at least six steps; increase your distance as you feel able.

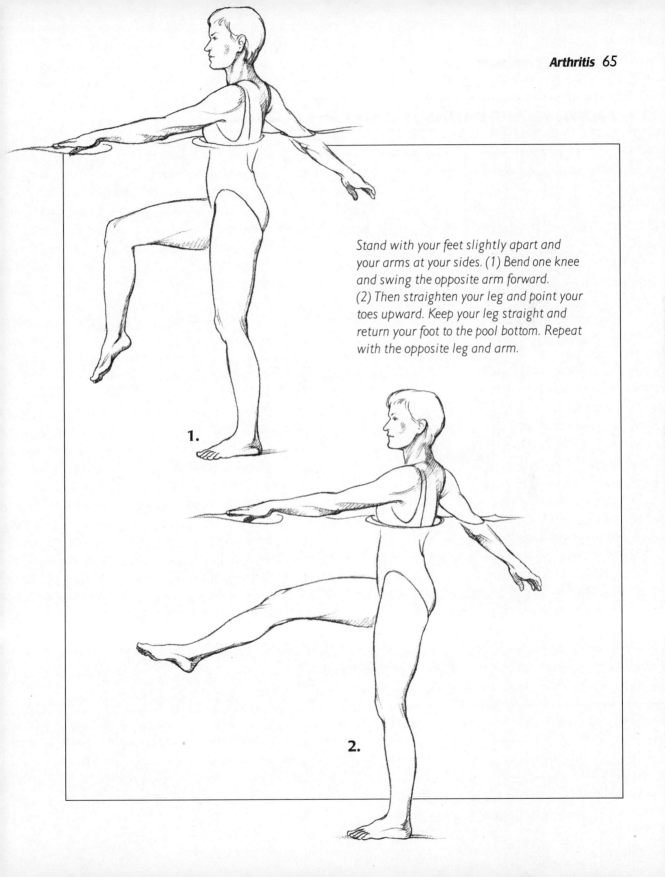

Stand with your feet slightly apart and
your arms at your sides. (1) Bend one knee
and swing the opposite arm forward.
(2) Then straighten your leg and point your
toes upward. Keep your leg straight and
return your foot to the pool bottom. Repeat
with the opposite leg and arm.

1.

2.

Warm Water Works Wonders—Continued

Hips and Feet

Stand facing the pool wall and grab on to the edge firmly with both hands. Bend your knees and begin to walk up the wall on the balls of your feet. Walk as high as you can, bringing your knees and chin close to your chest, then walk back down. (Do not do this exercise if you experience any discomfort or back pain.)

Stand with your arms relaxed at your sides. Lift one leg behind you, placing the ball of your foot on the pool bottom first and then continuing until your foot is flat on the bottom. Continue walking for a minute or two, backward, keeping your back straight and lifting your leg from the hip.

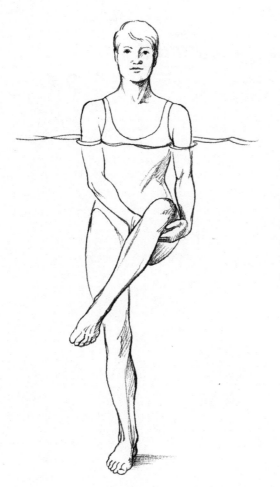

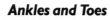

Knees

With your back firmly against the pool wall, lift one leg, bend your knee, and put both hands under the thigh, supporting it near the knee. Now circle your lower leg slowly, first in one direction, then in the other. Repeat with the other leg.

Ankles and Toes

Supporting yourself against the side of the pool, raise one foot and circle it, first in one direction, then in the other. Repeat with the other foot. (If you feel tingling or cramping, stop.)

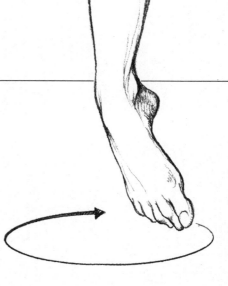

Warm Water Works Wonders—Continued

Feet

Stand with your feet about 6 inches apart and your arms spread for balance. You can hold on to the edge of the pool with one hand if you need to. (1) Roll forward onto your toes, tensing your leg and stomach muscles and keeping your back and head straight. Hold for a count of six. (2) Roll back onto your heels, raising your toes slightly. Hold for a count of six, then return to the starting position and repeat.

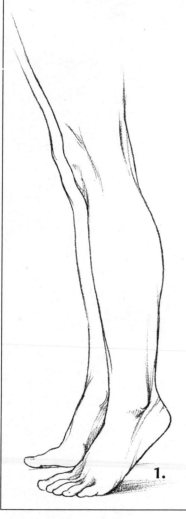

1.

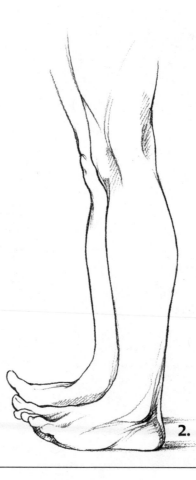

2.

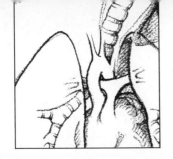

Asthma

*I*f you have asthma, you live with the ever-present fear of having an attack that could leave you breathless any time you exert yourself. That's a high price to pay for a little recreational bicycling or a game of tennis. It's a fear that forces many people to become exercise dropouts.

"It was scary not knowing when my chest would begin to tighten or if my breathing would get so bad I'd have to go to the hospital," says Mark Luetkemeyer, a St. Louis librarian who has had asthma since infancy. "I'd start wheezing 5 minutes into any physical activity. I had to sit out gym class and quit Boy Scouts because I couldn't keep up on camping trips. Eventually, I avoided all physical activity."

Experts theorize that exercise-induced asthma works like this: Upon exertion, your breathing deepens. The air rushes into your airways without a chance to become properly warmed and humidified through your nasal passages. For people with sensitive airways, an onslaught of relatively cold, dry air triggers (among other things) the release of high doses of histamine. This substance causes the muscles surrounding the small airways of the lungs (the bronchioles) to go into spasm and squeeze down. Histamine also causes the airway linings to swell and produce

mucus, which plugs the narrowed air passages, producing that awful chest-tightening sensation that people with asthma come to dread.

Fortunately, Mark (and many others like him) has discovered that with medication and monitoring, he can enjoy exercise without frightening symptoms—in fact, that regular exercise actually *improves* the breathing problems of asthma.

At the urging of his doctor, Mark enrolled in an exercise program for people with asthma at the St. Louis University Medical Center. Three times a week, he bicycles or walks on a treadmill under close supervision.

"Working out helps my chest feel more open, and I can breathe easier," he says. "I don't need as much asthma medicine as I did before I started exercising."

Mark is also thrilled with the confidence and control he's gained from exercise. "Now I know how my body reacts during exercise and what to do if I start to get in trouble," he says. "What's really wonderful is that I can go up to my father's cabin on the Lake of the Ozarks and take walks through the woods without wheezing."

More Efficient Breathing

The key to exercise's effectiveness as an asthma therapy is that it makes breathing more *efficient*.

"We've found that if an asthmatic person breathes 100 liters of air per minute before aerobic training, for example, he'll breathe less after training," says Francois Haas, M.D., Ph.D., director of the Pulmonary Function Laboratory at New York University Medical Center in New York City. "With less air coming in and out, there's less of the stimulus that triggers asthma."

Other scientific evidence shows that exercise may affect the airways directly. "We also found that when a physically fit asthmatic person breathes in a greater amount of air, his exercise-induced asthma is still less severe than it was before training," says Dr. Haas. "This may indicate that exercise helps make the airways less sensitive."

The Best Exercises for Asthmatics

Any exercise that raises your heart rate and increases your respiratory rate is helpful. But some forms of exercise are ideal.

"If I had to pick the best exercise for asthma sufferers, it would be swimming," says David Orenstein, M.D., director of pediatric pulmonary medicine at Children's Hospital in Pittsburgh. Swimming has been shown to cause fewer episodes of exercise-induced asthma than other activities. "One explanation is that swimmers inhale warm, humid air, which is less likely to trigger an asthma attack," he says.

People with asthma may also find that tennis, baseball, and other start-and-stop exercises may induce fewer symptoms than continuous kinds of activities like running or bicycling. By engaging in shorter bursts of exercise and then stopping, you may be less likely to provoke an attack, says Stanley Wolf, M.D., clinical professor at George Washington Medical School in Washington, D.C. If you're looking for a safe way to get regular aerobic exercise, however, he recommends brisk walking in an indoor shopping mall.

"It's easy, and you don't have to worry about cold air, pollen, or other asthma triggers," says Dr. Wolf. Plus, you can usually find a companion to walk with who can add fun to your jaunts.

Special Precautions

For the majority of people with asthma, any exercise should be safe as long as you take certain precautions, says Ellen Garibaldi, M.D., director of the Adult Asthma Exercise Program at St. Louis University Medical Center.

"If your asthma is under control, and you premedicate before exercising, there is no physical activity you can't—or shouldn't—do," she says.

Premedication means taking two puffs of inhaled bronchodilator a half hour before exercising. Studies show that this precaution protects against exercise-induced asthma in 95 percent of all cases.

Your doctor may have you use a bronchodilator along with cromolyn sodium, an oral medication that helps reduce airway sensitivity.

And be sure to keep your inhaler handy *while* you exercise, says Dr. Garibaldi, who recommends that you use it at the first sign of discomfort.

If you want to be extra careful, particularly if you have a history of asthma attacks while exercising, try a group exercise program for people with breathing problems.

Dr. Wolf has had success with group sessions that put emphasis on reaching and other upper-torso movements. "The exercise is aimed at stretching and strengthening the diaphragm, which is the major breathing muscle," says Dr. Wolf. "The diaphragm becomes weak and inefficient in people with asthma, who breathe rapidly and shallowly. People in the program felt the exercises made their breathing 'open' and 'clean.' "

A big plus for participating in specialized programs is that you can have your heart rate and breathing tolerance monitored and learn ways to handle those symptoms of tightness in the chest, says Dr. Wolf.

In the program Mark Luetkemeyer attended, for example, he learned how to use a peak flow meter, a device used to measure breathing. "This gadget was a big help in letting me know when I should stop exercising and when it was okay to get back up to speed," he says.

Gentle Exercise for Stress Relief

There's a special type of exercise that's particularly good for asthmatics—exercises that let them relax. Like yoga.

Nashville administrative assistant Laura Clendening uses yoga postures to avert asthma attacks in the same way some people use massage to abort a migraine headache.

"If I drape myself backward over a bolster at the first hint of pressure in my chest, I can fully relax," she says. "Yoga helps open up my passageways so I feel more comfortable and can breathe easier. This helps me pull out of the attack before it gets really bad."

Experts agree that performing yoga can be a good way to feel in control when dreadful symptoms occur.

"An asthma attack can feel very much like a panic attack," says Mary P. Schatz, M.D., a pathologist at the Centennial Medical Center in Nashville, an instructor of therapeutic yoga, and author of *Back Care Basics: A Doctor's Gentle Yoga Program for Back and Neck Pain Relief.* "When you fear your air supply is shutting off, your muscles tighten up. Tense muscles make you have to work harder in order to breathe. This extra work uses up more oxygen. Yoga can be an easy and effective way to relax tense muscles."

When you feel a twinge of chest tightness, a "passive backbend" yoga posture may help bring relief. Fold one or two blankets into a pile 4 to 10 inches high. Sit on the very edge of the pile, keeping your knees bent and your feet flat on the floor. (Adjust the height for comfort.) Gently lie back, allowing your shoulders and the back of your head to rest on the floor. The blankets will support the small of your back. Breathe gently and evenly. As you exhale, slowly slide one leg straight out on the floor in front of you, then slide the other. Hold the posture for 1 to 4 minutes.

Learning how to breathe deeply and gently is a major benefit of yoga. "During an asthma attack, the airways clamp down, making exhaling harder," says Dr.

Schatz. "Learning to exhale fully keeps your airways open and helps your lungs empty, enabling you to inhale more deeply."

Studies show that relaxed deep breathing—like that taught in yoga classes—may also help shore up resistance against asthma attacks.

British researchers had one group of people with asthma practice a yoga breathing technique involving an extended exhale; another group was told to breathe normally. Each group practiced breathing for 15 minutes, twice daily. After two weeks, the researchers found that it took twice the amount of histamine to cause the airway to narrow down in the yoga breathers as it did in the normal breathers.

What this might mean in practical terms is that your body may still produce histamine when you exert yourself—that's what happens in people with asthma—but your airways may not react to the histamine by narrowing down.

To do an abbreviated form of this type of yoga breathing, simply sit or lie in a comfortable position. Close your eyes. Inhale easily and slowly through your nose. Now exhale the same way through your nose, then pause at the end of the inhalation while counting to yourself, "one thousand one, one thousand two." Then inhale again. Continue breathing this way for a minute or longer. (See "Yoga" on page 480.)

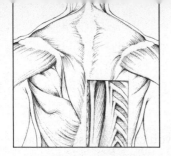

Back Pain

Almost anyone who owns a wrench knows about WD-40. You spray some of this solvent on a stuck nut, work it a little bit, and before you can say "@*!+&$*" the nut's unstuck, and life can go on.

Well, exercise has been called "WD-40 for the back," and with good reason. Properly done, exercise lubricates the joints of the spine, loosens and restores flexibility to a multitude of spine-shoring muscles and ligaments, restores or improves blood flow to back muscles, helps strengthen the muscles surrounding and supporting the spine, and helps strengthen the thigh muscles, which should be doing most of the work when you lift that bale.

Exercise can do so much good for your back that many doctors agree it tops the list of back pain prevention strategies. (Improperly done, though, just about any kind of exercise can *hurt* your back. More on that later.)

Properly done, certain exercises may also ease acute back pain caused by a muscle spasm. Knee-to-chest stretches (see the illustration on page 83), shoulder shrugs and neck rolls (see "Neck and Shoulder Pain" on page 239), or certain yoga positions (see "Yoga" on page 480) may help, depending on the location of your pain.

Exercise programs are often prescribed to restore an injured back. Later, that rehabilitation program might be modified to a maintenance plan to keep the back from sustaining another injury. That's important, since once you've had one episode of back pain, your chances of being laid up with a second bout are high.

Exercise programs may even prove to be a successful alternative to surgery for certain back problems.

One study, done by doctors at the San Francisco Spine Institute and the SpineCare Medical Group in Daly City, California, looked at 64 people with low back pain and leg pain caused by one or more herniated disks pressing against nerve roots. Some 90 percent of those who went through an aggressive physical rehabilitation program that included stretching and strengthening exercises and posture training reported that they had good or excellent results. Most were able to return to their previous jobs, according to Jeffrey Saal, M.D., the study's main author.

Fifteen of the 18 people in one group, who had been advised by a surgeon that they needed surgery as soon as possible to avoid long-term complications, reported that they also had good or excellent results with their exercise program. Of the 6 people in the program who failed to improve with exercise and went on to have surgery, 4 were found to have an additional prob-

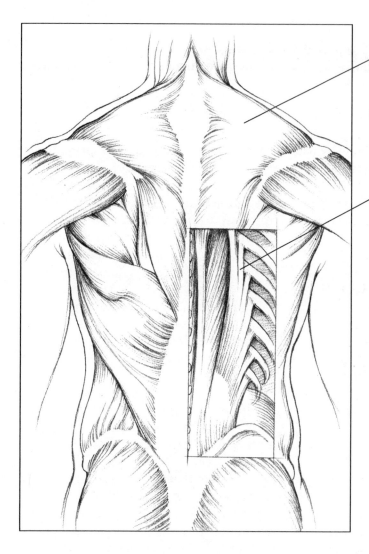

Superficial muscles

Trapezius (upper fibers, middle fibers, lower fibers): supports your shoulders Latissimus dorsi: anchors on your lower back and pulls your arm back

Deep muscles

Erector spinae: 3 columns of muscle that extend your back

Your back is an intricate network of bones, ligaments, and muscles. Muscles anchored to the back support and move your shoulders and upper arms. Others anchor the back to your pelvis and vice versa. They all work together, performing a balancing act so you can stand, twist, and bend. With so many delicate working parts, it's no wonder the back is a frequent source of trouble for many people.

lem—stenosis, a narrowing of openings in the spinal column, which can pinch nerves.

These findings, that the right kind of exercise can ease even severe back pain, should be good news for a fairly large percentage of the population. Eight out of ten people experience back pain at some point in their life.

Hazards of a Pampered Life

We may think of our back simply as neatly stacked bones. But open an anatomy book to the "back" section and you'll be impressed by pages and pages of—you guessed it—muscles.

They include the *erector spinae* muscles, the long muscles on both sides of the spine that stretch from the very bottom all the way up to the base of the skull. There are also dozens and dozens of muscles in at least five crisscrossing layers, serially arranged so that each connects a small group of vertebrae.

Together, all of the muscles of the back, not to mention assorted muscles in the abdomen that help to support the back, allow you to defy gravity. They give the body the ability to stand upright, to bend forward, backward, or side to side, to twist, to jump high hurdles, and to dance until dawn. And when strained, insulted, or injured, many of them can lay you flat on your back in pain.

Being physically inactive—sitting all day at a desk, driving to and from work, spending the evening in an easy chair— allows the muscles that support the back to shorten, tighten, and weaken.

Tight back muscles mean that when you twist, turn, or lift, you can easily tear muscles that have been stretched beyond their limit. Weak muscles elsewhere in the body can tax the back, too. If your quadriceps (the muscles on the front of your thighs) are weak, you may be unable to perform a bent-knee lift. Instead, you'll bend at the waist and strain your lower back muscles. If you tear *them,* you'll know it—sudden, intense pain will convey an unmistakable message.

As any chicken farmer can tell you, leading a cooped-up life makes it easier for you to plump up. If the additional poundage comes in the form of a potbelly, your lower back will suffer disk compression.

Being flabby can also make it harder to maintain good posture. (Strong muscles, though, don't guarantee good posture.) Bad posture sets the stage for additional

weakness and injury by promoting muscle imbalances, especially when you place strenuous demands on muscles that haven't been challenged for some time. (Did you really *have* to move that dresser yourself?) (See "Posture Training" on page 387.)

Lumbar Lube-Job

With all this talk of weak muscles and flab, it sounds as though there's a good reason why exercise is so helpful in preventing and curing back pain. Actually, it helps in *lots* of ways.

There are two basic types of joints in the spine—the disks (the cushiony material between vertebrae) and the articular facets (the cartilage-lined bits of bone sticking out from each vertebra, which help the vertebrae stay aligned).

"Both of these joints have the ability and the need to slide over one another as the body twists and bends," says Charles Steiner, D.O., chairman of the Department of Osteopathic Sciences at the University of Medicine and Dentistry of New Jersey in Stratford. "Otherwise there is joint rigidity and back pain."

The ability to slide depends on joint lubrication, just as it does with any joint, Dr. Steiner says. With movement, the membranes that line the joints are stimulated to produce and distribute lubricating fluid throughout these joints, helping to keep them healthy.

The best lube-job for back joints is provided by range-of-motion exercises, Dr. Steiner says. For people prone to back pain, he recommends rolling from side to side, then slowly bending and straightening the knees, for about 5 minutes before getting out of bed in the morning. He also recommends breaking up any lengthy period of sitting or inactivity with a motion his students call "the Steiner Sway." Standing, put your feet about shoulder-width apart. Then gently twist your trunk from side to side, from your hips, allowing your arms to hang freely, for about a minute. Your arms will flap back and forth like a rag doll's when you're doing the movement correctly. "This loosens your entire back—hips, lower and middle back, shoulders, and neck," Dr. Steiner says.

Paying more than lip service to a warm-up routine can also prevent back injuries, Dr. Steiner says. He urges his patients to slowly go through all the motions they expect to make, for at least 5 minutes, before they start playing. If you are planning to play tennis, for example, you would do several slow-motion swings (including backhand), serves, and reaches to strike a ball. "Studies show that the best way to protect your muscles during athletic activities is to do repetitive small movements that gradually increase in length until the muscles, ligaments, and tendons are at full extension," Dr. Steiner says. And when you're warmed up, you should feel warmed up.

Walking, not with arm-pumping rigidity but with a free, swinging motion that allows your hips and arms to move freely and your spine to undulate, is also a super-luber. Do it for 20 minutes or so, with correct posture, and you'll feel back tension just melting away.

Stretch, Flex, and Elongate

T'ai chi, an ancient Chinese art that emphasizes slow, dancelike movements (including squats, lunges, twists, side bends, and arm, leg, and trunk circling) can also knock the rust off your spine, Dr. Steiner says. (See "Martial Arts" on page 370.)

Some doctors also recommend yoga to help ease certain kinds of back pain. Yoga involves gentle, full stretching movements. If you are under a doctor's care for back pain, check with your doctor before doing yoga, however.

Yoga poses designed to encourage deep, relaxed breathing are particularly helpful at relaxing back muscles, even those deeply buried, says Larry Payne, Ph.D., director of Samata International, a yoga school in Los Angeles. Deep breathing relaxes your whole body, and it stretches the muscles of the rib cage and the muscles connecting ribs with the back, he explains.

One particular yoga pose—rather graphically known as "the corpse"—is particularly helpful. Simply lie flat on the floor with your feet shoulder-width apart and your arms at your sides. (You can put a rolled towel under your shoulder blades to open up your chest.) Then breathe deeply by allowing your exhalation to continue a few seconds longer than you normally would. Remain in this pose for 5 minutes or as long as it feels comfortable, says Dr. Payne.

The same range-of-motion exercises that help to lubricate the back joints also loosen and lengthen the muscles and ligaments that keep the body upright. That's important because tight muscles and ligaments are prone to tear even with a simple twist or bend, especially as we get older. (For appropriate stretches, see "Stretching" on page 440.)

Get in Circulation

Exercise also restores or improves blood flow to the back muscles. "Some studies have shown that back pain comes from ischemia, or poor circulation to the muscles," Dr. Steiner says.

Aerobic exercise, such as walking, swimming, or bicycling, increases blood flow throughout the body and floods the back muscles with blood. In a large, nationwide survey, 98 percent of people with back pain agreed that regular walks were very helpful in providing long-term pain relief. Swimming also fits the bill, providing an impact-free workout while gently working back muscles.

Both walking and swimming strengthen and stretch back muscles as well as relaxing them. And neither exercise is overly taxing, so they're good choices if you're weak *and* stiff. If you choose walking, dress warmly for cold weather. Wear a coat that covers your buttocks. It'll help your lower back muscles loosen up. If you prefer swimming, exercise therapists say you should plan to work out at least three times a week, for a half hour or more. Find a pool with balmy water—at least 83°F. The warm water will help relax back muscles, and you won't have to swim like a shark is after you in order to stay comfortable. (See "Walking" on page 458 and "Swimming" on page 449.)

If you plan to bike to strengthen your back, make sure your bike is custom-fit to your body. Otherwise, you could be fueling back pain. (See "Bicycling" on page 327.) Some physical therapists prefer walking to biking, since biking puts people in the same on-your-butt position they already spend so much time in. Walking, on the other hand, extends range of motion in the back. Exercise therapists have mixed feelings about rowing machines, however. Used incorrectly, or too enthusiastically, rowing machines can strain back muscles.

If you enjoy other sports, learn to do them in a way that protects your back, cautions Dr. Steiner. A number of sports require specific movements that can trigger back pain if not done with a great deal of care—the arch during a dive into water, the twist while driving a golf ball or swinging at a baseball, the up-and-down bumps of horseback riding, the rigid extension of legs and torso required to steady a heeling sailboat. If your sport of choice seems to be taking its toll on your back, you might want to consult a sports medicine specialist to help you pinpoint and alter the specific movements that are causing the problem.

Reinforced Support

Along with general aerobic exercise, there are any number of specific exercises that can be helpful. These can strengthen the muscles of the back and stomach to help prevent injury.

Any group of muscles can become weak, but among people with backaches, there seem to be certain patterns. Stomach muscles and quadriceps may be flabby in people with low back pain, while their back muscles are tight. People with upper back pain sometimes have weak trapezius muscles. These are the diamond-shaped groups of muscles that extend from the base of the head, across the shoulders, and down between the shoulder blades. When weakened, they allow the shoulders to hunch over and the head to hang forward.

So many muscles are involved in supporting the back that it's important to assess your own muscle weaknesses—or better, to have a health professional do so—and then do exercises specifically designed to address those weaknesses, says physical therapist Tom Lorren, director of rehabilitation services at the Texas Back Institute in Plano, a suburb of Dallas. "Strength may not be important for one person, but for someone else it may be the whole basis for what they need to do to start moving forward and functioning," he says. "We usually first look at the obvious things, and it's fairly easy to tell if someone is out of shape."

Two sets of stomach muscles usually need strengthening: the rectus abdominis—a long, flat muscle that extends right down the center along the whole length of the abdomen—and the obliques—side muscles that help you bend forward or backward with a twist.

Numerous exercises promise to strengthen the key muscles of the abdomen, but people with low back problems need to be especially careful about which exercises they choose and how they do them.

Partial curls and rotational curls may be your safest, most effective choice of tummy-tightener. (See the illustration on page 90.)

Properly done, these exercises also give the muscles of the lower back a safe, much-appreciated stretch.

Exercise machines can also safely and quickly strengthen these muscles, says Lorren. If you are using weight machines in a gym, don't overdo it, Lorren cautions. Use a weight you can control through the *entire* movement.

Can you rise easily from a chair, without having to push yourself up with your arms? If not, you may need to work on your quadriceps, the thigh muscles that allow you to use your legs rather than back muscles when you stand.

The biceps, the muscles on the front of your upper arms, help you to draw objects toward your chest. You use these muscles to lift and carry a box or bag of groceries, for example. Strong biceps take some of the load off your upper back muscles. (To learn how to strengthen the quadriceps and biceps, see "Resistance Training" on page 404.)

Building Better Backs

Why wait until moving day to build up your back? Staying in shape with regular exercises, properly done, will help save your back from injury whether you're getting out of a car, picking up grandchildren, or just chasing butterflies. The exercises presented here will help you safely stretch and strengthen the muscles that support your back. Flexible muscles are less likely to tear.

When doing any kind of back-stretching exercise, come out of position carefully. Slowly unwind your spine upward. Or if you're lying on the floor, first roll over to your side, then push up to a sitting position with your arms.

This pelvic tilt is a fundamental exercise in correcting a major cause of low back pain. It should be maintained while doing the exercises that follow. (1) Lie on your back. (2) As you exhale, pull in your abdominal muscles as you press your lower back into the floor. To accomplish this, you will need to tighten your buttocks and rotate your hips slightly upward. You can also do this exercise while standing by pulling in your abdomen and tightening your buttocks as you press your lower back into an imaginary wall. Your knees will bend slightly.

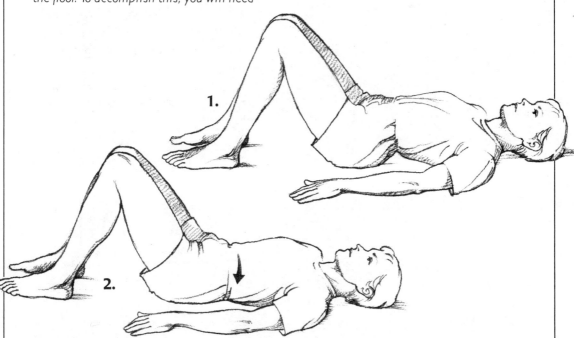

Building Better Backs—Continued

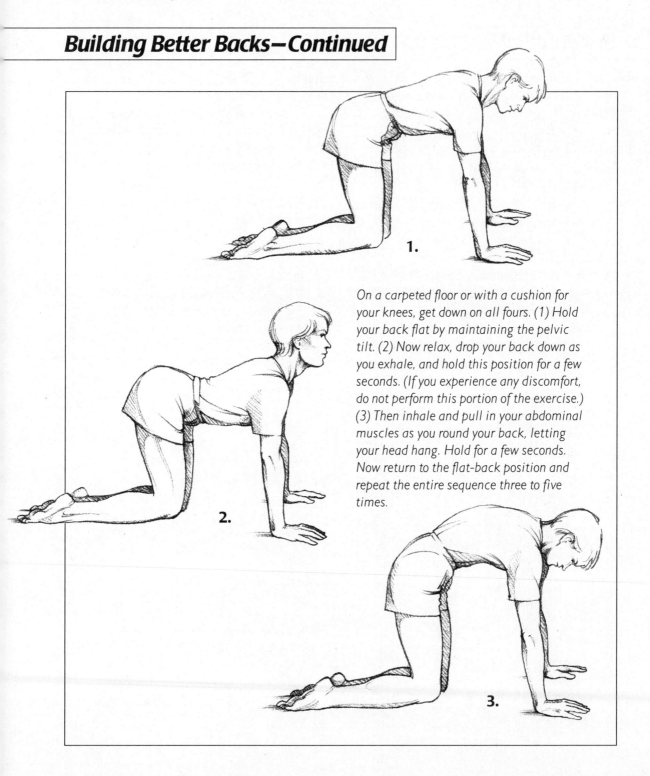

On a carpeted floor or with a cushion for your knees, get down on all fours. (1) Hold your back flat by maintaining the pelvic tilt. (2) Now relax, drop your back down as you exhale, and hold this position for a few seconds. (If you experience any discomfort, do not perform this portion of the exercise.) (3) Then inhale and pull in your abdominal muscles as you round your back, letting your head hang. Hold for a few seconds. Now return to the flat-back position and repeat the entire sequence three to five times.

Stand with your feet comfortably apart, clasp your hands together, and bend your knees until you're in a squatting position. Keep the motion smooth. Rest your arms on or between your knees. If you can't maintain your balance at first, you can hold on to the front of your lower kitchen cabinets. Practice until you can do the squat with your feet flat on the floor. When it becomes comfortable, remain in this position for a few minutes.

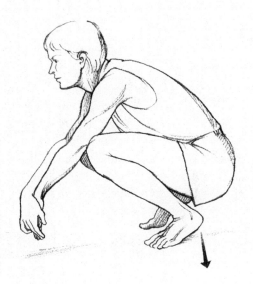

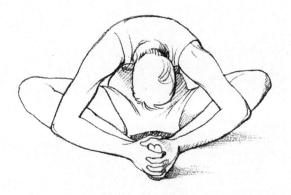

Sitting on the floor, bend your knees outward and bring the soles of your feet together. Without forcing your heels into your groin, grasp your feet with both hands. Keep your back straight, bend at your hips, and gently bring your body down as far as you can comfortably. You will feel a good stretch in your hips. Hold for as long as you can without strain and return to an upright position. Repeat for a total of 30 seconds of stretching. Your goal is to bring your head down to your feet.

Building Better Backs—Continued

Sit squarely on a chair and spread your feet apart so they are parallel to the chair legs. Keeping your back straight, lean forward with your upper body as far as you can, and then allow your back to relax. Hold for a few seconds. Don't lean forward past the point of discomfort. You will benefit from this exercise even if you can only lean halfway down.

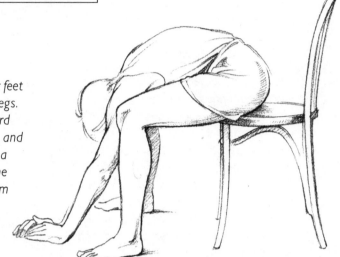

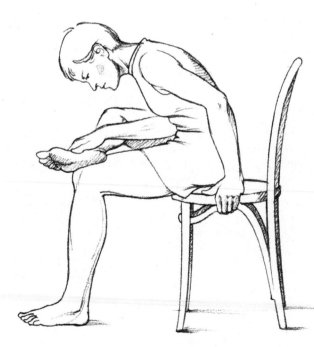

Sit squarely on a chair with your right ankle resting on your left knee. Hold on to your right ankle with your right hand and the chair with your left hand. Keeping your back straight, slowly lean forward from the hips. You will feel a deep stretch in your right hip. Stretch only as far as it is comfortable. Hold for a few seconds, then sit upright with the aid of your arms. Switch legs and repeat.

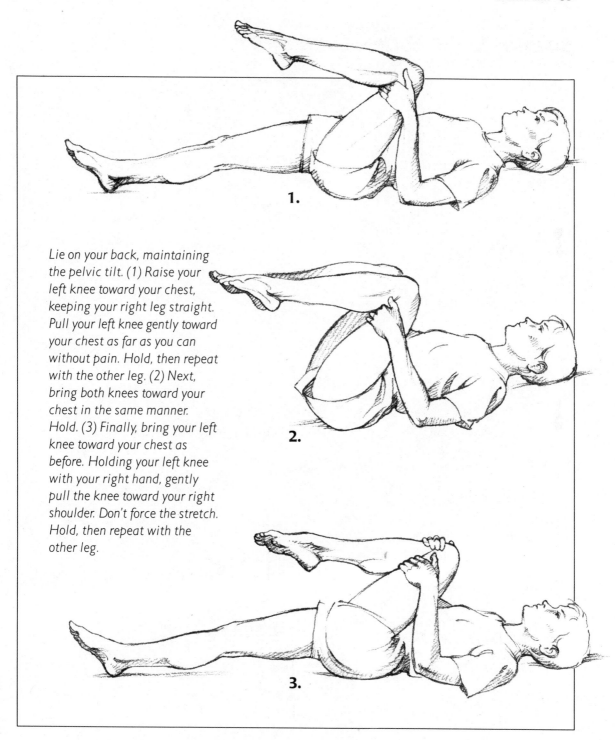

1.

Lie on your back, maintaining the pelvic tilt. (1) Raise your left knee toward your chest, keeping your right leg straight. Pull your left knee gently toward your chest as far as you can without pain. Hold, then repeat with the other leg. (2) Next, bring both knees toward your chest in the same manner. Hold. (3) Finally, bring your left knee toward your chest as before. Holding your left knee with your right hand, gently pull the knee toward your right shoulder. Don't force the stretch. Hold, then repeat with the other leg.

2.

3.

Building Better Backs—Continued

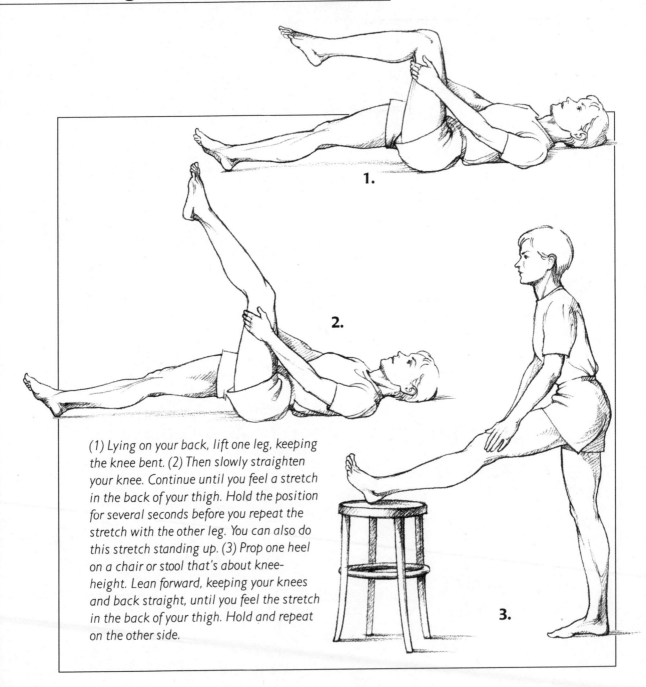

1.

2.

(1) Lying on your back, lift one leg, keeping the knee bent. (2) Then slowly straighten your knee. Continue until you feel a stretch in the back of your thigh. Hold the position for several seconds before you repeat the stretch with the other leg. You can also do this stretch standing up. (3) Prop one heel on a chair or stool that's about knee-height. Lean forward, keeping your knees and back straight, until you feel the stretch in the back of your thigh. Hold and repeat on the other side.

3.

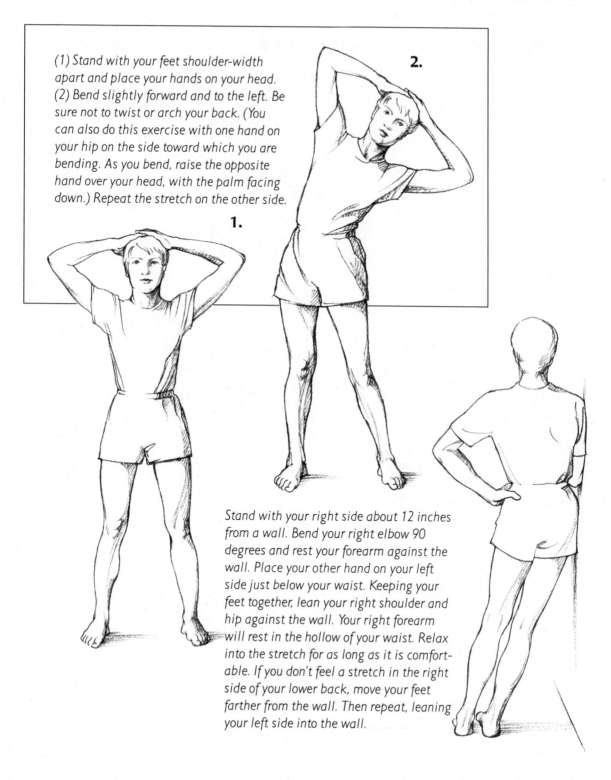

(1) Stand with your feet shoulder-width apart and place your hands on your head. (2) Bend slightly forward and to the left. Be sure not to twist or arch your back. (You can also do this exercise with one hand on your hip on the side toward which you are bending. As you bend, raise the opposite hand over your head, with the palm facing down.) Repeat the stretch on the other side.

1.

2.

Stand with your right side about 12 inches from a wall. Bend your right elbow 90 degrees and rest your forearm against the wall. Place your other hand on your left side just below your waist. Keeping your feet together, lean your right shoulder and hip against the wall. Your right forearm will rest in the hollow of your waist. Relax into the stretch for as long as it is comfortable. If you don't feel a stretch in the right side of your lower back, move your feet farther from the wall. Then repeat, leaning your left side into the wall.

Building Better Backs—Continued

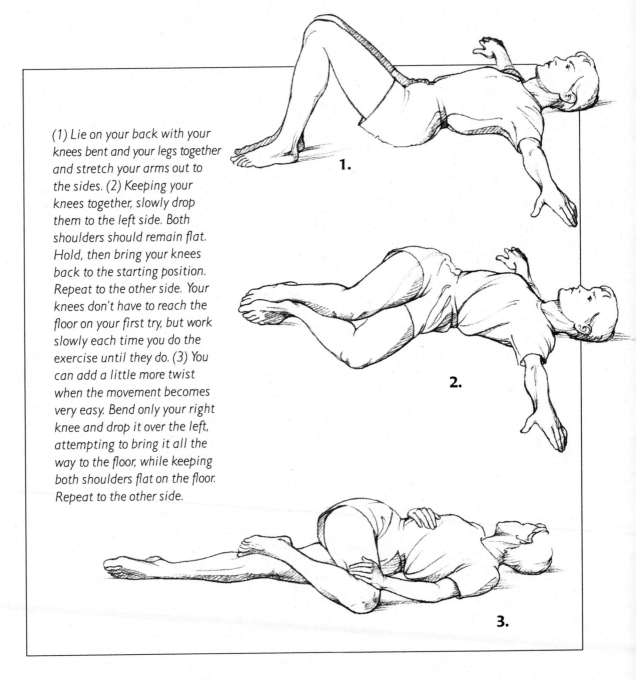

(1) Lie on your back with your knees bent and your legs together and stretch your arms out to the sides. (2) Keeping your knees together, slowly drop them to the left side. Both shoulders should remain flat. Hold, then bring your knees back to the starting position. Repeat to the other side. Your knees don't have to reach the floor on your first try, but work slowly each time you do the exercise until they do. (3) You can add a little more twist when the movement becomes very easy. Bend only your right knee and drop it over the left, attempting to bring it all the way to the floor, while keeping both shoulders flat on the floor. Repeat to the other side.

1.

2.

3.

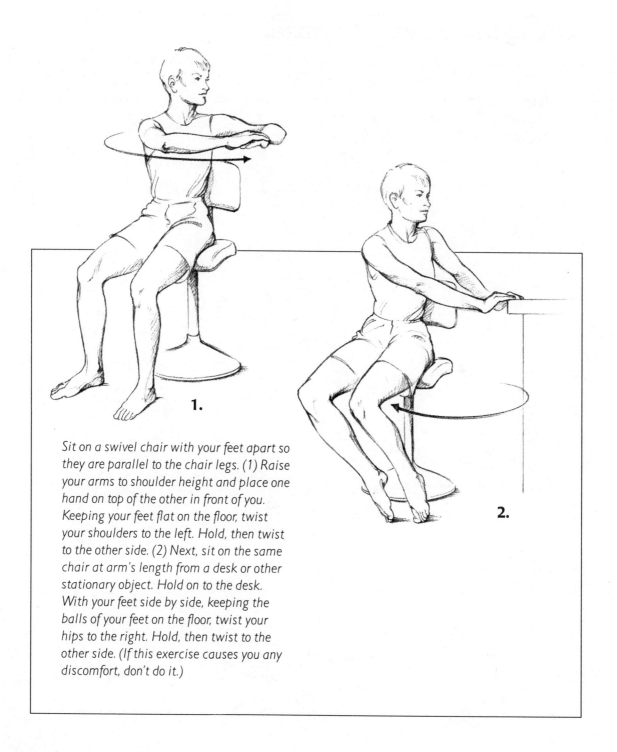

1.

2.

Sit on a swivel chair with your feet apart so they are parallel to the chair legs. (1) Raise your arms to shoulder height and place one hand on top of the other in front of you. Keeping your feet flat on the floor, twist your shoulders to the left. Hold, then twist to the other side. (2) Next, sit on the same chair at arm's length from a desk or other stationary object. Hold on to the desk. With your feet side by side, keeping the balls of your feet on the floor, twist your hips to the right. Hold, then twist to the other side. (If this exercise causes you any discomfort, don't do it.)

Building Better Backs—Continued

(1) Lie on your stomach with your arms at your sides, palms up. (2) Lift your head and shoulders off the floor as you exhale. Don't strain. Hold for 10 seconds, but don't hold your breath. Then bring your chin slowly to the floor. (3) Still lying on the floor, turn your head toward your right shoulder as you lift that shoulder off the floor. Keep your hips flat and don't strain. Hold for 10 seconds and lower your shoulder. Repeat on the other side.

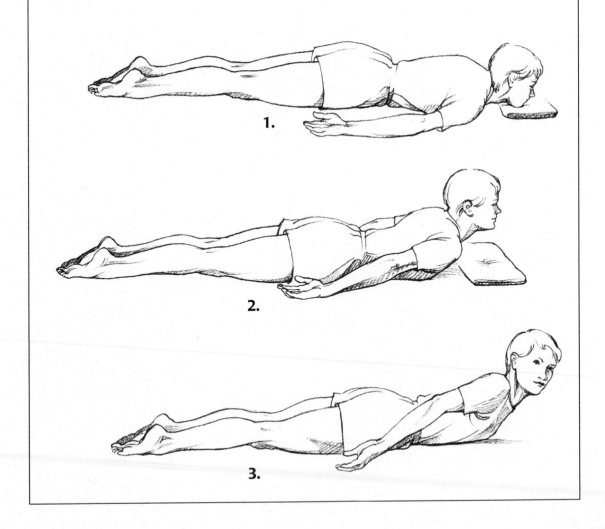

1.

2.

3.

Lie on your stomach. With your knees bent 90 degrees, lift your right hip a few inches off the floor, keeping your right thigh in line with your hip. Don't strain. Hold, lower, and repeat with the left hip.

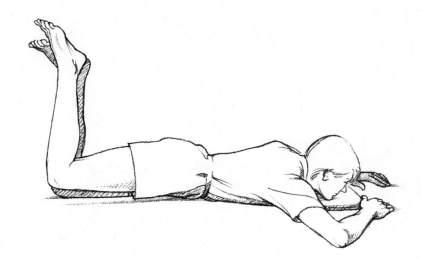

Lying on your stomach, bend your right knee. Keep your hips flat as you lift your knee off the floor as high as you can.

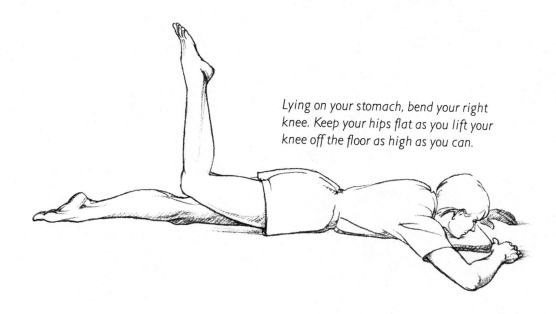

Building Better Backs—Continued

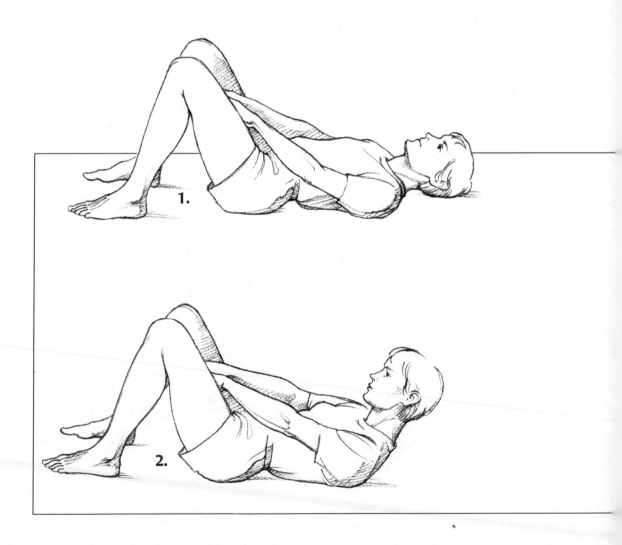

1.

2.

It's very important to maintain the pelvic tilt while doing this exercise. You will have to tighten your lower abdominal muscles to keep your back pressed against the floor.

Lie on your back with your knees bent. Lift one foot about 6 inches off the floor and lower it slowly. Repeat with the other leg. To make this exercise more challenging, before lowering each foot to the floor, extend your knee.

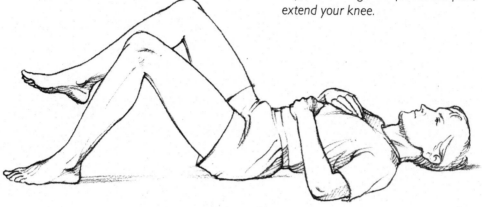

This exercise is like doing a sit-up, but only halfway. (1) Lie on your back with your knees bent and your arms extended between your thighs. (2) Tuck in your chin and curl your upper body just enough to lift your shoulder blades off the floor. Hold, then lower your upper body slowly to the floor.

(To make the curl more difficult, hold your hands at the sides of your head. Do not pull your head forward as you curl your upper body, but let it come up naturally.) (3) Now put your feet together and cross your arms over your chest. Twist your right shoulder toward your left hip as you curl up; hold. Repeat, twisting to the other side.

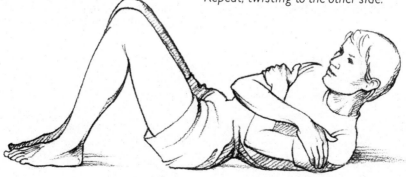

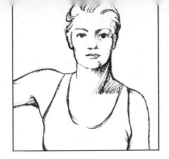

Bursitis and Tendinitis

Couldn't resist showing off your basketball dunking skills to the neighborhood kids, and now your Achilles tendon is killing you?

You're suffering from tendinitis.

The kitchen floor is gleaming from the hands-and-knees scrubbing you gave it—but your knees are curiously and grotesquely swollen?

This is bursitis.

Spent the weekend painting your garage and now your shoulders are so stiff and sore you can hardly move them?

You may have both tendinitis *and* bursitis.

These conditions are swellings—*-itis* just means "inflamed"—of tendons or of bursae, the little sacs that provide cushioning so your tendons and bones can move smoothly. Because tendons and bursae are so close together, what affects one can affect the other, and both can become inflamed simultaneously, says Patrick Guiteras, M.D., family practitioner and clinical faculty member of the University of North Carolina at Chapel Hill School of Medicine.

"You'll see this condition in people who go out without any preparation and begin to hoe their garden or play golf," he says.

The key word here is *preparation*.

"The only thing that causes any part of your body to break down is that you have challenged it beyond the strength of your abilities," says William D. Stanish, M.D., associate professor of surgery at Dalhousie University and director of the Sports Medicine Clinic of Nova Scotia, both in Halifax. In cases of tendinitis and some types of bursitis, he says, what's important is that you prepare your body ahead of time—specifically with exercises to improve strength and flexibility.

What Goes Wrong

It's ironic that bursae can cause so much pain when their purpose is to make things move smoothly. They're situated at the friction points in your body—between tendon and bone and between skin and bone. You can think of them as collapsed little balloons with mineral oil in them, says James Richards, M.D., an orthopedic surgeon at Matthews Orthopedic Clinic in Orlando, Florida. You have about 150 throughout your body.

When injured, however, they fill with fluid and swell, with painful results. The damage can come from an external trauma, such as a blow to the knee by falling, or from overuse, such as sitting or kneeling too long. Here's where the colorful names associated with some types of bursitis come in: housemaid's knee, weaver's seat, and tailor's bottom. People who kneel or sit for long periods of time suffer from these conditions when the bursae of the knee, buttocks, or hip become inflamed from constant pressure. And wearing shoes that exert too much pressure on the back of your heels may cause "pump bump"— inflammation of the heel bursae.

The problems can also come from within the body. Bursae that are used over and over again, such as those in the shoulders of swimmers, baseball pitchers, or house painters, can become inflamed from the constant use. Runners may suffer from bursitis of the knee or from trochanteric bursitis, a painful condition resulting from inflammation of the bursae around the hip.

In some cases bursae become inflamed because of the condition of the tendons around them. When tendons—particularly those in the shoulder and hip—swell, they can cause pressure on nearby bursae.

Tendinitis is caused by stress on a tendon that just isn't strong enough or flexible enough to withstand it, and it may involve small tears of the tendon as well. Areas where you may suffer include your heel, upper arm, elbow, hip, wrist, and hand.

A common site of bursitis and tendinitis is the shoulders. Shoulders are capable of an astounding range of motion, notes Dr. Guiteras. Because the system of tendons, muscles, and bursae that allows all that motion is so intricate, when a problem does occur, the entire shoulder is affected.

One particular bursa of the shoulder— the subacromial—can become inflamed from overuse or repetitive motions such as swimming or raking. This kind of bursitis is often caused by swollen shoulder tendons.

When tendons or bursae in the shoulders become inflamed and painful, the body stops using the muscles in the affected area and tries to use other muscles instead. The joint then moves inefficiently, which can result in still more damage and pain, points out Thomas W. Harris, M.D., author of *The Sports Medicine Guide for the Everyday Athlete.*

Dealing with the Problem

Once you develop a painful, stiff joint, you may not be sure if you have bursitis, tendinitis, or a combination of the two. But not to worry: "From a clinical standpoint, the treatment is pretty much the same in the initial stages," says Dr. Guiteras.

As long as the pain isn't disabling and you aren't running a fever, experts recommend basic home treatment: Cut back on activity involving the affected part, use an ice pack, and take an anti-inflammatory medication such as aspirin. You should cease the offending activity for several days, stretch gently until you are free of pain, and gradually build back to your previous activity level, says Dr. Guiteras.

Although you shouldn't force yourself to continue your customary exercise through pain, experts agree it's important that you don't stop moving during your time off— particularly with injured shoulders. A certain amount of gentle exercise is not only advisable, it's often crucial. A joint that is not used will become stiff and lose mobility, notes Dr. Guiteras, and in extreme cases scar tissue forms that can severely impede normal motion. If your shoulder pain is severe or lasts more than a few days, consider seeing a physician, says Dr.

Guiteras. You may need additional treatment or very specific muscle exercises.

"People just aren't aware of the complications that could result," says Dr. Guiteras. "The longer I'm in practice, the more organized and aggressive I am in getting formal physical therapy started."

Physical therapists prescribe a wide array of shoulder exercises to help build strength and improve range of motion. Here are some you can try at home. They may also help you avoid further problems.

For upper-body flexibility, stand with the hand of your unaffected arm on the painful shoulder to help support it. Bend your torso at the waist and let your affected arm hang loosely. Rest your head on the edge of a dresser or the back of a chair. Slowly swing the arm backward and forward for 30 seconds, then from side to side for 30 seconds. Circle your arm clockwise for 30 seconds, then counterclockwise for 30 seconds.

To stretch shoulder muscles, stand with your hands clasped behind your head. Bring your elbows together in front of your head, then push your elbows backward as far as you can without causing pain or arching your back. (For other exercises, see "Neck and Shoulder Pain" on page 239.)

Bursitis, unlike tendinitis, can result from an infection, and infected bursae require medical treatment. Bursae may get infected through a microscopic break in the skin, explains Dr. Guiteras, or through an infection in the bloodstream. If you have infected bursae, you'll probably know it: There will be fever, severe pain, and a great deal of swelling. Treatment may involve antibiotics or surgical drainage.

In some cases, exercising your tendons and muscles may be the key to avoiding these painful scenarios. While stretching and strengthening exercises can't do anything for bursitis or tendinitis caused by outside forces such as a fall to the floor or too-tight shoes, they can help prevent many tendinitis problems and bursitis caused by inflamed tendons or muscle imbalance.

The Preventive Power of Exercise

Here's how exercise can help. Your tendons connect muscle to bone, and they stretch as your muscles contract. According to Dr. Harris, two things contribute to tendon injury: applying a lot of tension to the tendon without adequate warm-up, and having a muscle stronger than the attaching tendon. Because muscles strengthen more easily than tendons, he points out, this is fairly common.

This means that being in wonderful cardiovascular shape or having bulging muscles by no means makes anyone immune to tendinitis or bursitis.

"People shouldn't assume that because they are exercising a lot they are having a beneficial effect on their tendons. The exercise has to be quite specific," says Sandra Curwin, Ph.D., assistant professor in the School of Physiotherapy at Dalhousie University. She designs individual exercise programs to treat patients with tendinitis by progressively putting more stress on the tendon to make it stronger and more elastic.

"The tendon will become a stronger structure—so you can put the same load on the tendon without injury," says Dr. Curwin.

When the stress that inflames the bursa is caused by muscle imbalance, strengthening and improving coordination of the muscles that support that joint will help, says Dr. Curwin.

Fending Off Recurrences

Muscle strengthening and flexibility exercises also help avoid reinjury of bursae in shoulders and arms, according to Stanley A. Herring, M.D., of Puget Sound Sports Physicians and associate professor of rehabilitation medicine and orthopedics at the University of Washington in Seattle. Because you'll need to know exactly which muscles to stretch and strengthen and when and how to do it, these exercises should be prescribed by a physical therapist or sports medicine specialist.

In some cases, you can develop your own exercise routines, and sometimes what's needed is a change in *how* you exercise.

Inflammation of the Achilles tendon, one of the most common sports injuries, can often be prevented by consistent, careful stretching and appropriate strength training. Using properly fitted shoes appropriate for your particular sport also helps.

To stretch your Achilles tendon, lean against a wall with your front leg bent, your back leg straight, and both feet flat on the floor. Hold for 20 seconds for each leg. For a strengthening and stretching exercise, stand on a step with your toes near the edge. Raise up on your toes, then slowly lower your heels until your heels are lower than your toes.

Flexibility exercises for hamstrings and quadriceps are often the answer for avoiding inflamed knee tendons that plague people who run and jump a lot. (See "Knee Problems" on page 195.)

Tennis players who suffer from tennis elbow often need to improve stroke technique. Because of poor position and timing, you may be using only your arm muscles on backhand strokes, and the stress on the muscles on the outside of the wrist causes inflammation. The solution is to hit the ball with your wrist and elbow extended so your trunk and upper arm provide the power, not your wrist. Or you can switch to a two-handed backhand, which spreads out the stress.

Swimmer's shoulder, a tendinitis or bursitis problem caused by muscle imbalance or overuse, is related to the amount you roll in the water as you swim. Elite athletes with flexible muscles may be overusing their shoulder muscles rather than rolling enough with each stroke. Less experienced swimmers with less flexible muscles, however, tend to roll *too much*, using the wrong muscles to pull themselves through the water.

Some bursitis treatment is particularly simple: You remove the problem. If you suffer from "pump bump" bursitis caused by too much pressure on the back of your heel, try another pair of shoes or a heel lift. Likewise, if your bursitis is caused by shoes that are too tight in the toes, ditch the shoes. For bursitis that results from external pressures such as kneeling, the use of knee pads or cushions will help reduce pressure on your joints.

Reach for It

Many tendinitis and bursitis problems are caused by a lack of flexibility. You can help avoid these problems by working on limbering up—but you have to be consistent. For best results, do these stretches three times a day.

Hold each stretch for several seconds and repeat once unless otherwise indicated. Keep your motions slow and gentle, and don't stretch to the point of pain.

Shoulders

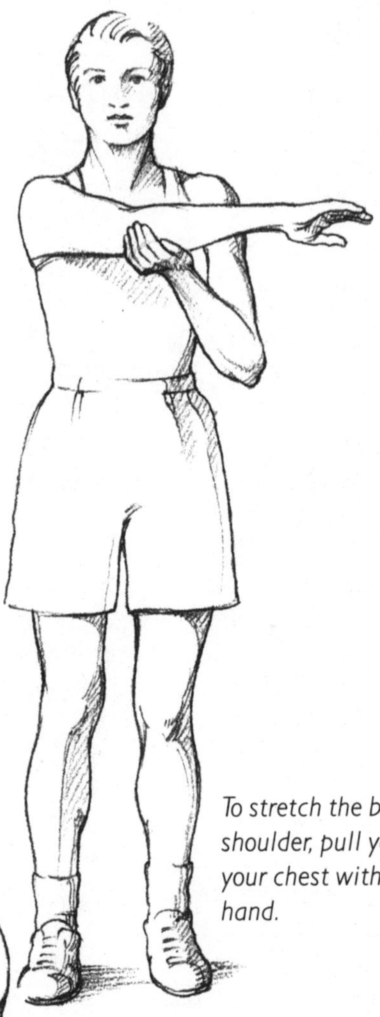

To stretch the back of your shoulder, pull your elbow across your chest with the opposite hand.

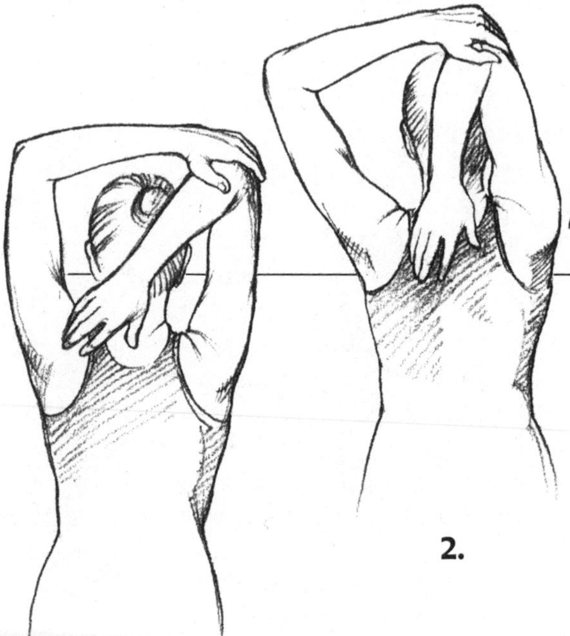

2.

1.

(1) To stretch the shoulder joint, put your arms behind your head and grasp one elbow with the opposite hand. (2) Gently pull the elbow toward the opposite side until you feel the stretch. (It's okay if you can't bring your elbow all the way behind your head.)

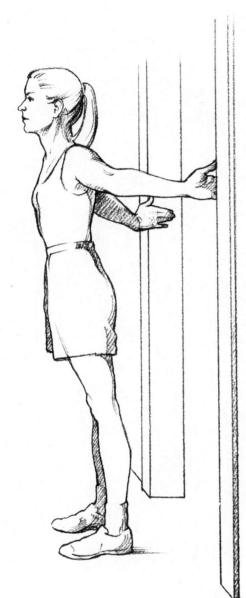

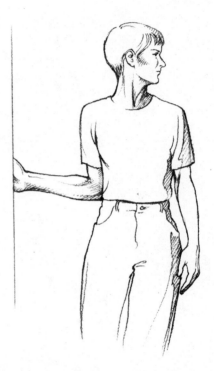

Stand in a doorway. Bend one elbow 90 degrees and place the palm of your hand behind you on the door jamb, keeping your elbow at your side. Holding on to the door jamb, turn your body away from your hand and feel the stretch in your shoulder.

Stand in a doorway and hold on to the door jamb at shoulder height. Lean forward through the doorway until your elbows are straight.

Reach for It—Continued

Shoulders

*Here's another deep shoulder stretch.
(1) Sit beside a table and rest your forearm
on the table with your palm down. (2) Lean
forward from the waist and slide your arm
straight out. The goal is to to bring your
head down level with your shoulder.*

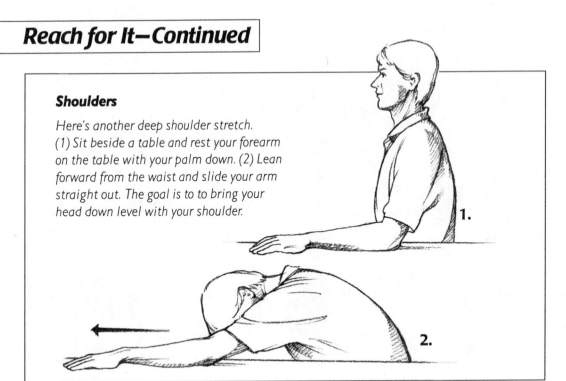

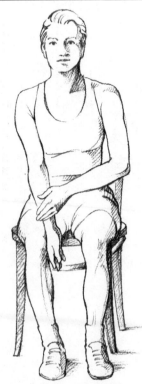

*While sitting, rest your forearm on your
thigh. To stretch your biceps, push your
forearm into your thigh with your other
hand as you straighten your elbow.*

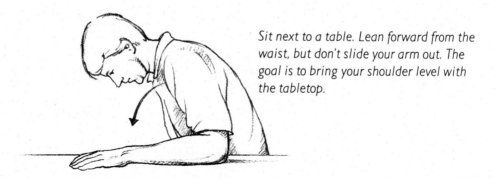

Sit next to a table. Lean forward from the waist, but don't slide your arm out. The goal is to bring your shoulder level with the tabletop.

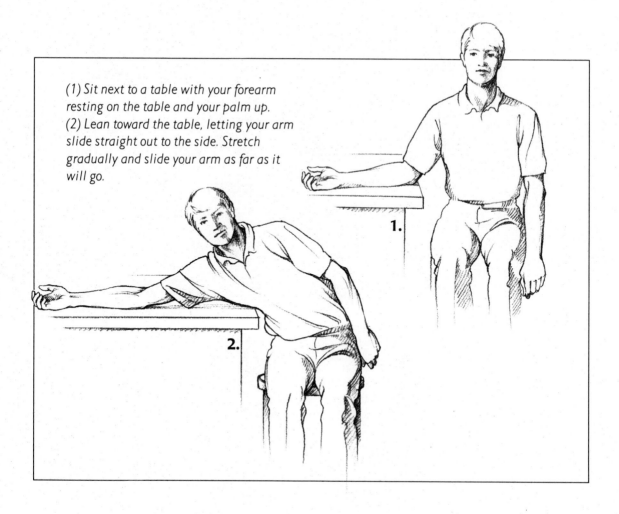

(1) Sit next to a table with your forearm resting on the table and your palm up.
(2) Lean toward the table, letting your arm slide straight out to the side. Stretch gradually and slide your arm as far as it will go.

1.

2.

Reach for It—Continued

Shoulders

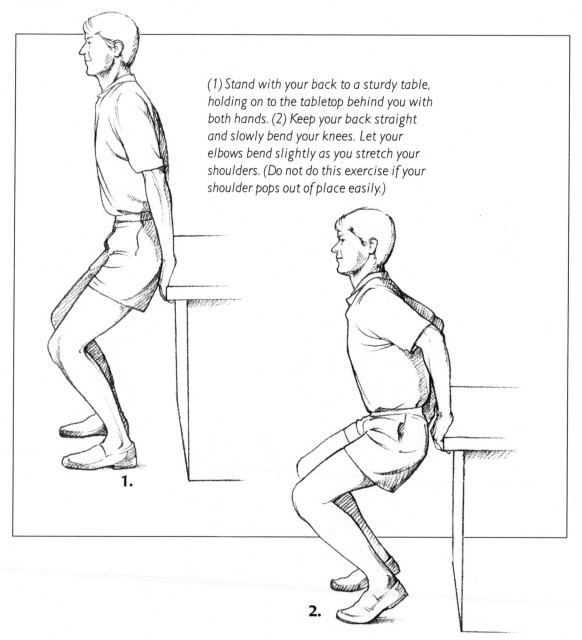

(1) Stand with your back to a sturdy table, holding on to the tabletop behind you with both hands. (2) Keep your back straight and slowly bend your knees. Let your elbows bend slightly as you stretch your shoulders. (Do not do this exercise if your shoulder pops out of place easily.)

1.

2.

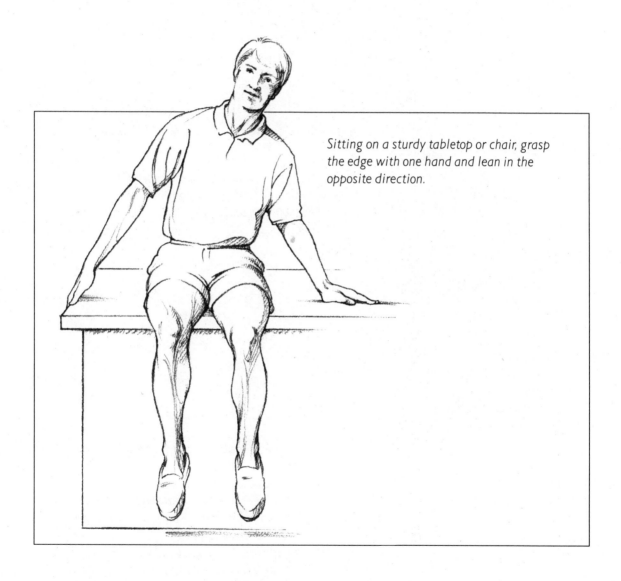

Sitting on a sturdy tabletop or chair, grasp the edge with one hand and lean in the opposite direction.

Reach for It—Continued

Shoulders

Lie on your back and prop yourself on your elbows. Let your weight rest between your shoulders. Hold for as long as it's comfortable.

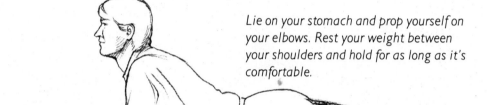

Lie on your stomach and prop yourself on your elbows. Rest your weight between your shoulders and hold for as long as it's comfortable.

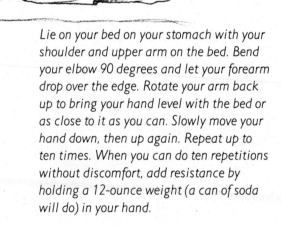

Lie on your bed on your stomach with your shoulder and upper arm on the bed. Bend your elbow 90 degrees and let your forearm drop over the edge. Rotate your arm back up to bring your hand level with the bed or as close to it as you can. Slowly move your hand down, then up again. Repeat up to ten times. When you can do ten repetitions without discomfort, add resistance by holding a 12-ounce weight (a can of soda will do) in your hand.

Triceps

(1) Lying on your back, raise your affected arm and bend the elbow 90 degrees toward your head. Hold the back of your other hand against the elbow. (2) Keep your upper arm perpendicular to the floor as you straighten your elbow. Do up to ten repetitions. When you can perform this exercise without discomfort, add resistance by using a 12-ounce weight, such as a can of soda.

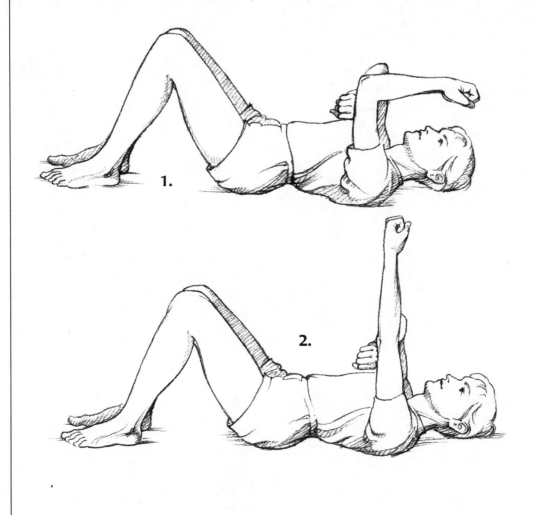

Reach for It—Continued

Elbows

*This exercise will help relieve tennis elbow.
(1) Stand sideways next to a wall at arm's
length. Extend your arm out to the wall and
bend your wrist so that the back of your
hand is against the wall and your fingers
are facing down. (2) Move your arm up the
wall until you feel a stretch in your
forearm.*

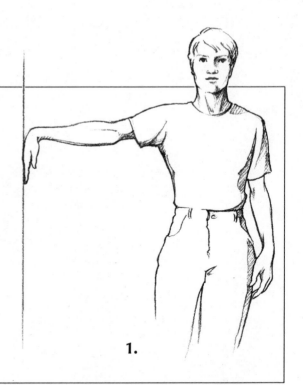

1.

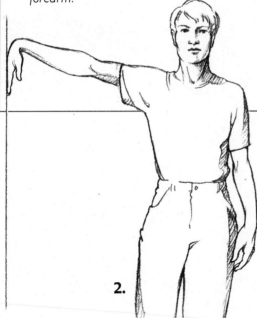

2.

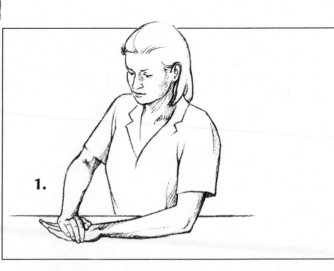

1.

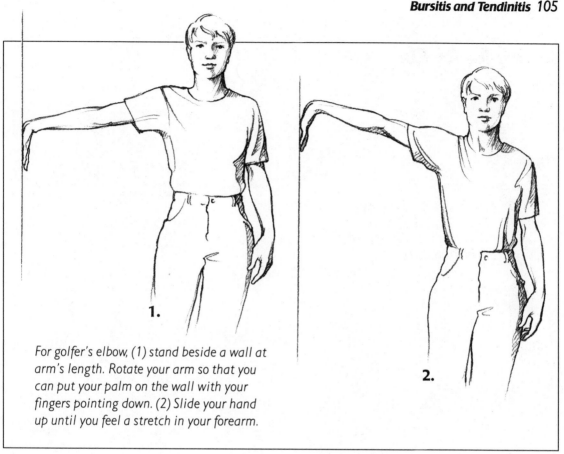

For golfer's elbow, (1) stand beside a wall at arm's length. Rotate your arm so that you can put your palm on the wall with your fingers pointing down. (2) Slide your hand up until you feel a stretch in your forearm.

(1) Rest your left forearm on a tabletop with your palm down and your elbow bent 90 degrees. Place your right hand on top of your left, then pull up from your left wrist as you push down with the right hand. (2) As you progress, gradually extend your elbow until you can do the exercise with your arm straight.

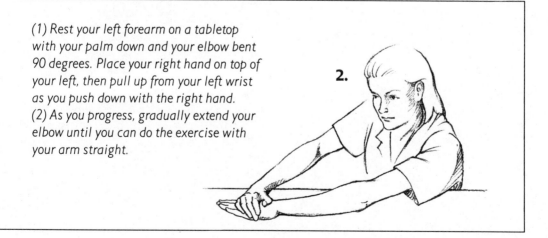

Reach for It—Continued

Hips

Stand at arm's length from a wall with the side of the affected hip facing the wall. Place your hand on the wall to brace yourself. Cross your outside leg over the other and keep that foot flat on the floor. Lean your hip toward the wall. You'll feel a good stretch along the outside of your hip and thigh.

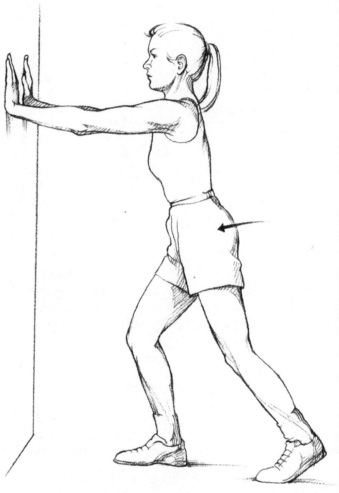

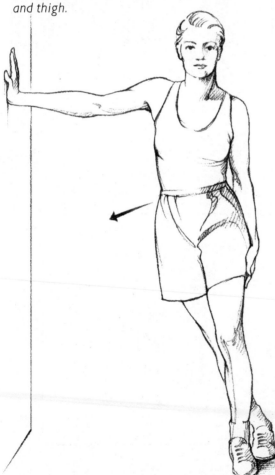

Stand at arm's length from a wall and place your hands flat on the wall. Take a step forward with the unaffected leg. Lean forward as you bend your knees slightly. Lift the heel of your rear leg off the floor, but keep the ball of your foot on the floor.

Heels

While standing, place your hands on a tabletop and take one step forward with the unaffected leg. Bend your knees and lean forward, keeping your feet flat on the floor. You will notice a stretch at the heel and calf of your rear leg.

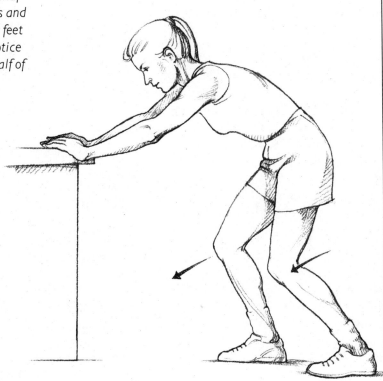

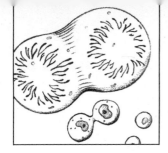

Cancer

I have no doubt that exercise pulled me through my cancer. I was strong enough to get through even my sickest times. Now I tell people, "Do something that's fun. Do something that's crazy." As far as I'm concerned, that's the best antidote for cancer gloom.

—Adele Podgorny, a Hodgkin's disease patient who sneaked out of her hospital room to ride an exercise bicycle in the staff gym, wearing a long-sleeved sweatshirt to hide her patient I.D. bracelet, and who recently took up Rollerblading.

There's no doubt that regular aerobic exercise can help reduce most people's risk of developing heart disease. But what about our nation's number two killer, cancer? Can a few hours a week of pedal pushing or pavement pounding keep us out in front when the race is against this nasty disease?

There's evidence that it may, at least for some kinds of cancer. In fact, some studies suggest that activity, even at low levels, plays as strong a role in preventing certain types of cancer as it does in keeping heart disease at bay.

Several population studies done during the last ten years or so that examined large groups of people over a period of years suggest that people who get regular, long-term physical activity—either through physically demanding jobs such as carpentry or mail delivery or through participation in sports—are less likely to develop some of the most common forms of cancer.

So far, studies show that exercise does its best against colon cancer and cancers of the female reproductive organs (endometrium, cervix, uterus, and vagina) and breast.

Athletes and Laborers

One study, for example, done by researchers at Harvard University, found that women who had been active in basketball, swimming, tennis, track, gymnastics, volleyball, or other sports in college later developed significantly less breast cancer than their inactive peers. Their relatively sedentary classmates had *twice* the risk for breast cancer, as well as 2½ times as much cancer of the uterus, ovaries, cervix, and vagina. That's a potent argument in favor of collegiate sports.

Another long-term study, an analysis from the National Health and Nutrition Examination Survey (NHANES), compared physical activity with rates of cancer in a large number of men and women. It found that men who considered themselves inactive had nearly twice the risk of developing cancer as active men. And inactive women had an approximately 50 percent higher risk than very active women.

In this study, inactive men were 60 to 70 percent more likely to develop colon cancer and lung cancer. And inactive women were 70 percent more likely to develop breast cancer after menopause and had a five times higher risk of developing cervical cancer than very active women.

These increased risks for cancer held steady even when other risk factors such as cigarette smoking and obesity were taken into consideration, says the study's main author, Demetrius Albanes, M.D., of the Cancer Prevention Studies Branch at the National Cancer Institute.

There's more: A dozen or more large population studies from around the world suggest that people who are physically active are less likely to develop colon cancer. In three recent studies, the risk of colon cancer was between 20 and 100 percent higher among men employed in sedentary occupations.

A study of Harvard University alumni found that highly active men (those who burned 2,500 or more calories a week engaging in sports and doing such activities as stair climbing and walking) had only half the colon cancer incidence of inactive men (those burning less than 1,000 calories a week on physical activity). But apparently it isn't necessary to knock yourself out with exercise to gain some measure of protection. The risk for moderately active men (burning 1,000 to 2,500 calories a week) was only slightly higher than that of the most active men.

Don't Overdo It

Research with animals also shows a connection between inactivity and cancer. It also shows that there may be a price to pay for overexercise.

A number of studies have shown that laboratory animals allowed to freely exercise on a self-propelled wheel are better at resisting breast cancer than animals not permitted to exercise. The exercising animals usually have significantly fewer tumors and less rapid growth of tumors compared to nonexercising mice, says Leonard Cohen, Ph.D., head of the Section of Nutritional Endocrinology at the American Health Foundation in Valhalla, New York.

Several studies, though, showed that lab animals and men who exercise to exhaustion have temporarily depressed immune function. (The immune system plays an important role in defending the body against cancer.) And in a few studies, exercise combined with a high-fat diet seemed to result in *accelerated* tumor growth.

Fighting Fat, Fighting Cancer

Researchers aren't yet sure how exercise cuts your risk of developing cancer, but it may work in several different ways.

One theory is that exercise helps keep you lean and at your ideal body weight. Being overweight is known to increase your risk for endometrial and gallbladder cancer, for breast cancer, and possibly for colon cancer. That's why the American Cancer Society recommends regular exercise: "We feel it's an important part of a program to help maintain ideal weight," says spokesperson Stacy Charney.

Fat seems to have a direct effect on a woman's hormones. The fatter you are, the more you convert androgen (a male hormone also secreted by women) to estrogen, says David Schapira, M.D., professor of medicine at the University of South Florida College of Medicine in Tampa. Also, more of the estrogen is converted to a "free" form of the hormone, which literally cruises the body looking for trouble. "Estrogen stimulates cells to divide in the breast and reproductive system, particularly the uterine lining. So excess or free estrogen may set the scene for cancerous growth," Dr. Schapira says.

In colon cancer, researchers are less sure what role body fat plays. But they think it might involve the body's manufacture of prostaglandins. These potent biochemicals are made from fats. Some cause an inflammatory response, which might be linked with cancer development.

Constipation, too, has been linked with colon cancer, and there's evidence that inactive people are more likely to be constipated, which increases the amount of time cancer-promoting materials in the bowel come in contact with the intestinal lining.

Exercise also affects the body's immune system and can help reduce the bad effects of stress-related hormones. Such hormones may be related to depressed immune system function, researchers say.

Is There an "Exercise Prescription"?

Do these studies show an optimum exercise level as far as cancer prevention goes?

"The gradient for cancer is similar to that for cardiovascular disease or any disease," says Steven Blair, P.E.D. (physical education doctor), an epidemiologist with the Texas Institute for Aerobic Research in Dallas and author of *Living with Exercise.* "It's a kind of dose/response relationship. Doing a little something is better than doing nothing at all. Being a little bit fit is better than being a couch potato.

"I tell people to try to get out of the least active group—those burning less than 1,000 calories a week on physical activity. That's where the risk is much higher. I typically recommend walking 1 to 2 miles in 30 to 40 minutes. And I tell people to do that on most days or to do an equivalent amount of some other kind of exercise."

For those who say they don't have time, Dr. Blair suggests they break their effort up into three 10-minute walks and throw in a few sets of stairs, some gardening, and a round of playing with the grandchildren. "For older people who normally don't exercise at all, I don't even mention target heart rates, aerobic training, or going to the gym," Dr. Blair says. "It just wouldn't make sense." Staying active is another matter, however. Given the connection between exercise and cancer, it *really* wouldn't make sense to just sit there in the proverbial rocking chair.

Cancer Patients Can Exercise

Yes, the evidence shows that regular exercise probably plays a significant role in *preventing* cancer. But what about all the people who already have the dread disease? Forty years ago, people were amazed and frightened by the idea of a heart patient exercising. But patients who went ahead and did it anyway often improved, and today, cardiac rehabilitation programs are considered a vital part of recovery.

For people with cancer, though, physical rehabilitation is usually limited to physical therapy for specific disabilities related to surgery or treatment. A woman who has had a mastectomy might need physical therapy to regain use of her arm, for instance; someone who has had a leg amputated because of bone cancer would also undergo therapy.

The person who is just plain worn out from fighting the disease and from treatment is really not addressed by most cancer rehabilitation programs, according to Maryl Winningham, R.N., Ph.D., of the University of Utah College of Nursing in Salt Lake City. Dr. Winningham is an exercise physiologist and a nurse specializing in the care of cancer patients. Many people who have cancer are out of shape from weeks of inactivity, stress, toxic treatments, and the cancer itself. They may live years longer—many do—in a vicious cycle, with inactivity and fatigue fueling each other, says Dr. Winningham.

What these people really need, she maintains, is the equivalent of cardiac rehabilitation—a program that helps them safely regain stamina and muscle strength.

"Lots of people with cancer assume their weakness is all due to their disease, when in fact it's due at least in part to inactivity," she says.

Her research has involved developing a "progressive aerobic interval training exercise program" for people with cancer, mostly women being treated for breast cancer. The program, which uses station-

ary bicycles, gradually increases over a period of weeks the level at which the people exercise and the amount of time they exercise. Each person in the program first has a series of tests, including heart function tests, to determine at what level and for what amount of time it's safe for him or her to begin exercising. Then they pedal away at a pace and time designed just for them.

Dr. Winningham was involved in a study of one group of women who participated in the aerobic training program for ten weeks. These women showed distinct advantages when compared to women doing only stretching and flexibility exercises or to a group instructed only to "do normal activities," she says.

Their energy capacity increased an average of 40 percent. All the women were undergoing chemotherapy at the time of the study. The energy boost meant they . were more likely to have the pep to continue their daily routines, according to Dr. Winningham. A similar group of people with cancer who did not exercise experienced a loss of their energy reserves. They showed a slow, steady decline in functional capacity. "They might feel like they had overexerted themselves doing even minor things," Dr. Winningham explains. Over the course of the study, nonexercisers lost 4 to 6 percent of their energy level.

The exercising breast cancer patients increased muscle mass, while the nonexercisers gained both weight and fat and also lost muscle. "It seems paradoxical, but many women undergoing treatment for breast cancer gain weight, even when they are nauseated and throwing up," Dr. Winningham says. "It is very distressing to them as far as body image goes, and the exercise helps to counteract the process."

Nausea associated with chemotherapy treatment was less in the exercising group. "Many said that within a few minutes of beginning exercise, nausea lessened and was less intense for hours afterward," Dr. Winningham says. (She cautions cancer patients to avoid exercise for 24 hours or more after intravenous chemotherapy, since heart irregularities are more frequent during this time.)

Positive moods were much more common in exercising cancer patients, who reported about two-thirds fewer episodes of feeling fearful, angry, or depressed compared to nonexercisers.

One participant in the program was Elly Castrodale, a 62-year-old woman who had ovarian cancer. She walks 2 miles at lunchtime, every day except Sundays, and rides a stationary bicycle some evenings for 15 or 20 minutes. "Mentally and physically, I feel like I am getting a real blast of fresh air and energy when I get out and walk," she says.

Does exercise, in fact, help people with cancer fight off the disease and live longer? Researchers don't know yet, but they do know that exercise can make a big difference in how a person feels. One researcher, Vickie Baracos, Ph.D., associate professor in the Department of Animal Science at the University of Alberta in Edmonton, is currently working with people who have lung cancer to see if an aerobic exercise program helps them live longer. "We have no results on that so far," she says. "But we have found that even people who are very weak after their cancer treatment can begin to exercise and to slowly increase their level of exercise. And, after a year, they have regained enough fitness to go about their normal daily activities."

BACK IN THE SWING

"Step on each other's feet, it doesn't matter. The point is not to do it perfectly, it's to have fun, to let go, to move." That's what Linda Simpson, creator of Ballroom Express, tells the cancer survivors who make up her Get Back in the Swing ballroom dancing workshops.

Since her own bout with cancer in 1988 (she had part of her jaw removed and replaced with bone from her leg), Simpson and her partner-husband David Canty have gone on to become the United States over-35 ballroom dancing champions. That feat was due in part to a love for dancing so strong that Simpson was back on the dance floor as soon as she could get out of her wheelchair.

Ballroom dancing is the perfect exercise and therapy for cancer survivors, Simpson contends. It's physical but not too strenuous. It's relaxing, sociable, and can help people feel better about their body. "At one dance, a man with a colostomy bag got up and did the Lindy. He said, 'I haven't done this in years. I didn't even think I should do this. But I feel great.' "

For more information on this program, contact Linda Simpson at Ballroom Express, 500 East 83rd Street, Apt. 7L, New York, NY 10028.

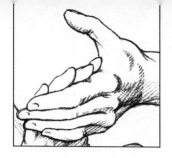

Carpal Tunnel Syndrome

From typing to gardening, knitting to driving nails, wringing out clothes to wrenching off rusty bolts— any lengthy, repetitive activity during which the forearm and hand are not kept straight can cause a number of arm, elbow, and wrist problems. One of the most prevalent problems is carpal tunnel syndrome.

The carpal tunnel isn't a new public works project through the Carpathian Mountains. It's the passage for the main nerve and tendons that govern finger motion. The bones in the back of the wrist form the floor and walls of the tunnel; the carpal ligament, spanning the wrist from below the lower knuckle of the thumb, serves as the roof. Inside the channel run the median nerve, which leads from the neck down into the hand, and the tendons that produce palm and finger movement.

Certain kinds of movements can translate into carpal tunnel pain—working with the wrists sharply bent up or down, long-term gripping or clutching, holding tools that vibrate or cause sudden jolts, and continually pinching or squeezing the fingers. The repetition, strain, and impact, coupled with insufficient rest from the activity, in effect rob the wrist of lubrication. Friction of the tendons causes swelling, which fills up the tunnel and causes compression. The good news is that the *right* kind of movement and the right kind of exercise can help prevent and relieve the stresses that cause carpal tunnel syndrome.

Women are five times more likely than men to develop carpal tunnel syndrome, according to Susan Isernhagen, a Duluth, Minnesota, physical therapist and an ergonomic consultant to industry. (Ergonomics is a science that involves designing healthful work environments.) Women are more slightly built, she says, so there is less room inside the carpal tunnel for the tendons and nerve to move. Because of hormonal ebb and flow, women are much more prone to fluid retention and swelling, which intensifies wrist pressure. Many women, in fact, acquire carpal tunnel syndrome while pregnant, and the symptoms disappear after they give birth. Finally, women also have traditionally had jobs requiring repetitive hand motions, Isernhagen says.

In the early stages of carpal tunnel syndrome, the compression on the median nerve causes numbness and tingling in the hand, specifically the thumb and the index finger, middle finger, and part of the ring finger. Initially, the sensation often appears only at night, and sleeping with the wrists bent and the hands curled can aggravate the problem, says Janna Jacobs, physical therapist and certified hand therapist with Baltimore Therapeutic Equipment Company in Maryland.

The symptoms soon appear during the day and intensify into more pronounced pain. People find themselves a little clumsier than they used to be, according to Jacobs: They drop things and cannot hold on to smaller objects. If the condition is left untreated, the median nerve and the muscles it controls eventually atrophy, causing permanent damage and loss of use of the hand.

"It's a shame so many people let it go that far," Isernhagen says. "The truth is, you don't have to get to that stage. For the most part, carpal tunnel syndrome is preventable."

Testing for Tingling

To determine whether you've acquired carpal tunnel syndrome, doctors normally perform several tests, two of which you can try yourself. To do Phalen's maneuver, put both elbows on a table with your forearm and hand in the air. Flex your hands down without forcing and hold for a minute or so. If tingling or pain develops, chances are you've got carpal tunnel syndrome.

For the other test, called Tinel's sign, hold your hand palm up and tap lightly on the middle of your wrist (that's where the median nerve is located). If your fingers begin to tingle, you may have carpal tunnel syndrome.

Exercise Handiwork

Prevention depends on many factors, including good posture (see "Posture Training" on page 387) and work environment.

But, says Isernhagen, stretching and strengthening exercises are equally important, to build up the muscles in the wrists and forearms and just to give your hands a break. As a preventive measure and during the early stages of carpal tunnel syndrome, Isernhagen recommends "pause breaks" for a minute or two every hour.

These stretching and strengthening exercises should be done two or three times a day for 5 to 10 minutes, says Jacobs. Both therapists also stress the importance of doing these movements as a warm-up before beginning hand-demanding activity.

Even for sitting in front of a computer terminal all day, "you need substantial muscle strength and endurance" in your upper body, arms, and hands, according to Jacobs. Before beginning a long session of crocheting or drilling, "you should be like an athlete warming up," she says. "Get the tissues and muscles of the hand, wrist, and arm more pliable and ready to work."

You should also do the exercises as soon as carpal tunnel symptoms manifest themselves.

None of these exercises should cause any discomfort. All can be done discreetly and in any order.

Move your elbow. If your elbows are bent for a good part of the day, you should always try to take a break and straighten your arms. Stretch them in front of you or let them hang at your sides. Then rotate your forearms, alternately turning the palms around and back.

Wrist stretches. Press both palms together at chest level, as if praying. Slowly lift your elbows up and away from the sides of your body as far as they can comfortably

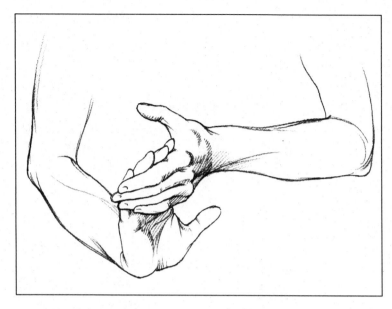

Gentle Wrist Bend

Rest your forearm on the affected side on a table. Gently bend back your wrist and hold the position for 5 seconds.

go and hold for several seconds. For a variation, spread out the palms but keep the fingertips touching, and press in.

Shoulder extension. Intertwine your fingers behind your head with your elbows pointed out. Gently move your elbows back and feel the stretch in your shoulders.

Finger stretching. Several exercises can strengthen the fingers and provide relief from cramping. First clench the hand into a tight fist, then release, stretching the fingers as far as they can go. Now flex each finger across the palm to touch the tip of the thumb. Repeat by curling the thumb over to touch the base of each finger. Finally, raise your arms over your head and stretch out the fingers as though attempting to touch the ceiling.

Knit One, Curl, Too

Certain resistance exercises can also help strengthen the fingers, wrists, and forearms. Those muscles are particularly important, Isernhagen says, for people who have to grasp a tool for a long time or repeatedly pinch something between their fingers.

Wrist curls should be done without weights at first, Jacobs suggests. Eventually, light dumbbells or a barbell can be incorporated into the exercise. Isernhagen recommends that the wrist movement in the curls be limited to a short arc—never fully flexed or stretched back.

To perform the curl, rest your forearms on your thighs with your palms up and your hands extending beyond the knees. Drop your hands slightly below the straight position and slowly curl up to just beyond even alignment with the forearm. Perform three sets of ten repetitions, then rotate your forearms so your palms are facing the floor and repeat the curling motions.

Curls also can beef up the fingers. With your forearms still on your thighs and a light dumbbell or barbell in your hands, let your wrists hang down over your knees. Slowly relax your fingers, letting the bar roll down almost to your fingertips. Just as slowly, curl it back up to your palms. (Make sure you don't drop the bar.)

When Not to Exercise

People who have advanced carpal tunnel syndrome—when numbness or pain may be constant—should *not* perform these exercises. "At that point," Isernhagen says, "it could be counterproductive. It's best to see a physical or occupational therapist to be evaluated."

For treatment, wrist splints and injections of anti-inflammatory medications may reduce the swelling and decrease the compression on the median nerve. But an operation may be inevitable. Various procedures exist, but the surgeon usually cuts the carpal ligament to allow for more room in which the nerve and tendons can move.

Following the operation, though, exercise assumes a new importance. "If you've had surgery," Isernhagen says, "one of the best ways to get function back in the hand is rehabilitation." Rehabilitation involves using the same routines that can help prevent carpal tunnel syndrome and treat its very early stages. "The earlier a doctor prescribes rehabilitative exercises," she says, "the more recovery you'll have."

Wrist Strengtheners

With your arm resting on the table, make a loose fist with the hand on the affected side. Use your other hand to resist the movements that follow. Keep your wrist straight and hold each position for 5 seconds. (1) First, with your palm up, try to push your fist against your other hand. (2) Then turn your palm down and try to push your fist up. (3) Now turn your fist sideways with your thumb facing up and again try to push your fist up. (4) Last, press the knuckles of your fist into the palm of your other hand. Repeat the sequence five times.

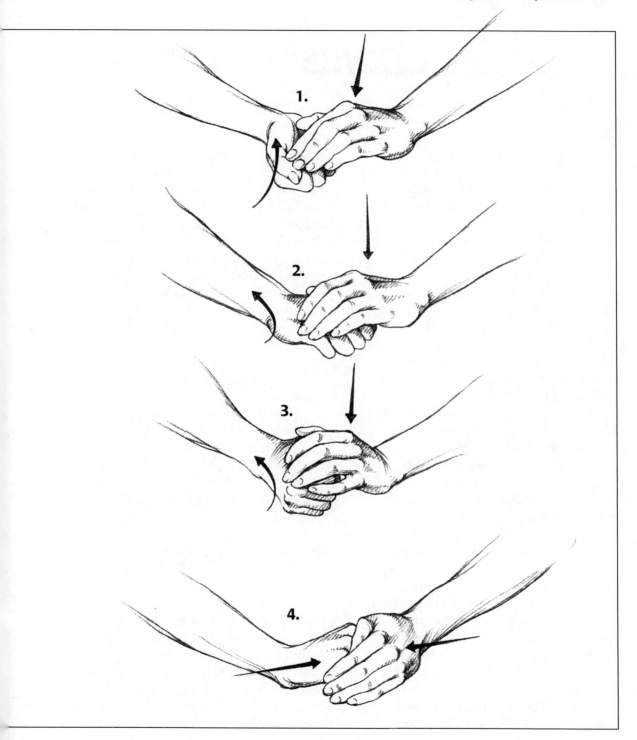

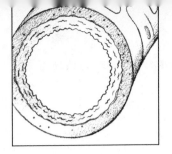

Cholesterol

Y ou can change your diet, you can quit smoking, you can even take medication—but if you don't exercise, you may be overlooking a simple yet mighty weapon in the struggle to keep your cholesterol down.

"For people who have high cholesterol, exercise can have an effect," says Roger Hughes, Ph.D., a professor of physical education at Cameron University in Lawton, Oklahoma, who has conducted several studies on exercise and its influence on cholesterol.

How dramatic an effect does exercise have? Well, in a one-year study of 264 people at Stanford University, researchers looked at a group of overweight men and women who were put on a diet low in saturated fat and cholesterol as well as a program of walking or running approximately 8 miles a week. After ten months, men lost 81 percent more body fat and women 38 percent more than people in similar groups who dieted but did not exercise. People who dieted and exercised experienced more positive changes in blood cholesterol levels than a similar group of people in the study who only modified their diet. Overall, those who only dieted saw their heart disease risk drop 20 to 23 percent. But the heart disease risk of those who dieted *and* exercised

decreased by a whopping 35 percent.

More proof that exercise can lasso cholesterol comes from Washington University in St. Louis, where researchers asked eight avid runners to stop working out for 16 to 22 days. The runners, who usually ran at least 35 miles a week, all had normal cholesterol levels at the beginning of the study—but not for long. Within three weeks, all of the runners who became sedentary showed increases in their blood cholesterol levels, including an 18 percent increase in lipoprotein, a blood fat that is linked to premature artery disease and stroke.

"What this study tells the average Joe is that even if he just runs 10 to 15 miles a week, his cholesterol levels would be better than if he did nothing," says Gustav Schonfeld, M.D., director of Washington University's Atherosclerosis and Lipid Research Center.

The Good, the Bad, and the Ugly

Medical science actually has a pretty good idea of how exercise affects cholesterol. Exercise combined with dietary changes provides a double whammy that changes your overall blood fat profile in a favorable direction. It can lower the "bad" cholesterol level and at the same time *raise* your level of "good" cholesterol. We know it sounds complicated, but you really don't need to carry around a medical encyclopedia to understand cholesterol and how you can use diet and exercise to control it. Here's the scoop.

Cholesterol is circulated through your blood wrapped up in lipoproteins, which are a gooey combination of triglycerides and protein molecules. (Triglycerides are yet *another* problematic blood fat.)

Low-density lipoprotein (LDL) is the "bad" kind because it carries large amounts of cholesterol and tends to stick to artery walls, much like snowflakes accumulate on the ground.

In contrast, high-density lipoprotein (HDL), the "good" kind, contains significantly less cholesterol than LDL. As HDL travels through the bloodstream, it picks up cholesterol and carries it back to the liver, where it is broken down and eventually excreted from the body.

The more LDL you have in your blood, the greater your risk of heart disease. (LDL levels should be 130 or lower.) The higher your HDL, the lower the risk. (HDL should be 50 or higher.)

In fact, it appears that for every 1 percent increase in HDL, there is a 2 to 3 percent drop in heart disease risk.

We have a kind of balancing game going on here, with your heart's health as the prize. The winning number is a relatively low LDL level—or a relatively high HDL level.

Keeping Your Lipids in Sync

Exercise has some effect on LDL, but dietary changes, weight loss, and in some cases medication are all effective ways to control that nemesis. But if you really want to increase your HDL levels, then listen up.

"You can't go to your doctor and ask for a pill to raise your HDL, because there isn't one. The only real way to raise HDL is through exercise," says Edward Palank, M.D., director of the New Hampshire Heart Institute in Manchester.

In a month-long study of ten endurance athletes in their mid-thirties who ran at least 29 miles a week, researchers at Brown University found the runners had 40 percent higher HDL levels and 45 percent lower triglyceride levels than ten sedentary men of similar ages.

Taking It Easy, Taking It Slowly

In fact, exercise may not have to be all that vigorous to produce results. It may be the duration of the activity rather than the intensity of the exercise that is important in influencing HDL levels, says Dr. Hughes.

In a ten-week study of 75 college students aged 18 to 24, Dr. Hughes found that those students who ran for 40 minutes at a moderate intensity three times a week had more changes in blood cholesterol levels than those who ran for 20 minutes at a high intensity.

"We're finding that intensity makes little difference and that duration is more important when it comes to cholesterol," he says. "So it's possible that you don't have to bust your behind to have an effect on cholesterol."

It is also becoming clear that lower-intensity aerobic exercise such as brisk walking can increase HDL, too. And that may be good news for people who are intimidated by the thought of huffing and puffing down the neighborhood jogging trail.

In a massive study of 3,621 adults, researchers at Brigham Young University in Provo, Utah, looked at the ratio of total cholesterol to HDL. They found that people who walked at least 2½ hours a week were 50 percent less likely to have a poor ratio compared with those who reported they did no walking or other exercise.

Thousands of miles away from the Utah desert, researchers in England followed the progress of 28 formerly sedentary women who participated in a one-year walking program. The women, who walked about 10 miles a week, had significantly higher HDL levels at the conclusion of the study than did a group of 16 women who didn't exercise. Researchers calculated that the walkers reduced their likelihood of having a heart attack in the next ten years by at least 50 percent.

Walking: Super Strategy for Cholesterol Control

More good news about walking and HDL cholesterol levels is emerging from researchers at Florida Atlantic University in Boca Raton. There, 20 women, ranging in age from 61 to 81, walked at a vigorous rate three times a week for two months. At the conclusion of the investigation, researchers found no changes in total cholesterol, but the proportion of HDL cholesterol increased, indicating a lowered risk of coronary artery disease.

Walking is a good moderate exercise that most people feel comfortable doing,

and it fits nicely into a comprehensive strategy to control cholesterol, doctors say. (See "Walking" on page 458.)

Bicycling, swimming, running, and dancing are other good aerobic exercises that can help boost HDL, says Dr. Palank, who advocates doing a variety of activities.

"I tell my patients—and they range in age from 7 to 95—to find an activity that they like and do it at least 30 minutes a day three times a week," he says. "For some people it's running, for others it's ballroom dancing. On the alternative days they do another activity.

"For instance, you might work out on a rowing machine three days a week, then golf, bowl, or play tennis on other days. The key thing is to find lifelong activities that you enjoy and will do on a regular basis."

Hoist a Few

Some researchers also are investigating the possibility that weight training might affect cholesterol levels.

"In a number of studies in which participants have done moderate- to high-volume resistance training, we've seen changes in lipoprotein profiles," says Robert Moffatt, Ph.D., a professor of exercise physiology at Florida State University in Tallahassee.

In a small, preliminary study, Dr. Moffatt and his associates asked ten men in their early to middle twenties to participate in two 30-minute weight-lifting sessions. During the first session, the men did high-volume resistance training, meaning that they lifted moderately heavy weights, did seven sets (at 8 to 12 repetitions) of each of the seven exercises, and rested no more than 1 minute between sets. In the second session, they participated in a low-volume workout. They lifted more weight, did fewer repetitions, and had 3-minute rest periods between sets.

Dr. Moffatt found no changes in the men's blood fat levels at any time after the low-volume workout. But blood tests taken 24 hours after the high-volume resistance training showed that the men's HDL levels had soared 11 percent. This study suggests that if you want to reap the benefits of weight lifting you don't have to hoist a lot of iron. More repetitions with less weight might provide better results. (See "Resistance Training" on page 404.)

Drop That Burger

Just because you start lifting a few weights or take several invigorating walks around your neighborhood doesn't mean you can forget about diet and other factors that contribute to cholesterol buildup.

"Exercise will help, but in most patients, you can't use it alone to modify cholesterol," says C. Noel Bairey, M.D., medical director of the Preventative and Cardiac Rehabilitation Center at Cedars-Sinai Medical Center in Los Angeles.

"For most people, LDLs will go down and HDLs will go up with the proper diet, the proper exercise, and stress reduction," she says. "But you have to do *all* those things if you really want to have an impact on cholesterol."

In other words, just because you exercise doesn't mean you can keep greasing up the frying pan.

"Even if you exercise you can't have steak and eggs every day," says Dr. Palank. "You can't eat fast food all the time. You still need to be conscious of your diet."

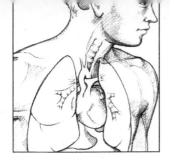

Colds and Flu

*A*t the first sneeze, many people reach for vitamin C. They should probably reach for walking shoes as well.

Moderate exercise, it seems, deserves more recognition than previously granted for activating the body's immune system, says Sandra L. Nehlsen-Cannarella, Ph.D., director of the Immunology Center at California's Loma Linda University Medical Center and a professor at Loma Linda University School of Medicine.

To get a handle on how exercise might help the body resist upper respiratory tract infections, she helped conduct a study that involved a group of 36 overweight, sedentary women. Over a 15-week period, half the women were asked to take a daily 45-minute walk; the other half did no exercise. The walkers provided "what we consider the proof that a relatively small amount of activity" can change how well people resist illness, reports Dr. Nehlsen-Cannarella.

Infection Protection

When the exercisers came down with colds, their symptoms—runny noses, fevers, and coughs—lasted about half the time it took the nonexercisers to get over their colds.

A bacteria or virus invading the body is like a finger flicking a light switch. It turns on the immune system, including a complex and intricate network of white blood cells that come to the body's defense. Macrophage cells engulf the intruding virus or bacteria and send an alert to other cells to step up the manufacture of antibodies. Lymphocytes—T-cells, B-cells, and natural killer cells—interact with each other to coordinate the attack and swarm in on the alien invader. Chemical messages flash through the bloodstream; chemical weapons targeted at the virus or bacteria are fired. The germs are destroyed.

Exercise prompts a protective immune response *without* the introduction of virus, bacteria, or any other offending substance. "What we're seeing with exercise is the same effect," Dr. Nehlsen-Cannarella says. "The immune system is turning on and activating more white blood cells just like it's reacting to something foreign."

Although many researchers in the past have noted this response, they've been reluctant to attribute any specific benefit to it. "Do more white blood cells mean a more efficient immune system and fewer illnesses? It may, or it may not," says Robert Jones, Ph.D., director of the Prevention and Health Promotion Program at Pennsylvania State University's College of Medicine in Hershey, Pennsylvania. What is certain, though, is that in sedentary people, "these changes do not occur," he says. "Their immune cells and resistance to infection, in fact, could be reduced."

Priming the Preventive Pump

Based on her research, Dr. Nehlsen-Cannarella has no problem making the connection between increased immune system activity and increased protection. During their study, she and her colleagues found that unlike the nonexercisers, the walkers showed an increase in the activity of natural killer cells and in the amount of antibodies in their blood. And they also experienced less-severe cold and flu symptoms.

Other studies have also found a link between exercise and an enhanced immune system. As a result of these studies, say the Loma Linda researchers, moderate workouts, particularly during the winter, may promote protection from infection "by priming the immune system before an infectious challenge takes place, with the result that duration of [cold] symptoms is reduced."

Dr. Nehlsen-Cannarella notes, however, that enhancement of the immune response continues only if the workouts do. "It'll go right back to where it was," she says, if you stop exercising. Whether the apparent boost in immunity builds long-term extra protection from viruses is unknown.

Moderation Makes Sense

The key word in the exercise-infection connection, however, is moderation. When exercise strides over the threshold from moderate to excessive—from, say, jogging to marathon running—you may be courting illness rather than preventing it.

"It's absolutely documented that when you overexert, you're having a detrimental effect on the immune system," Dr. Nehlsen-Cannarella says. Intense, sustained exercise stuns the immune system for both physiological and psychological reasons, she says.

Changes in the immune system after exhaustive exercise include a drop in natural killer cell activity and in the levels of antibodies. The pressure to endure and succeed leads to stress, which in turn increases the levels of cortisol, a hormone known to depress immunity.

Even the heavy, sustained breathing required during maximum exertion enhances the danger of infection. "You're exchanging a lot of air and with it more microbes," Dr. Nehlsen-Cannarella says. "That alone exposes you to a greater risk."

Meanwhile, the immune system is busy attending to the demands of extreme exercise and the internal repair of muscle cells damaged by extensive exercise, leaving the body somewhat unprotected from external infectious attack.

If you do engage in high-intensity exercise, you need to take special precautions to protect yourself for several hours afterward, according to Gregory W. Heath, D.Sc., an epidemiologist and exercise physiologist in the Cardiovascular Health Branch of the Centers for Disease Control in Atlanta. Dr. Heath has studied the relationship between respiratory infections and running.

"Not that everybody who exercises heavily will get a cold or the flu," he says. "But there's a window of vulnerability if you come into contact with an invading agent.

"Avoid people who are ill and kissing

TAKE YOUR COLD TO BED

Although regular workouts may condition the body to better resist the effects of a virus, it's not always wise to exercise in the midst of a cold or the flu, according to Sandra L. Nehlsen-Cannarella, Ph.D., director of the Immunology Center at Loma Linda University Medical Center in California.

During a mild illness, you may continue very light workouts—if you feel up to it. You might be better off if you rest, though, and resume exercising in a few days.

If, however, symptoms include fever, swollen lymph glands, fatigue, or muscle aches, steer clear of the gym and jogging path for two weeks to a month, she says. What an otherwise healthy body would

consider moderate activity soon seems strenuous under the influence of illness. Workouts—especially overly rigorous routines—can exacerbate cold and flu symptoms, lead to other viral infections, and possibly damage the heart.

Many common respiratory viruses, which tend to swim through the body and attack the heart, gain strength under the strain of demanding exercise, Dr. Nehlsen-Cannarella says. Attempting to work the illness out of the system drives the heart closer to the danger zone of potential cardiac damage or death through irregular heartbeats.

So feed a fever and starve a cold, if you want to abide by the old-fashioned adage. But don't invite either along for a run.

the kid who has a runny nose," Dr. Heath recommends. "And make sure you wash your hands really well, because generally, the primary mode of infectious transmission is from hand to mucous membrane."

And you might want to think twice about attending that postmarathon party, particularly if you notice that someone in the room has a cold. If an ill wind blows your way from a misdirected cough or sneeze, Dr. Heath says, "you could get the virus if the dose is high enough."

A Little Is a Lot

Where does all this leave you if you want to exercise to bolster your immunity?

Some exercise can apparently beef up

the immune system, while a lot of exercise can knock it down. "It's somewhat paradoxical," Dr. Heath says, "but it displays very nicely the life statement: 'In all things moderation.' "

Walking, lawn work, gardening—all can be considered moderate exercise that adds muscle to the body's immune response, he says. For a regular workout, Dr. Nehlsen-Cannarella suggests walking or jogging at 70 percent of your maximum heart rate. (To figure your maximum heart rate, see "How Good Is Your Workout?" on page 324.) "Do a little, even if it's just mild exercise—do something more than sitting around like a couch potato," she says. "As long as you're out walking, it's good." (See "Walking" on page 458.)

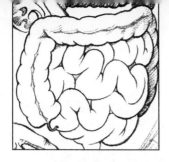

Constipation and Hemorrhoids

Nobody likes to talk about it. The straining. The aggravation. Even the pain. But constipation is a reality, a tiring, worrisome battle with what should be a simple, natural function.

Are you anxious about hearing nature's call? Then listen to this expert's advice: "Exercise and diet are the factors that promote better bowel movements," says Lester Rosen, M.D., associate clinical professor at Hahnemann University in Philadelphia. "People who keep a toned, fit body and eat a high-fiber diet usually aren't bothered by constipation."

Are You Constipated?

Before we talk about how to cure constipation, let's define the problem. It's important to remember that there is no "right" frequency of elimination. Constipation is a change from your bowel habits—you're constipated if your bowel movements are less frequent and more difficult than normal. A person who is constipated goes a number of days—not just a few—without having a bowel movement, and the resulting stools tend to be very hard.

Stress and drug side effects are common causes of constipation. But most people become constipated for three reasons: They don't get enough fiber, they don't get enough fluids, and they don't get enough exercise. Let's look at the dietary factors first.

If your diet is low in fiber, you produce small stools that don't adequately stimulate the walls of the colon, the last section of the intestine. When the colon walls aren't stimulated, the colon doesn't produce contractions, the muscular movements that move stool along. So the stool justs sits there, becoming hard and difficult to pass.

And if your diet is low in fluids, the stool dries out even more.

But if you have a high-fiber diet, and if you drink lots of fluids, you have bulky, soft stool that triggers colonic contractions—and easy elimination.

Regular Exercise for Regularity

High-fiber food and sufficient fluids are two-thirds of the equation. The third factor is exercise.

In a scientific study at Colorado State University in Fort Collins, researchers enrolled a number of students in a six-week running program, comparing the time it took meals to travel from the mouth to the rectum (a measurement called transit time) before, during, and at the end of the program. They found that running shortened transit time by 30 percent.

"A vigorous running program speeds transit time in normal students," says Loren Cordain, Ph.D., professor of exercise physiology and director of the Human Performance Research Lab at Colorado State University. "Whether moderate exercise can do the same for constipated people remains unproven."

How does exercise speed up the bowels? "My guess is that vigorous activity may boost the hormonal secretions that increase bowel movement," says Dr. Cordain.

But there may be lots of other reasons why exercise relieves constipation.

Sit-Ups Help Sluggish Bowels

"Any exercise that strengthens the abdominal muscles makes it easier to pass a stool," according to New York gastroenterologist Myron D. Goldberg, M.D., author of *The Inside Tract: The Complete Guide to Digestive Disorders.* "During defecation these muscles are voluntarily contracted, increasing intra-abdominal pressure. This pressure helps push the stool out of the body."

But weak abdominal walls can't do the job, says Dr. Goldberg. Instead of supplying pressure inward and down to help expel stool, they give way. Doing sit-ups, however, can strengthen the abdominal muscles so pressure goes where it's supposed to.

(Dr. Goldberg has another tip: If you are working up a sweat, or exercising in hot, humid weather, be sure to drink plenty of fluids. "Sweating draws fluids from your body and may dehydrate you to some extent," says Dr. Goldberg. "And dehydration contributes to constipation.")

Yoga: A Laxative with a Twist

Another type of exercise may help relieve constipation. The gentle twists and bends of yoga are often all it takes to coax a lazy colon into action, according to Richard Miller, Ph.D., co-founder of the International Association of Yoga Therapists. Yoga acts as a natural laxative for two reasons, he says. First, the physical movement creates intra-abdominal pressure, helping to move the colon contents. Forward bends, for example, compress the abdomen, facilitating bowel movement. Torso twists rotate the inner abdominal wall, pushing the stomach contents along the intestinal tract.

Yoga also helps you breathe more fully. "Breathing deeply lifts the diaphragm, massaging the intestine and promoting elimination," says Dr. Miller.

Use the following yoga postures for constipation relief.

Knee lift. This pose is called *apanasana,* meaning "wind-removing"—it helps remove both gas and the solid contents of the intestines. Lie down on your back, with your knees bent and your feet flat on the floor. Now lift your knees up toward your chest. Wrap your fingers lightly around your knees. Inhale. As you exhale, pull your knees down into your chest. Inhale as you return your feet to the floor. Exhale. Repeat six times.

Now lift your knees back up to your chest, wrap your arms around them once again, and hold the pose for six deep breaths.

Forward bend. This posture may be done while seated on the toilet. Keep your knees comfortably apart. Place your fists just below the bottom of your rib cage, on each side of your navel. Inhale.

As you exhale, gently press your fists into your abdomen and slowly bend over, bringing your head toward your knees. Inhale and return to upright position. Repeat six times.

Remain bent over for six deep breaths.

Torso twist. Sit with your arms hanging naturally at your sides. Inhale. As you exhale, rotate your abdomen, leading with your navel, to the left, letting your shoulders and head follow. Inhale and return to center. Exhale. Repeat the twist to the right. Return to center. Twist three times on each side. Then hold each twist for six deep breaths.

DON'T TAKE HEMORRHOIDS SITTING DOWN

If you've suffered chronic constipation for a long time, chances are you have another condition that exercise may help—hemorrhoids.

If your fiber and fluid intake is low and you strain while going to the bathroom, you're probably already familiar with the discomfort of hemorrhoids, which are blood-swollen veins that may protrude from the rectum.

Being sedentary can definitely aggravate the condition, according to Max Ali,

M.D., president of the Detroit-based Hemorroid Clinics of America. Driving long distances and sitting in front of a computer all day without taking a break can make the condition worse.

If you must sit for prolonged periods, get up frequently and walk around. "Almost any kind of exercise helps relieve pooling of blood in the veins," says Dr. Ali. An exception is heavy lifting. "Lifting heavy loads can make hemorrhoids worse," he says.

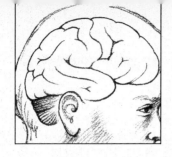

Creativity Blocks

Just for laughs, stand-up comic David Little runs. He knows that if he wants to make an audience giggle, chuckle, and howl with laughter, he needs to unleash his creativity. To do that, David jogs at least 4 miles each evening before he performs.

"Running seems to make me feel more creative and sharper on stage. I find I get ideas when I'm running. It clears my head, and often I'm able to work out a new routine for my show. If I don't run, I feel really sluggish," says David, a 32-year-old Dallas man who is on the road performing about 45 weeks a year.

Plodding along an unfamiliar street in a strange town might seem like an unusual way for a comic to write jokes, but experts say David may be doing the best thing he can to turn on his creative juices.

"A bout of exercise usually frees up creativity. It helps you get rid of the static in your mind. It literally helps you un-focus," says Keith Johnsgard, Ph.D, a psychologist at San Jose State University.

"For some people, the creative thinking that occurs during and after a run is quite pronounced," says Kenneth Callen, M.D., an associate professor of psychiatry at the Oregon Health Sciences University in Portland.

He recalls a composer who used run-ning to inspire himself to write music. "When he got to a point in his composi-tion where he didn't know where to go next, he'd go out for a long run. By the time the run was over, the next musical passage had come to him," Dr. Callen says.

Running Jogs the Mind

That's just one man's experience. But studies suggest he may well be on to something. In a survey of 424 runners conducted by Dr. Callen, about 59 percent reported feeling more creative while running. They felt they were able to develop ideas or unusual solutions to problems spontaneously. Many of the runners kept a pencil and notebook in their locker so they could write down their ideas immediately after their workouts.

In a study of 100 fourth- through eighth-grade students, Bruce W. Tuckman, Ph.D., professor of educational research at Florida State University in Tallahassee, found that the children who ran during their physi-cal education classes were more creative at the end of one semester than those stu-dents who participated in an athletic program consisting of volleyball and basketball.

But running isn't the only activity that may boost creativity. Researchers at the Baruch College of the City University of New York found that students who partici-pated in aerobic fitness and dance classes were able to think of more uses for an ordinary object, such as a pencil, than students who didn't do aerobic exercise.

"In all of our testing there was an extremely strong response, and it appears that aerobic exercise *does* increase creativity," says Joan Gondola, Ph.D., a Baruch College professor who conducted the study.

In yet another study, at the Veterans Administration Medical Center in Salt Lake City, 55- to 70-year-olds who regularly did speedwalking had faster reaction times and improved their creative thinking.

"My assumption would be that any type of aerobic exercise would facilitate creativity," Dr. Gondola says.

Balancing the Brain

Why aerobic exercise ignites the creative fires in some people's heads still isn't clearly understood. Some researchers believe that exercise increases oxygen flow to the brain. Others think that vigorous exercise may trigger the release of hormones in the brain that enhance mood and creativity.

Dr. Tuckman and Dr. Gondola believe that aerobic exercise may suppress activity in the left hemisphere of the brain, the half that is responsible for logical thought, and stimulate the right hemisphere, which regulates intuition and creativity.

"During the first half hour of exercise, you may exhaust the left brain. You think about what you're going to wear tomorrow or a specific task you have to do," Dr. Tuckman says. "But after the first 30 minutes of vigorous exercise, you get away from those kinds of thoughts, and you just let things start popping into your head. It's almost like dreaming when you're awake."

But while researchers are fairly certain that aerobic exercise can unlock your creativity, no one is really sure how much exercise is needed to reach that point.

In fact, studies indicate that overly intense exercise may have adverse affects on mood. Overexertion may inhibit creativity as well, says Dr. Callen.

"If you do a marathon, you're not going to feel very creative. You're going to be wiped out," he says. "The point is, doing a lot of exercise tends to stifle creativity. But a little bit of it is probably beneficial."

Dr. Tuckman, a runner for 21 years and a veteran of 40 marathons, agrees. "I don't think you have to exercise at a tremendous level of intensity. I think a 30- to 40-minute workout at a reasonable tempo would do it," he says.

Most experts who have studied the link between creativity and exercise suggest an aerobic activity—walking, swimming, biking, running—at a moderate pace at least three times a week.

"I would recommend walking for a number of reasons," Dr. Tuckman says. "It's the most socially acceptable form of exercise, and it requires the least amount of expert knowledge to do it."

He suggests beginning by walking about 1½ miles three times a week at a pace of 15 minutes per mile. Of course, before you begin any exercise program, you should consult with your family physician, particularly if you have a history of heart or pulmonary disease.

"You don't have to walk very fast, but you should feel like you're exercising," Dr. Tuckman says.

If you really want to get your creativity flowing, exercise alone and leave the cassette player at home, he says.

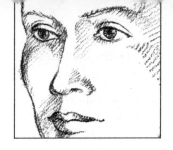

Dependencies (Alcohol and Drugs)

The spotlight shone on Rae Thrift early in life as a Rockette at Radio City Music Hall. The 15-year-old didn't get her kicks from the chorus line, though. She turned to alcohol and drugs, plunging herself into a black pit of addiction some 30 years deep. When she emerged, she danced her way into the sunshine of sobriety with the help of exercise.

Now the activity coordinator at the Betty Ford Center in Rancho Mirage, California, Thrift can't say enough about the value of exercise in overcoming a wide variety of chemical dependencies. Exercise and other activities haven't always been a mainstay of alcohol and other drug rehabilitation, Thrift says.

Back when she was in early recovery, treatment centers never advocated fitness in treatment because the traditional 28-day treatment program was too short and counselors didn't want patients to lose focus in the battle against the addiction, she explains.

She stumbled onto the healing properties of exercise many years ago during a time of desperation in her own life. These days many recovery experts share her enthusiasm for exercise as a critical component of effective treatment—and for good reason.

Working out turns out to be "an impor-tant piece of the recovery puzzle," says Teri Nelson, supervisor of the Recreation and Occupational Therapy Department at Hazelden Foundation in Center City, Minnesota. Drugs and drink devastate the user emotionally, physically, socially, and spiritually, she says, and exercise can be an integral part in the rejuvenation of each facet.

A Binge Too Far

Drinkers and drug users live an unhealthy lifestyle, and "a lot works against exercise" in both addiction and recovery, according to Robert L. Kaman, Ph.D., associate professor in the physiology and the public health and preventive medicine depart-ments at the Texas College of Osteopathic Medicine in Fort Worth. Many of the problems from which addicts and alcohol-ics suffer aren't directly the result of the chemical abuse. They typically smoke heavily and count coffee consumption in pots, not cups. They have an almost total lack of interest in their health and follow poor nutritional habits. "They're completely deconditioned," Dr. Kaman says.

Thrift can vouch for that. For her, excessive drinking and drug use didn't start immediately. "It's sneaky, you know. It didn't get bad until my twenties," she remembers. Thrift smoked marijuana daily for 15 years, adding alcohol, pills, and cough syrup. Dreams of dance died as she progressed further and further into her addiction. Twenty-two years later, at 38, she tried to clean herself up. Clean living, though, was difficult, and it lasted only 4 years. A relapse into drinking and drug use lasted for another 2 years.

"I was terrified I was going to die," she remembers, "but I wanted to live." She resumed the self-help meetings she once abandoned and, in 1976, entered a recovery house, where she stayed for 1½ years.

As recovering alcoholics and substance abusers often do, Thrift smoked heavily, drank too much coffee, and overate. When she left the recovery house, the once lithe and lively dancer was "thrown into the world middle-aged and with a big belly. I couldn't even breathe."

Frightened and directionless, Thrift started searching for an anchor. She thought about Radio City Music Hall. Through the haze of lost memories and dim visions of a gray past, "a part of me remembered how wonderful it was to be fit," she recalls. "A part of me knew about discipline and dance and knew how helpful it could be to my recovery."

In addition to her addiction therapy and self-help meetings, Thrift started to walk, first just 10 minutes a day, then 15 minutes, gradually building up to a half hour and then 45 minutes. After she began practicing visualization and taking aerobics classes, her body started to function normally for the first time in years. She could breathe and move and lift. She felt better about herself and her future. As a result of her recovery, she developed something she never before had: confidence and self-assurance.

How Exercise Helps Addicts in Recovery

Although individual chemicals abuse the body in different ways, many of the destructive consequences of habitual drug and alcohol use are similar. The symptoms intensify the longer the substance abuse continues, and they may become even worse during the initial withdrawal, as a battered body and mind try to cope with the loss of something they have come to depend on. And throughout it all, during both the dependency and the withdrawal process, stress exacerbates both the physical and emotional symptoms even more.

The depression and mood swings that addicts are subject to, experts say, occur because alcohol and other drugs destroy the brain's levels of norepinephrine, a neurotransmitter essential for emotional stability. Fluctuations of another brain chemical, dopamine, can cause paranoia, skewed perceptions, confusion, visual delusions, and memory loss. Depletion of other neurotransmitters produces anxiety, fear, and paranoia. One of the reasons exercise is such a potent recovery tool is because it helps restore depleted neurotransmitters.

People dumping their dependencies "report improvement right away" in emotional outlook when they exercise, Nelson says. "It's very common for them to say, 'Boy, I feel a lot better.'"

Motivating them to begin that first workout, though, requires patience, understanding, and constant encouragement, says Maxeen Vashro, consultant for substance abuse treatment centers and owner of Body to the Max in Minneapolis.

"They're very stressed out," she says, and often their bodies are so out of shape that even minimal exertion is difficult.

But when people persist and get through that first session, endorphins released by the body generate a feeling of euphoria and contentedness, she says. Other chemicals stimulated by exercise lighten the load of stress. "They reach a different plateau of attitude," says Vashro. "You can see a total change in personality right within an hour or half-hour class."

Booze It and Lose It

Physically, drug and alcohol use saps the immune system of its power to combat bacteria and disease, robbing it of its ability to fight off something as innocuous as a cold—or as deadly as a tumor. The skin looks ashen and becomes more susceptible to infections. Colds linger longer. Blood pressure rises, artery-clogging LDL cholesterol increases, and chances of an irregular heartbeat and stroke increase dramatically.

Appetite wanes markedly, leading to virtual malnutrition and depletion of vitamins and minerals, which further ravish the immune system. Muscles, including the heart, begin to weaken and atrophy, partly as a direct result of the chemical on the body, partly because people stuck in a stupor tend not to move about much. Reaction time is harmed; muscle coordination and motor skills are impaired.

Exercise counteracts all these destructive physical effects, says Dr. Kaman. Working out bolsters the immune system,

lowers blood pressure, and fights elevated cholesterol levels. It strengthens the heart and all other muscles in the body, reversing any atrophy, and improves dexterity and coordination by reintroducing people numbed by chemicals to how their body moves and feels.

The Dangers of the Exercise "High"

Exercise may seem like the perfect panacea for addiction, but certain precautions are in order, according to those who work with alcoholics and drug users. Because it stimulates endorphins, which commonly have been called the body's own opiates, exercise creates a natural high.

That's fine for those not genetically or behaviorally predisposed to addictive behavior. But it can be disastrous for recovering alcoholics and drug users.

A lot of chemically dependent people actually turn exercise into an addiction, says Nelson. You shouldn't switch one addiction for another, even if the substitute seems benign and beneficial.

No matter how ravaged their body is from alcohol or other drugs, "highly compulsive and addicted individuals tend to overexercise and can hurt themselves," Thrift says. Sometimes they'll run until they collapse. At a weight machine, they'll select the heaviest weight and try to lift it.

Substituting exercise for alcohol or drugs "can get in the way of a balanced, spiritual recovery," Nelson says. Take away the daily exercise for whatever reason—injury, illness, schedule alterations, holiday gym closings—and people end up lost, hungry for a fix, and much more vulnerable to falling back on the original addiction.

When Nelson hears from someone that exercise is making all the difference in his or her recovery, "I tend to get a little nervous," she says. But because the effects of a workout are so immediately beneficial, "it can be okay initially" to lean on exercise—as long as the person is under professional supervision.

"They're grasping, grasping for anything" that can help them feel better, she says. But through therapy and counseling, they eventually have to understand and accept the fact that exercise is only one part of a total readjustment of lifestyle; mutual-help groups such as Alcoholics Anonymous, counseling, stress management, relaxation training, and regular medical care by someone schooled in addiction treatment are also essential.

Just Say "Slow"

Recovering alcoholics and drug users can turn to a panoply of exercises—as easy as gentle stretching, as vigorous as racquetball and weight lifting. But it has to begin slowly. "Remember," Vashro cautions, "there's been a lot of damage. They have to rehabilitate both the body and the mind."

Walking probably is "the most beneficial way to start," Thrift says. Once the body begins to adjust to an increase in activity and nonchemical stimulation, a moderate calisthenics and aerobics pro-gram will improve coordination and revive the cardiovascular system even more, she says. Swimming and exercising in a pool also are therapeutic. And body conditioning with light weights will restore strength to weak muscles.

Group exercise and team sports help reintroduce recovering addicts to sober social interaction, experts say. The camaraderie provides emotional support, and if competition is not emphasized, people learn that even if they lose the game, they still win.

The stress-reducing impact of exercise, felt almost immediately, begins to feed on itself as the activity continues. And within weeks, outlook and self-esteem soar as people see the physical changes in their body, says Thrift. "It all comes back to self-esteem," she says, "one of the problems we alcoholics and addicts have." At the Betty Ford Center, she has seen recovering addicts and first-time exercisers "who look like they're going to die. But with abstinence from alcohol and other drugs, proper nutrition, and a proper balance of exercise, the body heals quickly," she says. A healthy hue returns to the skin, flab begins to melt away, muscle tone firms the body, and people begin to walk taller—physically and psychologically.

Once people begin to work out regularly, eat well, sleep well, and come to terms with their addiction through counseling and self-help, "they're going to start to bloom," Thrift says. "It's like a little flower. You've *gotta* look better. That's the miracle of recovery."

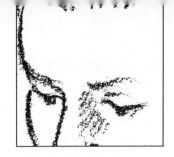

Depression

*I*f depression makes you feel like a boulder in a river watching life flow past you, don't just sit there — swim for shore.

"As human beings we're designed to get a daily dose of exercise. If we don't get it, then we just don't feel right," says Keith Johnsgard, Ph.D., author of the *The Exercise Prescription for Depression and Anxiety* and a psychologist at San Jose State University.

Running, dancing, swimming, bicycling, and walking may be among the best cures we have for depression, he says.

Exercise Jump-Starts Emotions

"Exercise really works," Dr. Johnsgard says. "It works as well as all psychotherapies."

He has many allies who support that notion. "I think that exercise should be part of every basic treatment program for depression," says Morris Mellion, M.D., president-elect of the American Academy of Family Physicians.

Even the American Heart Association (AHA) is convinced that exercise can affect attitude and outlook. (It's not uncommon for people who have suffered heart attacks to go through a period of depression as they try to pick up the pieces and get on with living.)

"Prescribed and supervised physical training may prevent or alleviate anxiety and depression in certain persons," states the AHA. "The physically trained patient is often able to show himself, his family, and his peers that he is capable of assuming his previous position in society."

Unfortunately, depression is becoming more common, according to researchers at Cornell University Medical College. They determined that since 1960 the rate of depressive disorders has increased in all age groups and has become more prevalent particularly among teens and young adults.

One in 20 American adults suffers from a depressive disorder, according to the National Institute of Mental Health. More than ten million people will have a depressive illness this year. In the next month, about 2 percent of all Americans will experience some symptoms of major depression.

Move into a Better Mood

Whether you're suffering from a serious depressive disorder or a simple case of the blues, exercise apparently can help you bounce back. "Depressed people seem to have a very good memory for unpleasant events. In fact, that's *all* they seem to remember," says Robert S. Brown, Sr., M.D., Ph.D., clinical professor of behavorial medicine and psychiatry at the University of Virginia.

In a University of Virginia study, researchers asked depressed students to memorize a list of adjectives that included words such as "pretty" and "ugly." Then 15 minutes later, they asked the students to recall those words. Most of the students remembered words that had bad or unpleasant meanings. Next the students participated in an aerobic exercise class. Afterward, the students were once again asked to recall the adjectives. This time, they remembered more of the pleasant words.

"Exercise seems to speed metabolism and get more oxygen to the brain, so it flushes out the body and mind," Dr. Brown says. "You get more circulation in the brain, so you're more likely to have normal recall instead of getting bogged down in unpleasant memories."

In another study by Dr. Brown, student athletes at the University of Virginia were given mood evaluation tests at the beginning and at the end of their sport seasons. The students were selected from a cross section of the university's athletic programs, including football, basketball, wrestling, and golf.

"The sports that required the least expenditure of energy produced the least amount of change on the mood tests, regardless of the team's win/loss record," he says. "The people on the wrestling team, for example, had a greater change in mood than those on the golf team."

Running from the Blues

That research, Dr. Brown says, supports his belief that aerobic workouts are the best type of exercise for relieving depression.

Research at the University of Pittsburgh also points to aerobic exercise as a mood enhancer. There, researchers studied 57 depressed women, some of whom participated in either aerobic dance or racquetball classes for ten weeks. A third group didn't exercise but attended an introductory psychology course. At the end of the study, the women in the psychology class had no noticeable mood changes, but those who participated in the exercise programs improved significantly. In addition, researchers concluded that "aerobic dance may be slightly better than racquetball for reducing symptoms of depression," according to Sanford Golin, Ph.D., associate professor of psychiatry and psychology at the University of Pittsburgh.

An hour of exercise can be just as effective—but more enjoyable—than an hour in therapy, according to one study. "Aerobic exercise is more effective than placebo or no treatment and not significantly different from other forms of treatment, including various forms of psychotherapy, in terms of outcome," according to Egil Martinsen, M.D., a Norwegian psychiatrist who was the principal researcher for a series of studies that examined the effects of various forms of exercise on anxiety and depression.

Weights May Provide a Lift, Too

Dr. Martinsen believes that nonaerobic exercise, such as weight lifting, also may influence mood. In a study of 99 patients at a Norwegian mental hospital, Dr. Martinsen determined that weight training and relaxation exercises were just as effective as running or walking in reducing depression. (See "Resistance Training" on page 404 and "Relaxation Training" on page 399.)

T'ai chi, a Chinese martial art that involves slow-motion exercise, is another type of nonaerobic activity that may significantly relieve depression, according to Australian researchers. In a study of 66 people who practice t'ai chi, researchers found that the exercise noticeably lowered the practitioners' levels of depression, tension, anxiety, and anger. (See "Martial Arts" on page 370.)

The Australian and Norweigan studies are backed by work at the University of Rochester in New York. Researchers there studied a group of depressed women who participated in running or weight lifting three times a week for eight weeks. The investigators concluded that women in both groups significantly improved their self-image and perception of their fitness.

How Exercise Combats Depression

If Dr. Martinsen and other proponents of nonaerobic exercise are right, they may be providing scientists with important clues about how exercise affects mood.

Some researchers, for example, suspect that aerobic exercise sparks the production of chemicals that increase brain cell activity and curtail depression. Others believe that aerobic exercise triggers the release of natural painkilling compounds, such as endorphins, that derail depressive thoughts.

But since nonaerobic exercise also seems to relieve depression, Dr. Martinsen suspects that exercise also may work because it distracts a depressed person from negative feelings or perhaps because it provides a sense of accomplishment.

However it works, many researchers believe exercise does help alleviate depression.

"The debate isn't whether exercise is an effective way to treat depression. The debate is whether there is enough evidence to use it as a *sole* treatment for depression," Dr. Mellion says.

While exercise may help most of us combat an occasional case of the blues, chronically depressed people may need more of an emotional lift than exercise alone can provide and should seek professional help, he says.

"Exercise has tremendous physiological and psychological benefits for the depressed patient. But I also believe it should be used in conjunction with other treatments such as counseling," Dr. Mellion says.

The jury's still out, however, on how effective exercise is in helping to elevate the moods of people who already feel good about themselves. Researchers at Duke University, for example, found no evidence that exercise can improve the sense of well-being in emotionally stable older adults. However, the researchers caution that their results aren't conclusive because measuring levels of happiness is difficult.

"As psychologists, we haven't really come up with good objective measures of well-being. Our measures tend to look at distress rather than at positive indicators such as happiness," says Charles Emery, Ph.D., a psychologist at Duke University Medical Center.

"A healthy person, instead of getting less depressed or anxious, may become happier and more outgoing because of exercise. We just don't have any good measures of something like that at this point," he says.

The Happiness Prescription

So how do you motivate yourself to exercise when you feel as lifeless as floor wax? First, remember that many therapists believe that motivation doesn't cause action; action creates motivation. In other words, if you wait until you're "in the mood" to exercise, you probably won't ever get around to it.

If you need an initial boost, ask a friend or acquaintance to work out with you. "There are days when you just don't feel like exercising," Dr. Johnsgard says. "You may feel depressed, de-energized, harried, or as if you are becoming ill. If a friend can get you out of the house and physically active, you'll soon learn that the times you least feel like exercising are the most rewarding times to do it."

Do an exercise that fulfills your emotional needs. If you tire of working out alone, for example, you may want to join a walking club or participate in a team sport.

"You have to tailor the exercise to the individual. Some people won't do it unless some social aspect or competition is involved. Others are terrified by those things. They need to be alone and have time to think," Dr. Johnsgard says.

However, he occasionally suggests his patients do several activities to combat exercise boredom, such as aerobic dancing three days a week supplemented by long walks or bicycle rides on weekends.

Walking is usually the best way to start

a program for physical and emotional wellness, Dr. Johnsgard says.

"Walking is the foundation, our bedrock life insurance policy. We may build on it if we choose, but for most of us it should constitute our basic health plan. There simply isn't anything else that fits the bill," he says. (See 'Walking" on page 458.)

Whatever exercise you select, begin slowly. Studies indicate that people who begin with high-intensity workouts are more likely to quit than low- and moderate-intensity exercisers.

How to Help Others

If a friend is depressed, Dr. Mellion recommends that you suggest exercise in a nonthreatening way, such as asking, "What do you think about trying some exercise?"

"You really can't tell someone to exercise. Ask, don't tell. Let them open up to you. Let them tell you what they think about exercise, and the answer might surprise you," Dr. Mellion says.

"Depression hurts," he adds. "Some people are experiencing so much pain from their depression that they're willing to try anything. It's amazing how willingly people comply with a routine when they're in pain."

Finally, keep in mind that even the experts get depressed every once in a while, and yes, they take a dose of their own medicine to shake off the doldrums.

"I run 4 to 5 miles a day to stay fit," Dr. Johnsgard says. "When I want to boost or improve my mood, feel good and super-relaxed, I pick up my pace and push even harder."

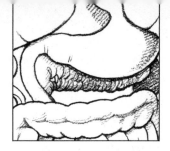

Diabetes

*I*f you have diabetes, you feel guilty if you take "just one teeny bite" from a candy bar or so much as look at a can of Coke. In fact, there are undoubtedly times you feel as if your life is controlled by an unyielding tyrant. Fortunately, these days medical science has a whole arsenal of weapons to keep that "tyrant" in check . . . including regular exercise.

For the overwhelming majority of people with diabetes, the right kind of exercise can help control the disease and reduce the risk of life-threatening complications.

Exercise can lower excess blood sugar levels, strengthen your muscles and heart, improve your circulation, and reduce stress. Studies indicate that all of these benefits can help decrease your risk of developing the complications linked with diabetes: heart disease, kidney disease, high blood pressure, nerve damage, blindness, and impotence. Amputations, caused by circulatory problems related to the disease, can also be avoided.

"For the majority of diabetics, exercise is a useful way to help control their disease," says molecular biologist David H. Wasserman, Ph.D., assistant professor at Vanderbilt University's department of molecular physiology and biophysics in Nashville. "It's simply a matter of doing it safely and properly."

Proceed with Caution

About 14 million Americans suffer from diabetes, a chronic disease in which the body can't produce or effectively use insulin, the hormone that helps transport glucose—a sugar that provides the body's basic fuel—into various cells to provide energy.

When your pancreas doesn't manufacture insulin properly or your cells can't use it, your body's metabolism is thrown out of balance. Glucose-hungry cells begin to starve, leaving muscles with little or no energy-producing fuel. You feel tired, and the unused glucose builds up in your bloodstream—creating a condition known as hyperglycemia—until it eventually spills into your urine. Unfortunately, excess glucose can be toxic and, in the long run, can ravage your body's delicately balanced ecosystem.

There are several different types of diabetes, but the most common are Type I (juvenile or insulin-dependent) and Type II (adult onset or non-insulin-dependent). Although people with either type experience similar symptoms and complications, experts agree they're actually two different diseases with very different causes and concerns.

Because of this, it's critical that any

SAVE YOUR EYES

Imagine going through life as though you were looking through a mud-splattered windshield. Or worse, if everything your eyes gazed upon—a stop sign, the TV screen, the fuzzy face of your beloved pooch—appeared to have a big, dark hole in the center.

This is what a person in the extreme stages of retinopathy might see. Retinopathy is an eye disorder caused by uncontrolled diabetes. The leading cause of new cases of adult blindness in America, this condition develops when tiny vessels in the retina rupture or burst because of a lack of oxygen and blood. The vessels die, forming tiny wool-like scar tissue. Ultimately, the retina may detach, causing blindness. In severe cases, new, fragile vessels grow sporadically, one on top of the other, hemorrhaging and leaking blood into the jellylike fluid that fills the eyeball. This increases the pressure in the eyes, which further aggravates the situation.

Keeping your diabetes under control should help you avoid retinopathy. If you already have the disorder, however, you must be particularly careful in the kind of exercise you choose. Exercises that increase blood pressure may encourage the rupture and hemorrhaging of blood vessels. Here are some exercises and sports that you should avoid.

Weightlifting, downhill skiing, scuba diving, and skydiving all can cause sudden increases of blood flow to the eyes and pressure in and behind the eyes, placing a sudden strain on the vessels.

Contact sports, such as basketball, football, and soccer, should be avoided. Any sudden pounding or jarring or quick movement of the head can cause the retina to pull away from the back of the eye and possibly detach.

This also holds true for jogging and diving into a swimming pool.

Before you begin exercising, discuss with your doctor any exercise limitations you might have due to your condition.

---

exercise program be designed in accordance with the type of diabetes you have and its severity. Despite the proven potential of exercise to lower blood sugar levels, medical experts say that some forms of exercise may not be beneficial for every person with diabetes. Indeed, certain exercises can be harmful. Studies show that if your blood pressure is even slightly higher than it should be, for example, it can rise even higher if you exercise at a level above 50 to 65 percent of your maximum heart rate. Because people with diabetes are prone to high blood pressure, their exercise regimen should be monitored closely, according to Lois Jovanovic-Peterson, M.D., senior scientist at the Sansum Medical Research Foundation in Santa Barbara and coauthor of *Diabetes Self-Care.*

In fact, before you begin any exercise program, experts urge that you be evaluated for heart disease, high blood pressure, nerve or kidney damage, retinopathy (see "Save Your Eyes" above), or any other condition that might be affected by an increase in physical activity. They also advise an exercise treadmill test (particularly if you're over 35). The test will enable the doctor to evaluate your physical endurance and to determine what level of activity is best for you. Failure to know and respect the limits set by the doctor could prove fatal for people with either type of diabetes.

If you have trouble finding a doctor who can help you develop an exercise program, call your local chapter of the American Diabetes Association. They can provide a nationwide list of 70 diabetes centers that can help. The kind of program that your doctor puts together for you will depend on the kind of diabetes you have and the severity of the condition.

Type II Diabetes: Pooped-Out Pancreas

Ninety to 95 percent of all people with diabetes have Type II. If you're one of them, you probably don't require insulin injections or oral medication to help lower your glucose levels. You may be obese— about 20 or more pounds overweight—and you probably acquired the disease at some point after you turned 40. And since Type II is usually hereditary, you most likely have a family history of the disease.

For you, the cornerstone of treating diabetes and normalizing your glucose level is pretty cut and dried—maintain a low-fat, low-sugar diet, lose weight, and by all means, *exercise.*

Working out is great therapy for the person with Type II diabetes. Indeed, experts agree that its benefits are so numerous that coupling it with proper diet and weight loss may be all you need to get the disease fully under control. In fact, if you're taking insulin, exercise may enable you to decrease the amount—*or eliminate it altogether.*

Unlike people with Type I diabetes, your pancreas does produce insulin—sometimes just enough to squeak by on, or sometimes too much. But no matter how much insulin your body makes, your cells aren't receptive to it. These "insulin-resistant" cells don't allow insulin to deliver its energy-giving load of glucose.

Some experts claim low insulin levels result from years of overeating, causing the overworked pancreas to poop out. It becomes too exhausted to continue producing enough insulin to help metabolize all that food.

But in addition to too many years of too much food, experts say too little exercise contributes to Type II diabetes. Studies have found that in groups of people where physical activity is high, the rate of Type II diabetes is low.

Exercise Cuts Your Risk by More Than Half

In a study of 87,253 female nurses conducted at Harvard Medical School, for example, researchers found that the more nurses exercised, the less likely they were to develop diabetes. Nurses who exercised hard enough to work up a sweat regularly reduced their risk of developing the disease by 84 percent compared to their sedentary sisters.

Moreover, nurses who were likely to develop diabetes because they were obese or genetically predisposed found that they had cut their risk by nearly three-fourths.

Not bad for a little sweat, eh? And the same is apparently true for men. In a study at the University of California, Berkeley, researchers examined the physical activity patterns of 5,990 male University of Pennsylvania graduates. The men answered questionnaires regarding lifestyle and risk factors for developing Type II diabetes such as family history, excess weight, and high blood pressure. Analysis over the next 14 years found that those men at highest risk who had engaged in leisure-time physical activity—sports, walking, or stair climbing, for example—were about half as likely to develop the disease.

In fact, the study revealed that for every extra 500 calories a week you burn with exercise, you lower your risk of developing diabetes by 6 percent.

"Not only is it clear that increased physical activity is effective in preventing Type II diabetes, but this protective effect of exercise is greatest among those people at highest risk for developing the disease," says the study's primary investigator, Susan Helmrich, Ph.D., at Berkeley's School of Public Health. Dr. Helmrich and her associates also found that the more vigorous a sport, the greater the decrease in risk.

Drop That Sugar

"So, all right," you might well say. "I ate too much. I didn't exercise enough. Now that I'm overweight, middle-aged, and already have diabetes, is there any hope for me?"

Absolutely. For one thing, studies show that exercise can lower excess sugar in your blood. One study of 300 people with Type II diabetes found that after a single 30-minute bout of moderately intense exercise, not only did glucose levels dra-

matically decrease, but in some cases, the beneficial effects of the exercise lasted for as long as 48 hours.

"Exercise helps transport glucose out of your bloodstream and into your cells where it can be used," says Dr. Jovanovic-Peterson. "It also increases blood flow to your body's organs and helps muscles use glucose independently of insulin." Furthermore, exercise helps lower the resistance that cells and tissues can have to the insulin.

And, of course, exercise helps you lose that excess weight, one reason you may have developed Type II diabetes in the first place. That's plenty of incentive to get moving.

One Step at a Time

If you haven't been exercising regularly, however, don't overdo it, experts warn. For one thing, studies show that if the physical activity is too intense, your blood sugar may *rise*, not fall.

That's why people with Type II diabetes should have an endurance test given by a physician before beginning an exercise program, recommends Dr. Jovanovic-Peterson. If you're already under a doctor's care, you might—with your doctor's approval—take the endurance test offered at most Y's.

Dr. Jovanovic-Peterson recommends this moderate step-by-step program to help people with Type II diabetes get maximum benefits from regular exercise.

"Three times a week, set aside 1 hour devoted to your exercise program. Try to space it out every other day. Spend 10 minutes doing warm-up and stretching exercises, followed by 20 minutes of moderate aerobic exercise such as cycling or brisk walking. Then take another 20 minutes for cool-down exercise such as stretching. Follow your routine with a relaxing, 10-minute shower." Eventually increase the duration of the exercise.

As you increase the amount of exercise you do, the rate at which your blood glucose level drops will increase.

"The key to stabilizing your blood sugar levels is prolonged, regular exercise," says Dr. Jovanovic-Peterson. "It's not enough to exercise sporadically."

The prolonged effect of regular exercise is that the uptake of sugar by the muscle is increased. Once your heart works at a faster pace with a more efficient use of oxygen, you become more cardiovascularly fit. Your muscles become so efficient, they use up their own stores of glucose as well as pull additional sugar from the bloodstream for about 8 hours after you exercise.

Excellent aerobic exercises for people with diabetes are brisk walking, swimming, rowing, cycling, dancing, and cross-country skiing, she says. (To learn how to start an exercise program involving any of these activities, see the appropriate chapters in part 2.)

Type I Diabetes: Balancing the Bod

About one out of ten people with diabetes is said to be Type I. Although you can get Type I diabetes at any age, children are far more likely than adults to develop it.

Scientists aren't sure what causes Type I diabetes—heredity plays a role—but studies suggest that something in the environment such as a virus or toxins may cause the body's immune system to go awry and attack the body itself. Antibodies mistakenly attack and destroy insulin-producing cells in the pancreas the same way they would a virus. Once the pancreas stops producing insulin, someone with Type I diabetes must take daily injections of the hormone to help carry glucose into the cells.

People with Type I, says Dr. Jovanovic-Peterson, should exercise for the same reason anyone with diabetes should exercise—to avoid debilitating complications. But following an exercise program is a lot trickier for people with Type I because of their dependence on insulin.

Because you control your body's sugar and energy balance by taking insulin, you must immediately compensate for the metabolic changes exercise makes by lowering the amount of insulin you would normally take or eating additional carbohydrates.

Keeping Your Energy on an Even Keel

Why? Think of your metabolism as a kind of internal seesaw. On one side of the seesaw there is insulin, on the other is glucose. For your metabolism to function effectively, they must be on an even level. If your insulin suddenly goes too high, it's out of balance with your blood sugar, which is now too low. If your sugar is too

POLICE YOUR FEET

If you have diabetes, paying attention to your feet is vital. It's even more important if regular exercise puts additional stress on your feet. That's because diabetes makes your feet particularly vulnerable.

Because high blood sugar levels interfere with your body's defense against bacteria, you're far more susceptible to infections. And if you have nerve damage (neuropathy), you may not have feeling in your feet.

"We saw a patient who had a tack in the bottom of his foot and he didn't even know it," recalls Barbara Campaigne, Ph.D., assistant professor at Children's Hospital Medical Center in Cincinnati.

She cautions that a simple blister or sore can become an infection that, left untreated, can lead to gangrene and possible amputation.

Here are some things Dr. Campaigne recommends to eliminate the potential for infection.

- Make sure you have properly fitted shoes that don't squeeze your feet and cause blisters.
- Keep your toes clean and your toenails clipped so that there are no sharp edges to perforate the skin during exercise.
- Always wear shoes around the house. Walking in your bare feet puts you at risk for getting serious cuts you can't even feel.
- Inspect your feet for cuts, sores, or blisters daily; use a mirror if you have to, so you don't miss a spot.
- Whenever you visit the doctor's office, insist he or she examine your feet.
- See your doctor immediately if you develop ingrown toenails, corns, calluses, or an infection.

high, your insulin level will be too low.

When you exercise, you burn sugar and the seesaw begins to tilt out of balance.

"At this point, you may not have enough glucose going to the brain," says Barbara Campaigne, Ph.D., assistant professor at Children's Hospital Medical Center in Cincinnati. "Obviously, if you're alone on a jogging trail somewhere and you develop very low blood sugar, the consequences can be very, very serious." (This could cause you to become confused or go into convulsions.)

That's why if you have Type I diabetes, it's extremely important that your physician and exercise specialist design a diet, insulin, and exercise program geared for your own particular metabolism, says Dr. Wasserman. This team will determine what you need to do to maintain ideal blood sugar levels during and after exercise. And they will help you figure out what you should eat and how much insulin you should take before exercise so that you can maintain ideal blood sugar levels.

The Pros Know

Some experts advise taking insulin at least 1 hour before you start exercising, for example, and eating a meal 1 to 3 hours ahead of time. This will allow time for carbohydrates to be absorbed as sugar into your bloodstream. (Carbohydrates metabolize into sugar.)

Maintaining a balance between insulin and blood sugar levels *during* exercise may seem complicated at first, but it's not. Ask any number of professional athletes, and they'll tell you their diabetes doesn't stop them from working out. The only difference between them and nondiabetic athletes is that they've learned to regulate their insulin/glucose balance to allow for every level of exercise. They've learned at what point in their exercise their glucose levels are dropping too far. Some compensate for this by drinking a small amount of fruit juice before they start exercising. Or during strenuous activity, they may eat a carbohydrate-packed snack every 30 to 45 minutes. Or, for example, between sets of tennis, they may sip diluted fruit juice.

There are a few additional precautions.

The American Diabetes Association recommends that you test your blood sugar level just before beginning a workout. But if your fasting blood sugar level exceeds 250 mg/dl, you shouldn't exercise. Beyond this level, your glucose may rise, not fall.

Other experts suggest that you should not start a strength-training program such as weight lifting unless you check with your doctor. Strength training is linked to increased blood pressure and could, among other things, put undue stress on your heart and the small blood vessels in your eyes.

So what kind of exercise *should* you do? The same as we described for Type II's: aerobic activities such as cycling, brisk walking, and jogging, depending on your age and how well controlled your disease is. In other words, hit the road, Jack. You've got nothing to lose and a chance to improve your control over your disease.

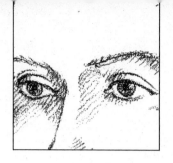

Eyestrain

*I*t can creep up on you at work when you least expect it—that stinging sensation in your eyes that makes them water, the persistent ache that starts in your head and spreads to your neck, shoulders, and back.

By midday, the images on your computer screen appear blurry or even doubled. It has become difficult and painful to follow words across the screen. And at the end of the day during your drive home, you notice that the buildings, signs, and trees you saw clearly that morning now appear fuzzy and out of focus.

If you experience these symptoms, you may be among millions of Americans struggling with eyestrain. Although more than 75 percent of people who use computers on the job experience eyestrain from long hours of staring into the video terminal, *any* activity or job that calls for intensive close-up work can cause this problem.

"A proofreader, an accountant, anybody with lots of paperwork can get it," says Lowell D. Glatt, O.D., of the American Optometric Association in Hicksville, New York. "Take the poor little clerk who's doing the books. For 8 hours a day, he's poring over papers a foot away from him. Sure, the boss may read for an hour or two, but then he's in a meeting. He gets to relax

his eyes while his clerk is seeing double."

Actually, it's not the eyes themselves that are being strained but the two sets of muscle systems that help the eyes function— the ciliary, or focusing, muscles, which control the focusing mechanism, and the eye movement muscles, which point the eyes toward whatever you are looking at.

"When you read, the ciliary muscles tense up and contract, turning the lens into a ball-like shape," explains R. Anthony Hutchinson, O.D., author of *Computer Eye Stress.* "When you look at the horizon, the ciliary muscles relax, and the lens is flattened. With close-up work such as might be found in an office or factory, the ciliary muscles are always tense and tire out very quickly."

Tiny Muscles Make Big Problems

Close-up work also taxes the eye movement muscles that control the position of the eyes. When your eyes focus on a close object, they must turn inward and converge. "The muscles that control the eye movement, when focused to stay in one position for sustained periods of time, may give us fatigue and stress symptoms," says Dr. Glatt. So working up close requires a continued effort that may cause fatigue.

And eyestrain itself causes even more eyestrain as your brain tells your eyes to correct the blurry vision. Says Dr. Hutchinson: "If you're reading along and suddenly what you're seeing is very blurred, your brain will say, 'Hey wait a minute, eye muscles, try to point both eyes at that line a little better. Ciliary muscle, let's get that word in better focus. Let's even try squinting a little and furrowing the brow to see if that helps make things any clearer.' So all of these muscles work a little harder on the blurred image."

Ease Your Eyes

So how do you solve the problem of eyestrain—particularly if your job involves lots of close-up work? For starters, make sure your office is well lit. And if you use a computer, the screen should be free of glare.

And remember to do a very basic eye exercise—blink! Normally, you blink once every 5 seconds. But sometimes you can concentrate so intensely on what you're doing that you "forget" to blink. The longer you go without blinking, the drier and more painful your eyes become, says Dr. Hutchinson.

Optimally, 9-to-5 folks who do close-up work all day long should spend 15 minutes each hour relaxing their eye muscles by looking at something far away—out a window, across the room. Obviously, that's not practical or even possible for most workers. But Dr. Hutchinson insists that you should take a 15-minute break every 3 hours.

Some eye-care experts recommend that as soon as you feel your eyes beginning to tire or burn, you should stop for a moment, focus your sights on something, *anything*, off in the distance—the tree outside the window, the wall on the other side of the office, anything that is beyond what you've been staring at. You've been exercising your eye muscles doing all that close-up work. Staring off into the distance helps them relax—and helps you get back to work without pain or discomfort. (And your boss thought you were goofing off!)

Dr. Glatt suggests this exercise to help "stretch" your eye muscles. Print two or three letters on four index cards. The print should be large enough so that when you put the cards on the wall across the room they are easily readable. The cards should be placed at the 12, 3, 6, and 9 o'clock positions on the wall. Now sit down at your desk and circle your eyes around the clock of cards a few times, then change direction. This should help alleviate some of your eyestrain.

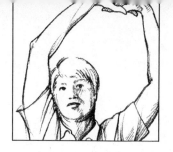

Fatigue

When insomnia looks in the mirror, it sees fatigue, its diametric double that works the day shift. While insomnia schemes to rob you of your rest at night, the menace in the mirror tackles you with tiredness when you should be widest awake.

Paradoxically, exercise not only helps you sleep better at night, it also stimulates and invigorates you, helping to boost your mental and physical performance during the day.

Exercise is "a wonderful antifatigue factor," according to Richard N. Podell, M.D., author of the book *Doctor, Why Am I So Tired?* Except in cases of serious physical illness, "everyone who is tired should consider exercise" as a treatment, he advises.

Why So Weary-Eyed?

The bad news is that almost anything—from stress and illness to vitamin deficiencies, depression, and poor posture—can cause fatigue. The good news is that many of the factors that can drag you down during the day can be reversed with the right kind of activity. Exercise can banish the fatigue-causing effects of stress, poor circulation and blood oxygenation, bad posture and breathing habits, and just plain being out of shape.

Framers of the Constitutional

Regardless of your level of fitness and no matter how frequently you work out, exercise frees body and mind from fatigue's tiresome touch almost within the blink of an eye. Something as simple as a vigorous 10-minute walk jump-starts the body's battery for at least an hour and can reduce tension, says Robert E. Thayer, Ph.D., author of *Biopsychology of Mood and Arousal* and professor of psychology at California State University, Long Beach. Exercise seems to instill a "subtle shift in mood, particularly feelings of optimism and the way people look at their problems," he says. A quick, brisk walk buoys the burdens people bear, turning pessimistic premonitions inside out and relieving the fatigue-causing aspects of stress.

A walk to shake off fatigue, whether it strikes at home or at the office, is "convenient, easy, usable," Dr. Thayer says. When you head out the door, your speed should be rapid, your posture comfortable but erect. Your arms should swing freely and easily at your sides. If leaving home or office is inconvenient or impossible, pace the place you're in. "You might walk around the halls or up and down some stairs," he recommends.

Dr. Podell also tells people to shake off fatigue by walking, but he prescribes a higher dose. Even 100 yards will help at first, he says, but you should slowly increase the distance you walk, building up to ¼ mile, then 1 mile and longer. The eventual goal, he says, should be 3 miles a day, although the exact regimen should be determined through consultation with a doctor. (See "Walking" on page 458.)

Regular exercise also ups your fitness level in general, an improvement that can help fight fatigue in yet another way. Obesity and poor cardiovascular conditioning can make everyday tasks extremely tiring. "Some people are chronically fatigued because they're so poorly fit that their daily activities fatigue them," says Steve Farrell, associate director of continuing education at the Institute for Aerobics Research in Dallas. Someone with a low fitness level may be taxed simply by walking through a parking lot with an armload of groceries.

"People with extremely low cardiovascular fitness levels may, in fact, be fatigued simply due to that," Farrell says. If they improve their fitness level, they'll function better without feeling so drained of energy, he says.

Regular, more intense exercise training generates a sustained, overall "alive" feeling, Dr. Thayer says. He warns, though, that there is an exertion level beyond which an exercise session transforms from a stimulant of energy to an ally of fatigue. This level differs from person to person and is often difficult to pinpoint. But it usually afflicts heavy exercisers—those whose goals go beyond general fitness.

Another Fine Breath

If walking is too pedestrian, more cultured tastes may prefer some nonfat yoga, either plain—a few simple stretches—or flavored with an infinite variety of postures. People who practice the ancient art of deep breathing and muscle control maintain that it can pump you up even if you're flat tired. It sends oxygen to the brain, says Barbara Musser, yoga instructor with the Preventive Medicine Research Institute in Sausalito, California. "Any yoga pose can be used to either relax or energize, depending on how you do it," she says. Postures performed slowly to relax can be done just a little more quickly to invigorate body and brain.

"The beauty of yoga is that anyone can do it, no matter how flexible or inflexible they are," Musser says. "Over time, flexibility and range of motion will increase." (See "Yoga" on page 480.)

Neck and shoulder rolls are particularly helpful in relieving the fatigue-causing tension that builds up over the course of the day. Shrug your shoulders up as close to your ears as possible. Roll them forward, then back. Then drop your shoulders and tilt your head to the side, straining *slightly* to try to touch your ear to your shoulder. Slowly drop your head down until your chin almost touches your chest, then gently roll your head up to the other side. Don't roll your head backward, Musser advises, because that places undue strain on the neck vertebrae. "You don't need any more pressure back there," she says. "You get all the tension-releasing benefits just going to the front."

Both for relaxing and for regenerating your energy supply, Musser says, the most important consideration probably is breathing. When you're tense, tired, or upset, respiration becomes shallow and short, depriving the brain of oxygen. Yoga advocates a rhythmic three-part deep-breathing practice called "deerga swasam." To perform it, exhale while contracting your abdominal muscles. Then inhale, expanding first the abdomen and then the lower lungs and upper chest. The preliminary abdominal tightening, she says, allows the diaphragm to drop down a little more than usual and the lungs to fill more completely with air. To finish, exhale slowly, first contracting your chest, then your abdomen. Inhale and exhale through your nose.

The Posture Factor

Yoga postures aside, the way you hold yourself when you sit and stand can have a big impact on how alert you feel. You are, of course, no slouch, but if your posture is, it could put both a figurative and literal slump in your day. The stoop-shouldered stand to lose a lot. "Certain types of posture restrict the lungs and oxygenation of blood," says Pueblo, Colorado, chiropractor David Walther, D.C. And less oxygen equals less energy.

Muscles under constant tension to prop up poor posture "give a tired feeling all over," Dr. Walther says. People whose work requires outstretched arms—seamstresses, for example, or car mechanics, or anyone who spends a lot of time typing at a desk—are especially susceptible to the kind of posture problems that feed fatigue. (See "Posture Training" on page 387.)

Tight chest muscles and weak neck, abdominal, and buttock muscles also inhibit breathing by taking the starch out of your stance. Exercises that strengthen

the muscles that work to hold you up can help banish tiredness in the long run.

To strengthen the trapezius muscles (which run from the neck, over the shoulders, and into the middle of the back), lie facedown and extend your arms out to the sides with your palms up, Dr. Walther says. Raise your arms up as high as they'll go and feel the tightening of the muscles in your upper and middle back. Repeat 8 to 12 times. Once the movement becomes too easy, you may want to increase the challenge by holding light weights in your hands.

Doing shoulder shrugs while holding dumbbells or other weights in your hands also will strengthen the trapezius muscles. To concentrate the effect on the proper muscles, hold the weights slightly out to the sides of your body and, with arms straight, raise your shoulders with just a touch of a backward lift, feeling the muscles at the base of your neck tighten.

Bolstering Your Back

Another collection of exercises to improve posture and facilitate breathing was devised originally to relieve back problems and correct a forward curvature of the spine. These exercises strengthen the muscles of the abdomen and buttocks and promote better posture.

First, lie on your back with your hands at your sides and your knees slightly bent. Flatten the curve in your lower back by pressing it against the floor and hold for a count of six. Repeat that pelvic tilt until you feel the exertion in your abdominal and buttock muscles. The exercise also can be done while standing against a wall.

Don't do these exercises if you experience any pain in your back.

For the second movement in the progression, remain on your back and bend your knees, keeping your feet on the floor. Then raise your knees as close to your chest as possible, hold for a count of six, return your feet to the floor, and repeat. In a variation that will work the lower abdominal muscles, raise your knees while at the same time trying to lift your buttocks from the floor and executing the pelvic tilt.

The next exercise directly strengthens the abdomen. With your knees bent while lying on your back, fold your arms across your chest and raise your head and shoulders off the floor. Keep your lower back flat on the floor as in the pelvic tilt. Repeat until you feel the exertion in your abdominal muscles. In a variation of this exercise that works the oblique muscles along the sides of your lower torso, raise your head and shoulders toward one knee, then toward the other.

To do another series of exercises that will strengthen the sides of your lower torso, lie on your back with your knees bent, your feet flat on the floor, and your arms at your sides. Rock both knees easily from side to side. Then intertwine your fingers behind your head and try to bring together your left elbow and right knee, then your right elbow and left knee. Repeat several times.

Next, extend your arms out to the sides and straighten your legs. Lift your right leg up over the left and attempt to touch your left arm. Keep your shoulders on the floor but permit your pelvis to twist easily. Repeat on the other side.

Two final exercises concentrate on buttressing the buttock muscles. Lie face-down, with a pillow under your stomach for comfort if necessary. Lift one leg as high as possible and hold for a few seconds. Repeat with the other leg. Work both legs in these exercise sets until you feel slight discomfort in the muscles of your buttocks and lower back. Next, put your hands behind your back and raise your head and shoulders off the floor. Hold the position, then repeat.

If you suspect that poor posture may be robbing you of energy, experiment with these exercises on your own. But also consult with a doctor or a physical therapist, just to ensure that you are performing the movements properly, and particularly if backaches have been a problem. If any of these exercises seem painful, avoid them until you've talked to a physician.

Brighten Up before Breakfast

For many people, waking up is hard to do. You yawn, you grunt, you rub the sleep from your eyes. And you stretch—haphazardly. You do whatever feels right, whatever twists and turns you into consciousness. Here's a series of gentle stretches that will ease you a bit more thoroughly into the waking world and won't leave you mourning for more sleep all day. All of them can be done flat on your back in bed before you arise.

This morning stretch will help align your spine for proper posture. Bend your knees, raise your arms back over your head, and inhale. To exhale, pull in your lower abdominal muscles while gently pressing your spine against the bed. At the same time stretch your arms and reach hard for the head of the bed. Relax, then repeat four times.

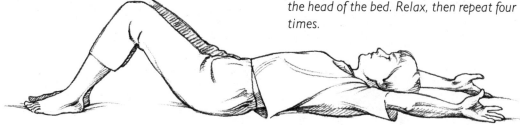

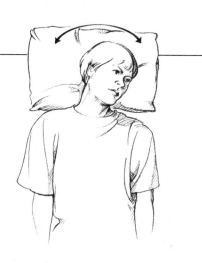

To limber up your neck, rest your head on the bed without a pillow, or with a very thin pillow, and roll your head gently from side to side 5 to 15 times. Keep your neck muscles relaxed and take deep, regular breaths in time with the head movement.

Brighten Up before Breakfast—Continued

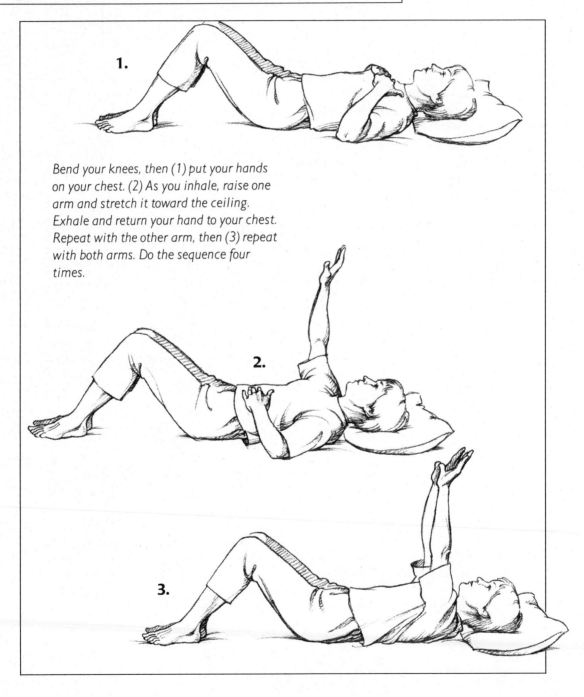

Bend your knees, then (1) put your hands on your chest. (2) As you inhale, raise one arm and stretch it toward the ceiling. Exhale and return your hand to your chest. Repeat with the other arm, then (3) repeat with both arms. Do the sequence four times.

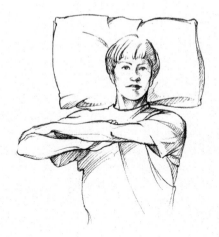

Now, grasp each arm just above the elbow with the opposite hand. Hold your arms above your chest. Without moving the rest of your upper body, roll at your shoulders and try to touch your right elbow to the right side of the bed. Repeat to the other side. Do this exercise 10 times at first, then gradually work up to 30 repetitions.

Place your hands together in the traditional praying position, then gently press the palms together. Relax. Repeat five times.

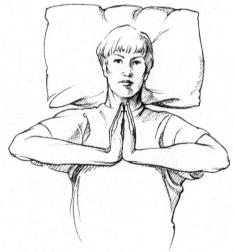

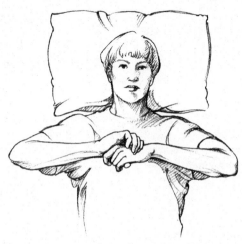

Imagine that you've been working in the garden and your hands are very dirty. "Wash" them by rubbing your hands and wrists vigorously for a minute or so. Then limber up your feet by pulling one knee at a time up to your chest and circling your foot.

Overcome Those Office Blahs

The computer screen is a blur of words as the keyboard crackles under your cramped fingers. You listlessly lumber through reams of reports and piles of papers. The neck is a knot of untangled tension. The eyelids lazily lower down to your cheeks. Whether it's 10:30 in the morning or 3:00 in the afternoon, the rest of the day hangs heavily from your shoulders.

If you can't go out for a 10-minute walk, you still can lose that load and refresh body and brain with several invigorating flexes and stretches that can be done anywhere—sitting at your desk or standing by the water cooler. These fatigue fighters stretch the muscles most likely to become strained and tense while on the job—the neck, shoulders, back, and hands.

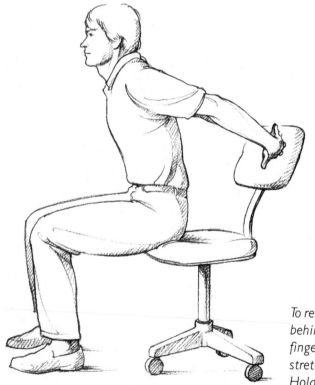

To relieve stiff shoulders, put your arms behind your back and intertwine your fingers. Raise your arms until you feel the stretch in your chest, shoulders, and arms. Hold for 30 seconds.

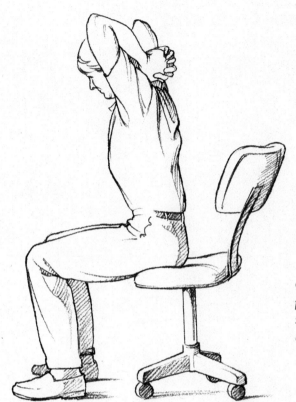

Clasp your hands behind your head and push the palms of your hands together. You should feel the effect in your chest and upper back muscles. Hold for 30 seconds.

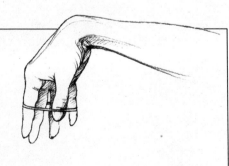

If you suffer from writer's cramp, here's an easy way to relieve it. Put a thick rubber band around the first joint of the fingers on the cramped hand. Then open and close your fingers, stretching the band as far as possible. Continue the movement for 10 seconds.

Overcome Those Office Blahs—Continued

This stretch relaxes the muscles of the lower back. (1) Spread your feet on either side of your chair, then lean over and grasp your ankles, letting your upper body sink between your knees. (2) Slowly bend to one side, attempting to touch your ear to your knee. (3) Then raise your arm sideways over your head and hold for 10 seconds. Repeat on the other side.

1.

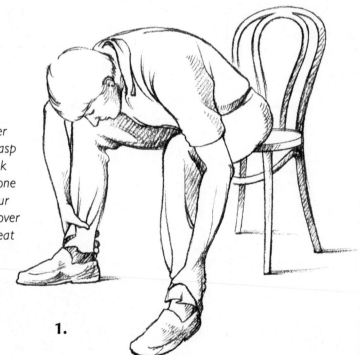

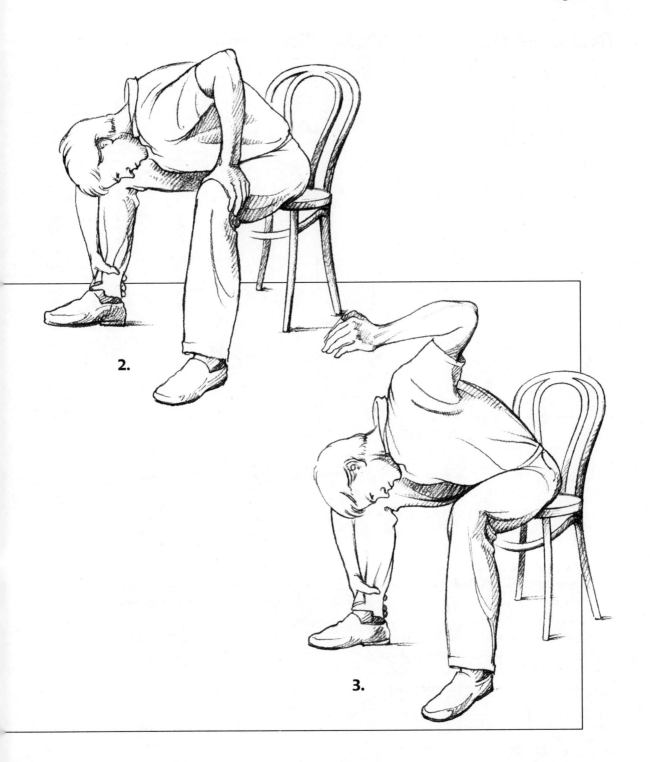

2.

3.

Overcome Those Office Blahs—Continued

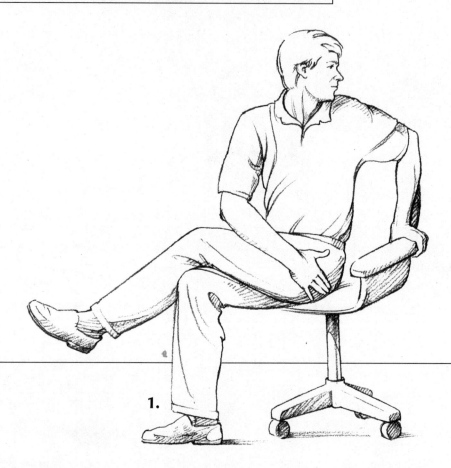

1.

Here are two simple versions of a yoga posture called the twist that will help stretch and relax the buttock muscles, which help to support the back. To do the twist while seated, (1) sit facing forward and cross your left leg over your right, then hook your right arm over your left knee. Hold on to the arm of the chair with your left hand. Exhale as you slowly turn your upper body to the left. Repeat on the other side. The other variation is done while standing. (2) Place your right foot on a sturdy stool or chair. Keeping the left leg straight, exhale and slowly rotate your upper body so that your left shoulder moves toward your bent knee. Repeat on the other side.

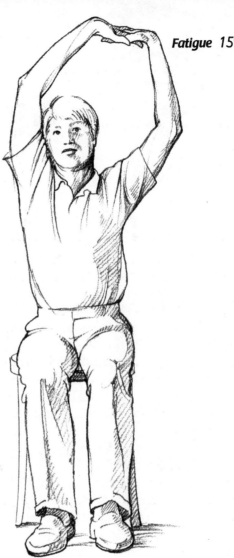

To help renew energy and get your circulation going, try this stretch. Sit straight, intertwine your fingers, and raise your arms overhead, palms up. Press your hands upward. Lean first to one side and then the other while continuing to stretch.

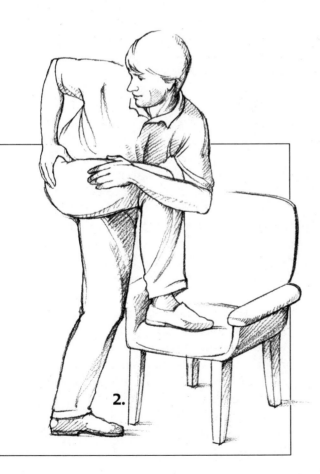

2.

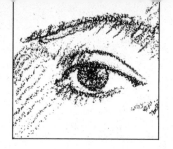

Glaucoma

New and startling research shows that exercise may be as powerful as a drug in preventing eye damage due to glaucoma, a serious eye disease that can impair vision and lead to blindness.

Normally the fluid in the eyeball drains out through small channels. In uncontrolled glaucoma, the fluid stays in the eye, causing high levels of pressure that damage or destroy the optic nerve, the part of the eye that transmits visual images to the brain.

While no exercise can reverse eye damage due to glaucoma, there's new hope for some people who are experiencing "intraocular hypertension"—the pressure buildup that heralds the onset of the disease.

Researchers at Oregon Health Sciences University studied a group of people with intraocular hypertension. The people rigorously pedaled stationary bikes for 30 minutes three times a week for ten weeks.

"The results were dramatic," says Linn Goldberg, M.D., associate professor of medicine and director of the university's Human Performance Laboratory. "Their intraocular pressure significantly decreased into the normal range." And that big drop in pressure was similar to reductions caused by a medication that is commonly used for that purpose, says Dr. Goldberg.

Once the group stopped riding the stationary bikes, however, in as little as two weeks their eye pressure rose to the same level it was before the training began.

Once proven, this research could add a powerful new weapon to medical science's antiglaucoma arsenal, according to Dr. Goldberg. Normally, when an ophthalmologist detects a buildup of pressure inside the eye, he or she is likely to prescribe eyedrops that contain a beta-blocking agent. While this medication causes an immediate drop in pressure, it may also produce unpleasant side effects, including weakness, confusion, memory loss, and depression.

A regular program of vigorous exercise now can be considered a natural alternative to drugs, says Dr. Goldberg. Vigorous exercise "looks wonderful in terms of preventive therapy," Dr. Goldberg explains. "What it says is that regular exercise can effectively reduce eye pressure—and, of course, that you must *continue* to exercise."

A word of warning is in order here. You absolutely cannot write your own exercise prescription. Glaucoma is the nation's leading cause of blindness in adults. Once a doctor determines that you have a pressure buildup inside your eyeballs, you *must* have the condition monitored for the rest of your life.

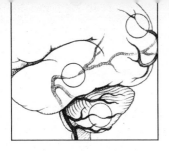

Headaches

Sometimes the pain slithers up the back of your head and slowly coils itself around the top of your skull like a python strangling its prey. Sometimes a pointy pain hammers rhythmically on your temple. And sometimes the pain surges through your head like an endless locomotive with an eye socket for a tunnel.

Whether a dull discomfort, a sharp slice, or a debilitating, pulsating pressure that lingers for days, headaches hit hard. But no matter what type of headache you have, the right kind of exercise often can play a role in preventing or eliminating the pain. That is, if exercise didn't cause your headache in the first place.

Exercise is "a two-edged sword in headache treatment," according to Seymour Diamond, M.D., director of both the Diamond Headache Clinic and the Inpatient Headache Unit at Louis A. Weiss Memorial Hospital in Chicago.

Depending on the type of headache, exercise can either bring on pain or relieve it. So part of the key to using exercise as a treatment, Dr. Diamond notes, is knowing what kind of headache you're dealing with.

That means that if you're plagued by recurring headaches, they should be diagnosed by a physician, preferably a headache specialist, who will consider factors such as when the headaches occur, how long they last, other physical symptoms, cyclical patterns, emotional state, and hormonal balance.

Improved Fitness Provides a Buffer for Pain

As a preventive program, exercise can have immediate and long-term effects on headache frequency and intensity. Headache sufferers who improve their physical fitness and muscle tone generally have fewer sieges, Dr. Diamond says.

People plagued by the various types of cranial crunch—tension, migraine, cluster, and exertion headaches—*all* can find some relief through improved fitness, headache specialists say.

Regular activity forces the brain to secrete more endorphins and enkephalins, the body's own opiate-like pain-dampening chemicals.

As the intensity and duration of the activity increase, so do the number of headache-slaying chemicals and the body's threshold for pain.

Regular exercise *between* headaches may prove helpful, experts agree. But for certain types of headaches, the right moves at the first sign of symptoms can nip the pain in the bud.

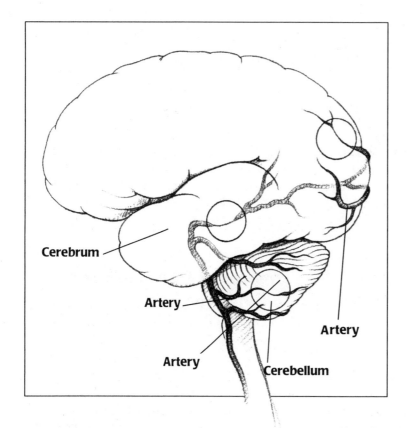

Cerebrum

Artery

Artery

Artery

Cerebellum

Vascular headaches can come in many forms—from a migraine to a cluster headache to an exertional headache. These headaches occur when the arteries supplying the brain go into spasm. Note how the blood vessels narrow in an individual who is suffering from a vascular headache.

Staving Off a Tension Headache

Tension- and stress-induced head pain is the most common type of headache, striking people who spend long hours hunched over their work or those who are bothered by anxiety and stress. The pain crawls up the back of the neck and envelops the entire top of the head, sometimes creeping back down into the neck, shoulders, and jaws. In fact, problems with the jaw, called temporomandibular disorder (TMD), often can cause tension headaches. (See "TMD and Bruxism" on page 311.)

Tension headaches can last as little as a few minutes or as long as a few weeks.

Some sufferers are beset six to eight times a month—at the least.

Exercising during a tension headache is very likely to offer some relief, says Robert S. Kunkel, M.D., who heads the headache center in the Department of Internal Medicine at the Cleveland Clinic. "General exercise—even if it's just walking—can help improve circulation, loosen up muscles, and give an overall better feeling," he says.

Jogging and pedaling a stationary bicycle can also bring relief, says Dr. Diamond.

In addition, there are a number of specific neck and shoulder exercises that can help ease the strain, Dr. Kunkel says. Moist heat or a cool compress should be applied to the neck and shoulders 15 to 20 minutes before the exercises, he advises, adding that an individual should experiment with the two temperatures to determine which is more soothing. For the duration of the headache, the exercises should be done in sets of five or six, twice a day, he suggests. Once the headache lets up, the exercises can be performed just once a day or every other day to help prevent recurrence.

Drop your head slowly forward so your chin touches your chest, keeping your mouth closed. Lift your head and repeat five or six times. Next, bend your head to the left, easing your left ear toward your left shoulder, then bend your head to the other side. Again, repeat five or six times. Afterward, slowly turn your head first to the right and then to the left so that your chin is positioned over your shoulder. Repeat the movement five or six times.

Now stand with your back against a wall and tilt your pelvis up so the arch in your lower back disappears and your body is pressed tightly against the wall. Place your hands behind your head and bring your elbows together in front of your face, then bring them back to touch the wall. Repeat five or six times. Next, lie on the floor on your stomach and raise your head and shoulders five or six times.

Stand straight and grab two books of equal size or some other light weights. Allow your hands to just hang at your sides. Now shrug, first with your shoulders pressed forward, then with your shoulders pushed to the back, then in a neutral position. Repeat each exercise five or six times.

Along with these exercises, Dr. Kunkel says, people should practice some form of relaxation training, such as deep breathing.

Just sit or lie down, close your eyes, and inhale deeply to a count of ten. Hold the breath for a slow count of five, then exhale just as slowly.

Against the Migraine

Migraines, one of the more painful kinds of headache, are less likely to be eased by an exercise regimen. In migraines, blood vessels in the head dilate, and the pain throbs with a nauseous disco stomp in sync with the heartbeat, usually on only one side of the head and almost always in the temple. Sufferers often see flashes of light before their eyes; they may vomit, tremble, sweat, and lose both balance and concentration. Almost invariably, someone mired in a migraine needs to lie down in a darkened room for the duration of the attack, which can last from a few hours to a few days.

Many factors can contribute to migraines, Dr. Kunkel says. Stress, disruptions in daily routines, and skipping meals can prompt an attack, as can certain foods, especially aged cheeses, red wine, and chocolate. Although men can get this type of headache, menstruating women are three times as likely to be sufferers.

Migraines are "by definition aggravated by physical activity," Dr. Kunkel says. Forcing exercise such as an aerobics class or jogging, in the midst of a migraine, only increases blood pressure and blood flow to the brain, intensifying the pain. Some people, however, have found that a gentle walk at the first sign of a migraine seems to lessen symptoms.

Exercising between bouts may ward off future attacks. Try a circuit weight-training program for improved muscle tone and better cardiovascular fitness, advises Dr. Kunkel. "Most of us feel exercise lessens attacks in people who are in fairly decent condition," he says.

Cluster Bluster

Cluster headaches are sort of like migraines for men, because they are ten times as likely to affect males as females. The pain, a steady surge that seems as if a concrete-crunching jackhammer is mercilessly burrowing its way out of the head through an eye socket, strikes one to three times a day for a couple of hours over the course of a couple of weeks or months. Then it disappears, only to return with renewed vengeance in six months or a year.

In contrast to migraines, clusters compel people to move. "The pain is so severe they can't sit still," Dr. Kunkel says. "They become very physically active," performing impromptu aerobic routines or running around the block a couple of times in the middle of the night. At the very least, they sit in a chair, uncontrollably rocking to and fro.

Clusters pounce at any time, although a significant number occur during the night. Most hit at the same time with an odd quartz-clock precision. The pain is maddening. "We've all had patients who have committed suicide because of the pain," Dr. Kunkel laments, noting that the malady has been dubbed the "suicide headache."

"Sometimes they just lose control," he says. "Sometimes they bang their head and hands against the wall. I've had two patients who broke their hands hitting the wall during an attack. There was one guy who tore his bathroom door off its hinges—twice."

There is no explanation for the inexorable need to move about or for the uncontrollable violence during a cluster headache, says Dr. Kunkel, but apparently people think it helps ease the pain.

Rather than banging their head and hands against the wall, Dr. Kunkel advises, cluster headache sufferers should engage in strenuous exercise to satisfy the need for an active diversion, concurrently strengthening the body to cope better with future attacks. If you feel compelled to run around the block, do it. Hop on the stationary bicycle, if you have one, or do some jumping jacks in the middle of the room.

Beyond Exercise

The effectiveness of exercise in soothing all kinds of headache pain may be enhanced if used in conjunction with biofeedback and relaxation training, says Dr. Diamond. In biofeedback, people are wired to machines that let them see a moving needle or a dial or hear variations in sound pitch that indicate how tense or sore their muscles are and how they actually can influence their headaches, willing them away through conscious relaxation. Dr. Diamond has employed the exercise/biofeedback combination for some 19 years to banish headaches from thousands of people who, often after years of agony, finally can become their own dragonslayers against pain. Ask your physician about where to go for biofeedback training.

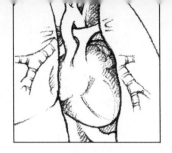

Heart Disease

Wouldn't it be nice if only love could break your heart? Unfortunately, nature isn't that kind. While you may be emotionally shattered by a wilted romance, it is more likely your heart will be devastated by cholesterol, high blood pressure, stress, smoking, poor diet, and a sedentary lifestyle.

Fortunately, you have a secret weapon on your side: exercise.

"Studies show that people who exercise live an average of 2 to 2½ years longer than people who don't. If you exercise on a regular basis, you're at least 20 percent less likely to suffer a fatal heart attack," says Renae Guiterrez, Ph.D., a fitness expert and patient education specialist at the Mayo Clinic Scottsdale in Arizona.

The positive effects that exercise has on the heart are widely recognized. Studies consistently show that exercise is the cornerstone for reducing the impact of major heart disease risk factors and that it can help prevent heart attacks.

"Exercise promotes many changes that are beneficial to us," says Linn Goldberg, M.D., director of the Human Performance Laboratory at the Oregon Health Sciences University in Portland.

Exercise decreases body fat, and by doing that you lower your cholesterol, especially LDL, the so-called bad cholesterol, he says. The greater your percentage of body fat, the more likely you are to have high cholesterol levels.

"Exercise also helps lower blood pressure and tends to make the body more sensitive to insulin so the body doesn't have to produce as much of it," Dr. Goldberg says. "We now know that increased insulin levels are a risk factor for high blood pressure and heart disease.

"Just by doing those simple things, exercise may lead to reductions in coronary and cardiovascular disease," he says.

Making a Better Pump

Regular exercise does two important things that affect the heart, says Gregory Kay, M.D., a cardiothoracic and vascular surgeon at the Hospital of the Good Samaritan in Los Angeles.

First, exercise makes muscle more efficient at extracting oxygen and nutrients from your blood. As you get your muscles conditioned, there is a lower demand on the heart to pump the blood through your body.

At the same time, exercise increases your heart's pumping capacity, Dr. Kay says.

"There is actually an increase in the heart size so that the heart is ejecting more blood with each squeeze. Because it's

RECOVERING THAT GOOD BEAT

If you do suffer a heart attack or have coronary bypass surgery, exercise can play a vital role in your recovery.

"Cardiac rehabilitation is still based on exercise. It's still the cornerstone that we use to modify all the other risk factors," says C. Noel Bairey, M.D., medical director of the Preventive and Cardiac Rehabilitation Center at Cedars-Sinai Medical Center in Los Angeles.

"If you exercise, you're likely to quit smoking," Dr. Bairey says. "If you exercise, your cholesterol is easier to manage. If you exercise, your diabetes and high blood pressure are easier to control."

There is a 20 to 25 percent reduction in death rates among people who participate in cardiac rehabilitation programs after suffering a heart attack, says Martin Juneau, M.D., medical director of cardiac rehabilitation at the Montreal Heart Institute.

The first few days after a heart attack you probably will be allowed to walk around the floor at the hospital. Then you'll gradually increase your activities, says Dr. Juneau. As soon as you leave the hospital, usually on the seventh or eighth day, you can start on a walking program. Then three or four weeks later, you can start on a more intensive rehabilitation program.

The timing of exercise after bypass surgery is just slightly different because doctors have to make sure the chest wound has healed, Dr. Juneau says.

In fact, if you do have heart surgery, it may be 8 to 12 weeks before you can begin your rehabilitation program in earnest, notes Gregory Kay, M.D., a cardiothoracic and vascular surgeon at the Hospital of the Good Samaritan in Los Angeles. (You'll be urged to start walking right away, though.)

---

ejecting more blood, it doesn't have to squeeze as often," he says.

The net result is a lowered heart rate and, in turn, less wear on your cardiovascular system. The average heart, for example, beats 70 to 75 times a minute. A heart conditioned through exercise can beat 45 to 50 times a minute but pump the same amount of blood as the average person's heart. That means a well-conditioned heart can beat 36,000 fewer times a day and 13.1 million fewer times a year than the average person's heart.

In fact, when it comes to preventing heart disease, the positive effects of exercise are so tremendous that being seden-tary is equal to smoking a pack a day or having a cholesterol level in the dangerous 300-plus range, Dr. Guiterrez says. Yet it's estimated that fewer than one-third of Americans exercise regularly enough to keep their heart healthy.

Time to Make a Change

"In the twentieth century, we've gone from being a very vigorous society to a very sedentary one. With that change has come an increase in cardiovascular diseases," Dr. Goldberg says. "We all know that our dogs need exercise, but many people won't do exercise for themselves."

Your exercise prescription will depend on a number of factors, including your age, the type of medications you're taking, and your sports interests.

But the most important aspect determining your prescription will be an exercise tolerance test. Your doctor will ask you to walk on a treadmill or ride a stationary bicycle while monitors attached to your body record your blood pressure and your heart's response to exercise. During the test, your doctor will be looking for any heart abnormalities.

The test also will give your doctor and therapist an idea of your physical capabilities and what type of workout program would be right for you.

"In our rehabilitation program, patients walk, run, bicycle, swim, and play volleyball and badminton," Dr. Juneau says.

"There are really very few limitations on the type of activities they can do if their treadmill test is good."

However, some activities are off-limits.

"There are a few sports that I don't recommend, particularly in the first few months," Dr. Juneau says. "I don't suggest that they do very intense, competitive exercise such as soccer, hockey, or squash because coronary patients tend to be very aggressive when they play competitively. When they do that, they go beyond the target heart rate set for them."

The majority of patients who've had a heart attack recover very, very well. These patients can recover a normal functional capacity after a few months of cardiac rehabilitation. Very often, they get in better shape than they were before because many patients who have their first heart attack haven't done strenuous exercise for many years.

Many of the 1.5 million heart attacks that occur in the United States each year could be prevented if people became more physically active, he says.

Even if you've been sedentary since you were a child, the good news is that it's never too late to start an exercise program that will improve cardiovascular fitness, Dr. Guiterrez says.

"If you're a fit 70-year-old, good for you. If you're an unfit 30-year-old, you still have a lot of time to change your lifestyle," she says.

A number of studies bear that out. Consider the reduction in cardiovascular risk factors in 39 sedentary Swiss men aged 30 to 50, who began jogging 2 hours a week. After four months, researchers found that the exercise had helped reduce the men's cardiac risk significantly by lowering their blood pressures, slashing their cholesterol and triglyceride levels, and trimming body fat.

Even less-intense exercise might help an unfit person fight heart disease, says Jean-Pierre Despres, Ph.D., a professor of exercise physiology at Laval University in Ste. Foy, Quebec.

Dr. Despres studied a group of sedentary, moderately obese Canadian men in their twenties and thirties who began exercising. The men, who had been inactive for most of their lives, did prolonged, low-intensity exercise such as walking 2 hours a day. At the end of 100 days, the men showed substantial weight loss, significantly lower total cholesterol levels, and increases in their levels of HDL cholesterol (the good kind).

"Absolutely, you can combat heart disease even if you've been inactive for many years," Dr. Despres says. "Heart disease takes a long time to develop. If you've been sedentary for many, many years, obviously you're at greater risk. But there is still time for you to reduce your risk by being more active on a daily basis."

More Good News

Over the years, researchers have gathered other impressive evidence that physical activity is a vital weapon in combating heart disease.

In a classic study of 16,936 Harvard alumni, for example, researchers concluded that middle-aged men who regularly exercised slashed their heart disease risk dramatically and possibly added up to two years to their life expectancy.

The men who expended at least 2,000 calories a week exercising had 39 percent less risk of developing coronary heart disease than their less active classmates. If every man in the study had exercised regularly, the researchers estimate that there would have been 16 percent fewer deaths from cardiovascular disease.

That research is backed up by a similar study, done at the University of Pittsburgh, of 541 women who had not yet gone through menopause. One group of women, who burned at least 1,000 calories a week

doing physical activities, had higher "good" cholesterol levels and lower blood pressure readings than sedentary women. In addition, a group of women who burned 2,000 calories a week had even lower levels of total cholesterol and triglycerides. The results suggest that physical activity significantly reduces the risk of heart disease among middle-aged women.

Researchers also have studied the deaths of 62,000 Iowa men aged 20 to 64 and concluded that physically active farmers had approximately 10 percent fewer fatal heart attacks than relatively sedentary nonfarmers.

In Puerto Rico, researchers followed a group of 8,793 men for a period of 8½ years. They found that the men who had vigorous exercise habits were half as likely to develop heart disease as the sedentary men.

The Clot-Dissolving Factor

Meanwhile, part of the mystery about *how* exercise protects the heart may be unraveling, according to researchers at the University of Washington School of Medicine in Seattle. They believe that regular workouts may prevent blood clots that can cause heart attacks and strokes.

They conducted a preliminary study of 10 young men, aged 24 to 30, and 13 physically fit older men, aged 60 to 82, all of whom participated in six months of intensive walking, jogging, and bicycling at 80 to 85 percent of their maximum heart rate. The researchers found that the older men significantly increased blood levels of a clot-dissolving substance called tissue plasminogen activator (TPA) in their blood.

RUN FOR YOUR LIFE

The first time it made big news was 2,500 years ago, when a runner raced 25 miles from the plains of Marathon to Athens to announce the defeat of the invading Persian army. Then he collapsed and died.

Over the last several years, you've occasionally read similar stories about famous and not-so-famous people who collapsed and died while running. And you wonder if it could happen to you. The answer? Probably not.

"In general, your risk of having a fatal heart attack is greater if *don't* exercise regularly than if you do," says C. Noel Bairey, M.D., medical director of the Preventive and Cardiac Rehabilitation Center at Cedars-Sinai Medical Center in Los Angeles.

"The benefits of exercising vastly outweigh the risk of dying while exercising," she says.

Doctors stress that the overwhelming majority of people who have died of heart attacks while exercising had undetected coronary disease. That includes Jim Fixx, the author of *The Complete Book of Running,* who suffered a massive heart attack and dropped dead at the age of 52 during an afternoon jog along the shoulder of a Vermont highway in 1984.

"Jim Fixx had garden-variety coronary artery disease, and a bypass operation almost certainly would have saved him," says Gregory Kay, M.D., a cardiothoracic and vascular surgeon at the Hospital of the Good Samaritan in Los Angeles.

A treadmill test is one important tool that doctors use to detect heart abnormalities. But Fixx avoided doing that.

"We offered to do an exercise test on Jim Fixx a couple of months before he died, and he refused. If we had done that, we could have learned about his heart disease and possibly could have done something about it," says Linn Goldberg, M.D., a heart researcher and director of the Human Performance Laboratory at the Oregon Health Sciences University in Portland.

Dr. Goldberg recommends that anyone over the age of 40 who hasn't exercised for several years—or any person who knows he or she has a coronary risk factor such as high blood pressure, elevated cholesterol levels, smoking, or a family history of heart disease—have a treadmill test before starting any exercise program.

When you do exercise, make sure that you warm up and cool down properly.

"More than 70 percent of cardiac complications occur during warm-up or cooldown," Dr. Kay says. To avoid complications "you have to *slowly* warm up and *slowly* cool down. You just can't abruptly start or stop."

You also should monitor your body very carefully when exercising, Dr. Goldberg says.

Chest pain, undue fatigue, indigestion, breathlessness, or dizziness are all signs that you should see a physician.

But even if your doctor does find evidence of heart disease, that doesn't mean your days of running, walking, or jumping are over. It does mean, however, that your physician must help you put together your exercise program.

Fred Pattle, for example, a 70-year-old former television weatherman, used to run 5 miles a day. In 1978 he started feeling chest pains during his runs.

But unlike Jim Fixx, Fred consulted a cardiologist and underwent heart bypass surgery. Today, 13 years later, he walks 3 miles twice a day near his home in Newport, Oregon.

"We're really excited about this study. It certainly indicates that exercise is a positive thing," says Wayne Chandler, M.D., a coauthor of the study and an assistant professor of laboratory medicine at the university. "This may be the first evidence that if you exercise, you can alter proteins in your blood that affect your heart attack risk."

The young people in the study didn't show the same dramatic increase in TPA, but they had been in better physical shape than the older people when they started. For that reason the training probably had less effect on their blood-clotting systems, Dr. Chandler says.

"I suspect that if we went out and found some 25-year-olds who were real couch potatoes, who did no exercise at all, we would have seen a positive change after training," he says.

Aerobic exercise also yielded dramatic effects in 101 previously sedentary people at Duke University Medical Center in Durham, North Carolina. Researchers there found that the men and women, aged 60 to 83, who completed the program increased their levels of good cholesterol significantly and increased their aerobic performance by at least 10 percent after 14 months of cycling, walking, and jogging.

In another Duke University study, 36 men, aged 31 to 59, who displayed aggressive (Type A) behavior such as impatience and hostility, which is associated with an increased risk of heart disease, did 12 weeks of walking and jogging. They not only increased their aerobic capacity by 15 percent, they also lowered their heart rate and blood pressure and reduced obvious signs of Type A behavior.

Hearts Need More Than Love

While exercise may be one of the best things for your heart, doctors stress that it's not the only thing.

"If you try to exclusively exercise, and you don't modify your diet, don't lose weight, don't quit smoking, and don't manage your high blood pressure, then exercise isn't going to save your life. But exercise done in conjunction with changes in those other risk factors can have a significant impact," says C. Noel Bairey, M.D., medical director of the Preventive and Cardiac Rehabilitation Center at Cedars-Sinai Medical Center in Los Angeles.

"There has to be a balance. It's very seldom that one factor will cause or prevent heart disease," agrees Peter Wood, Ph.D., associate director of the Stanford University Center for Research in Disease Prevention in Palo Alto, California.

Healthy Hearts Need Aerobics

Most experts agree that to strengthen your heart and improve your overall fitness level, you need to do aerobic exercise at least three times (but preferably five times) a week for at least 20 minutes a session.

But before you walk or run to the nearest gym, you may want to check with your physician, particularly if you are 40 or older, overweight, smoke, or have a family history of heart disease. You should see a doctor immediately no matter what your age if you have chest pains or prolonged shortness of breath—these may be symptoms of heart disease. (For more information, see "Angina" on page 14.)

Aerobic exercises such as running, swimming, bicycling, stair climbing, and cross-country skiing are all good ways to get your cardiovascular system in shape, Dr. Bairey says. But of all the aerobic exercises, walking may be the best one to get into shape with the least amount of trauma to your joints.

Walk Away from Heart Disease

Brisk walking at a pace of 3½ to 4 miles per hour is probably the simplest aerobic workout to do and provides most of the cardiovascular benefits of more strenuous workouts such as jogging or bicycling, Dr. Bairey says.

"Numerous studies have shown that you get 80 percent of the cardiovascular benefits by simply taking a brisk walk three to five times a week," she says. "Just getting people up off the couch and getting them to walk to the store three times a week will provide *tremendous* benefits."

Perhaps the best evidence of the heart-protecting power of exercise like walking comes from a study conducted by Lars G. Ekelund, M.D., Ph.D., an associate professor of medicine at the University of North Carolina at Chapel Hill. Dr. Ekelund and his colleagues put 3,106 healthy men aged 30 to 69 through a treadmill test. Each man was assigned a fitness rating based on his heart rate during exercise and the length of time he was able to stay on the treadmill. The researchers kept tabs on the men for a number of years. Over the next 8½ years, 45 of those men died of cardiovascular disease. Although age, smoking, cholesterol, and blood pressure did contribute to those deaths, the researchers

believe the study confirms that a low level of fitness also is a major independent risk factor for heart attack and stroke. Similar results came from a recent study that concentrated on women, adds Dr. Ekelund.

In effect, *not* exercising ages you and tacks many years of wear onto the heart, according to Dr. Ekelund. But a simple program of aerobic exercise, such as vigorous walking about 30 minutes three times a week, can reclaim those "lost" years.

"I think brisk walking is the best form of exercise for middle-aged and older adults. You probably can get as much benefit from 40 minutes of brisk walking as you can from more strenuous activities such as jogging, with less risk of cardiac or orthopedic problems," says James Barnard, Ph.D., a professor of kinesiology at UCLA and a consultant to the Pritikin Longevity Center in Santa Monica. (See "Walking" on page 458.)

But that doesn't mean you shouldn't be doing more, Dr. Bairey says.

"You are going to get most of the cardiovascular benefits by walking," she says. "But if you want to get more benefits, you need to do a higher level of physical activity. So if a person wants to do something like jogging and they can do it appropriately, they should be encouraged to do it."

Jogging has been among the most popular high-intensity aerobic activities for many years. It increases your heart's pumping ability, involves more muscles, and burns more total calories and more body fat than walking. In fact, jogging at a pace of 5½ miles per hour burns about 740 calories an hour. That's more than you can burn during the same amount of time by walking, swimming, or bicycling. Burning those extra calories while jogging is important because it might stimulate your body to create more HDL cholesterol, a substance that helps lower your heart disease risk, according to researchers at the University of Missouri. (See "Running" on page 421.)

Of course, jogging and running don't appeal to everyone, but there are plenty of alternatives.

Stair-climbing machines, for example, provide many of the aerobic advantages of jogging, but with less strain on your knees and other joints, experts say. A 30-minute workout on a stair-climber three times a week can burn off about 2,000 calories weekly. That's the threshold exercise level that some scientists believe leads to cardiovascular fitness and contributes to longevity. (See "Stair Climbing" on page 429.)

If you want to do something more challenging, you might consider jumping rope, says Kathleen Hargarten, M.D., medical director of AthleticForce at Columbia Hospital's Sports Medicine Center in Milwaukee. A 30-minute jump-rope workout can be the equivalent of running an 8½-minute mile. (See "Jumping" on page 358.)

Swimming is a total-body workout that uses nearly all your major muscle groups. It challenges the heart and lungs to work hard, yet causes fewer injuries than other aerobic exercises.

"Swimming is an enticing workout because you can get some great cardiovascular benefits from it," says Dr. Guiterrez. "It's a non-weight–bearing exercise, so it doesn't put undue stress on the knees, back, or hips." (See "Swimming" on page 449.)

Cycling is another terrific aerobic exercise that gives the heart and circulatory system a dynamite workout. It conditions your legs and, like swimming, can increase aerobic capacity with less stress on the joints. It's also a convenient exercise because you can do it at home on a stationary bicycle. (See "Bicycling" on page 327 and "Stationary Bicycling" on page 434.)

Rowing and cross-country skiing are another pair of excellent workouts that you can do on home exercise equipment, Dr. Kay says. These total-body exercises work out muscles in the arms, legs, back, and abdomen, Dr. Kay says. (See "Rowing" on page 418 and "Cross-Country Skiing" on page 341.)

In addition, both rowing and cross-country skiing give your upper body a better workout than other aerobic exercises such as jogging or stair climbing, Dr. Kay says. He believes that's an advantage that shouldn't be overlooked.

"If you're neglecting your upper body, you're really missing out on something," Dr. Kay says. "If you think about it, most of what we do each day involves only the upper body. So if you don't exercise your arms or upper body, those muscles won't be conditioned, and you'll be increasing the strain on your heart."

Don't Forget the Weights

Weight training is a good way to condition your upper body, strengthen your heart, *and* supplement your aerobic workout, Dr. Bairey says.

"Increasingly, people are turning to strength training," Dr. Bairey says. "It's been demonstrated that heart patients can do low-weight, high-volume repetitions. We're not pumping iron here, but we're finding that this type of weight lifting confers some aerobic conditioning and also improves upper body tone and helps the patient maintain flexibility."

That notion was supported by a preliminary ten-week study done in Canada of 18 men suffering from coronary artery disease. The researchers found that the men who did weight training in combination with aerobic exercise had greater improvement in aerobic performance and strength than those who did aerobics only.

"Not only did their strength go up, but their aerobic performance went up as well, which suggests that weakness of the muscles was limiting their maximum aerobic capacity," says Neil McCartney, Ph.D., author of the study and a professor of physical education and medicine at McMaster University in Hamilton, Ontario.

But strength training isn't just for heart patients, Dr. Kay says. Healthy people can benefit from it, too.

"Strength training is an important part of conditioning for everyone, but you have to do it right," Dr. Kay says. "If you think you're on muscle beach and try to lift 250 pounds the first time you're in the gym, you're going to have difficulties."

Dr. McCartney suggests doing a variety of strength exercises such as arm curls, leg presses, calf extensions, and knee extensions. (See "Resistance Training" on page 404.) If you have heart disease, you should get your doctor's permission before beginning to work out with weights.

How heavy should the weights be? You can safely start with one set of repetitions at about 40 percent of your maximum one-lift load and gradually work up to three sets at 80 percent of your lifting capacity, Dr. McCartney says. In other words, just because you *can* hoist 100 pounds doesn't mean you should. Lighten up. During each set, he says, do about 12 repetitions for arm exercises and 15 repetitions for the legs. He recommends that you rest 2 to 3 minutes between sets.

Keep Moving

But how *much* exercise do you need to do to improve your heart's health? "The short answer is the more, the better," Dr. Wood says. "I think it's only reasonable that the more you put into your exercise program, the more benefits you'll get out of it."

But while a planned exercise program is best, experts agree that doing *some* activity is better than doing nothing.

"It doesn't matter so much what you do but that you do it, and do it regularly," Dr. Bairey says. "You can really improve your risk a great deal simply by doing low-intensity things that shouldn't put you out that much."

In fact, some intriguing research supports the notion that just being more active in your leisure time can help prevent heart disease.

In one long-term British study, for example, 9,376 male civil servants aged 45 to 64 were divided into four groups depending on their self-reported level of activity.

OUR CHILDREN: FAT OR FIT?

Years ago, most children played hide and seek. These days you'll most likely find them hiding out on the couch in front of the television.

"It's a real problem. Habits learned early in childhood are leading to real disease," says C. Noel Bairey, M.D., medical director of the Preventive and Cardiac Rehabilitation Center at Cedars-Sinai Medical Center in Los Angeles. "There's compelling evidence that suggests we need to start preventing heart disease at an early age."

If distaste for exercise seeps down to our children at an early age, it could have surprisingly dire consequences, according to Bernard Gutin, Ph.D., a professor of pediatrics at the Medical College of Georgia in Augusta.

In a study of 216 five- to six-year-old, primarily Hispanic children in New York City, Dr. Gutin and his colleagues found the children who had low levels of fitness and high body fat tended to have high blood pressure, a risk factor for coronary heart disease.

"It's astonishing that these relationships were showing up at a very early age," Dr. Gutin says.

"It's worrisome because for those children who are unfit or fat, there will be a lot of unnecessary morbidity and mortality on down the line."

Some experts blame children's growing addiction to television for much of the problem. The average two- to five-year-old watches about 28 hours of television a week, and many kids are glued to the screen up to 40 hours a week. And that doesn't include time spent playing video games or watching videocassettes.

The connection between television viewing and the risk factors for heart disease (including a lack of fitness) is truly amazing. Researchers at Harvard School of Public Health and Tufts New England Medical Center have concluded that every additional hour a kid watches television each day makes him 2 percent more likely to be fat.

In addition, University of Texas researchers determined that the snack foods children tend to eat while viewing TV contain high levels of fat, saturated fat, and/or sodium. So it isn't too surprising that University of California, Irvine, researchers concluded that 2 or more hours of TV a day is the strongest predictor of high cholesterol levels in children.

Even worse, watching television saps energy from our children, says pediatrician Kurt V. Gold, M.D., one of the California researchers.

"They're sitting, but they're not really relaxing. They may be expending tremendous amounts of mental energy processing the audiovisual messages TV is throwing at them," he says. The upshot of that exhaustion is that our children may not have the energy to go out and play later.

Fortunately, there is still time to make changes that will reduce risk of heart disease among our children, experts say.

You need to have plenty of healthful snacks available and limit your children to 1 or 2 hours of television daily, according to the American Academy of Pediatrics. Help them plan their viewing. Flipping the channel only encourages more viewing. The set should go on for specific programs and go off when those shows are over.

"Given the proper environment—good food and not a lot of TV—children will do the right thing," Dr. Bairey says. "The natural inclination for children is to play. They're just naturally very physically active."

The most active men—those who burned more than 3,000 calories a week doing brisk walking or vigorous cycling, swimming, stair climbing, or rowing—had less than half the number of heart attacks and deaths as sedentary men during the following nine years. But the men who did less intense walking for 30 minutes a day also had a lower mortality rate and fewer heart attacks than the least active men.

In another long-term study of 3,043 railroad workers aged 22 to 79, researchers found that after 20 years of follow-up, those men who were the least active were more likely to die of coronary heart disease than men who expended 1,000 calories a week doing activities such as golf, dancing, gardening, softball, and volleyball.

Then there's the classic Honolulu Heart Program study of 8,006 Japanese-American men aged 45 to 69. After 12 years of follow-up, researchers concluded the men who had an active lifestyle had 30 to 60 percent less incidence of coronary heart disease than their sedentary peers.

"The evidence clearly suggests that just some amount of activity is beneficial. In other words, you don't have to be a marathoner or triathlete to lower your heart attack risk," says Richard P. Donahue, Ph.D., an epidemiologist at the University of Miami School of Medicine and author of the Honolulu study.

More evidence that leisure activities can strengthen your cardiovascular system comes from Italy, where researchers studied 100 male factory workers.

The workers who were active in their leisure time— doing things such as running, tennis, soccer, handball, and gardening— had a slower pulse rate and improved cholesterol levels compared to their sedentary counterparts, who spent their spare time reading, watching television, and going to movies.

"The best advice for people is to keep active," Dr. Wood says. "Exercise is a fairly powerful factor that will prevent or at least delay the nasty consequences associated with heart disease."

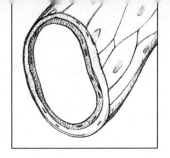

High Blood Pressure

Ray Watts had had high blood pressure since the age of 46. And with treatment that included medication, his pressure stayed at a respectable 150/90. A little high but—as far as his doctor was concerned—okay.

Then somewhere around his 53rd birthday, his world started falling apart. His wife had a heart attack, his daughter left home, and a political scandal threatened his career.

Ray's blood pressure went through the roof. His doctor increased the medication, but it didn't do much good. His uncontrolled pressure cost him three "ministrokes," a couple of blackouts, and headaches that left him pale and shaking. For the next five years his blood pressure bounced back and forth between high and higher.

Until, that is, he met his second wife. An Iowa-bred farm girl, she believed in walking a couple of miles every morning and dancing every night. And if he wanted to be a part of her life, she told Ray, he'd better get with the program.

He did. He walked every morning, danced every night, and even took to riding a bike. And his blood pressure dropped to its lowest point in 15 years and stabilized. He still needed medication, but now the medication could do its job.

A Good Swift Kick

Can exercise actually "cure" high blood pressure? Scientists aren't really sure, but studies indicate that even if exercise can't eliminate the condition, for most of us it can certainly give it a good swift kick in the right direction.

People with mild or borderline high blood pressure—what doctors call hypertension—may be able to reduce their dependence on drugs or even wean themselves completely off medication with something as simple as regular, vigorous walking, says Mark B. Effron, M.D., assistant professor of medicine at Johns Hopkins University and director of the Coronary Care Unit and the Cardiovascular Research Laboratory at Sinai Hospital in Baltimore.

Others, those like Ray Watts whose blood pressure ranges from moderately to severely high, may find that exercise will simply help their medication do its job.

How High and Why

Before you rush out to do three laps around the block, however, let's take a look at exactly how high your blood pressure should be to begin with—and why it sometimes goes higher.

Your body needs some degree of blood pressure to fight gravity, doctors explain. Without it, blood would slosh around

176

HOW HIGH IS HIGH?

Anyone with a resting systolic measurement (the top number of a blood pressure reading) of more than 140 has high blood pressure.

Diastolic measurements—the numbers on the bottom of blood pressure readings—determine the degree of severity of the condition.

Someone with a diastolic reading between 90 and 104 has mildly high blood pressure, doctors say, while a diastolic of 105 to 114 would indicate moderately high blood pressure. A diastolic reading of 115 or higher would be classified as severely high.

Fortunately, 70 percent of those with high blood pressure have only a mild condition.

inside your body—rushing from your head and pooling in your feet as you stand, or forming a blood puddle on the side closest to the floor as you lie in front of the TV.

Both the pumping of the heart and the condition of the arteries determine blood pressure. Each beat of the heart propels blood through the body. The force of the pumping action is measured as *systolic* pressure, the top number of a blood pressure reading.

Between heartbeats, healthy arteries constrict in order to maintain enough pressure on the blood to prevent it from draining away. The amount of force necessary to do this is measured as *diastolic* pressure, the bottom number of a blood pressure reading.

Arteries preprogramed by heredity, hardened and clogged with fat and cholesterol, beaten up by diabetes, or constricted by cigarette smoke are not flexible enough to do a good job of dilating during a heartbeat or constricting afterward. And their rigidity causes both systolic and diastolic readings to rise.

Flexible blood vessels equal a healthy heart and low blood pressure. Rigid blood vessels equal an overburdened heart and high blood pressure.

Sodium intake and kidney function also figure into your blood pressure equation. Tissues swelled and stiffened by water retention compress the arteries, forcing the heart to pump harder through narrower openings. And obesity also causes high blood pressure, because the heart has to pump a greater volume of blood through an increased tissue mass.

A person who has high blood pressure wouldn't necessarily be aware of it, however, as symptoms don't develop until major damage has been done. That's why it's important to have blood pressure readings taken as part of a regular checkup. Normal blood pressure is usually measured at 120/80 mmHg (millimeters of mercury) by a sphygmomanometer—the blood pressure cuff. In high blood pressure, one or both of those numbers could increase.

In general, doctors agree, the lower the readings, the better for your body. The higher the readings, the harder your heart has to pump—and the higher your chance of dying from heart disease. Untreated, high blood pressure leads not only to such relatively minor problems as headaches and visual impairments but to such major killers as heart disease, kidney disease, and stroke.

Take One Walk and Call Me in the Morning

Until relatively recently, most physicians would have simply scribbled out a prescription for one drug or another as the primary method of managing high blood pressure, says family practioner Jeffrey L. Tanji, M.D., an assistant professor at the University of California's Davis Medical Center.

No longer. For the treatment of mildly high blood pressure, many researchers now advocate that exercise be the treatment of choice. They point out that the heavy-duty drugs used to treat high blood pressure have equally heavy-duty side effects and may be unnecessary when exercise frequently has the same beneficial effect.

"Instead of taking a pill, you take exercise," says John J. Duncan, Ph.D., associate director of exercise physiology at the Institute of Aerobics Research in Dallas. "Exercise *is* basically a pill, because it causes physiological changes. One is man-made; the other is natural."

Setting the Proper Tone

Initially, says Dr. Tanji, physical activity increases arterial flexibility two ways. It reduces the level of stress-related chemicals in the bloodstream that constrict arteries and veins, and it also increases the

release of endorphins—the body's own natural painkillers—that themselves reduce pressure.

Exercise also increases the amount of "good" HDL cholesterol. This further increases the flexibility of blood vessels, since the HDL cholesterol flushes away the "bad" LDL cholesterol, which tends to accumulate on arterial walls and stiffen them up.

Over time, adds Dr. Effron, physical conditioning lowers your resting heart rate and improves the responsiveness of your blood vessels so that you literally reset their tone and improve their flexibility.

The weight reduction that frequently accompanies exercise also contributes to reducing blood pressure, says Dr. Effron, but exercise lowers blood pressure even if people do not lose body fat, he adds.

The Evidence

How much can exercise actually reduce blood pressure?

That depends. In a joint study done at the Johns Hopkins University Medical Center and several other Maryland medical facilities, scientists found that exercise reduced blood pressure 13 to 14 points in a group of 52 men. The men, all of whom were sedentary and taking medication for mildly high blood pressure, began the study with an average blood pressure reading of 145/97. After ten weeks of weight training and walking, jogging, or biking, they finished with an average blood pressure reading of 131/84.

In a second study, this one at the University of California, San Diego, ten men with mildly high blood pressure (a mean reading of 136/94) knocked their collective blood pressure readings down to a respectable 130/85 with a ten-week program of walking, jogging, or stationary bicycling.

Not bad. A third study, however, indicates that maybe not all of us can obtain these benefits. In that study, scientists from Duke University, Vanderbilt University, and Boston's New England Deaconess Hospital worked with 92 men and women with blood pressure readings that ranged from mildly high to moderately high (140/90 to 180/105). After a 16-week exercise program similar to those used at both the University of California and Johns Hopkins, there was no reduction in blood pressure.

Does this rule out the theory that exercise can help lower your blood pressure? Not necessarily. Since this third study measured people who had different characteristics from those in the previous studies, it means that the differences between people—sex, weight, age, aerobic capacity—may determine whether or not exercise can reduce blood pressure.

As the researchers from Duke, Vanderbilt, and Boston concluded in their study, further research is necessary to identify the very specific and individual characteristics that will tell us just who is most likely to benefit from a workout.

Going for the Glow

Until scientists come up with an exercise prescription that's as individual as your blood type, doctors generally suggest that the best way to see if exercise can reduce your blood pressure is to lace up your sneaks and give it a shot.

Researchers argue over the precise degree of exercise necessary to affect high blood pressure, but most agree it's not a whole heck of a lot. By walking, jogging, or bike riding at 50 to 60 percent of your maximum heart rate, says Dr. Tanji, many people can reduce their diastolic blood pressure by 15 to 20 points. (To learn how to determine your maximum heart rate, see "How Good Is Your Workout?" on page 324. And for information on how to start a walking, running, or bicycling program, see the appropriate chapters in part 2.)

You should exercise hard enough to get your heart pumping, says Dr. Tanji. But keep in mind that exercising close to the maximum of which your body is capable is counterproductive and potentially dangerous.

That's because a vigorous workout that pushes you to use somewhere between 70 and 90 percent of your capability can constrict your arteries and send your blood pressure through the roof.

When workouts are done week after week at the proper intensity, however, the pressure-lowering effect of exercise shows itself immediately after the activity, lingers into the following day, and remains as long as the workouts continue, says Dr. Duncan. Following even a single exercise session, he adds, "there's a 3- to 5-hour afterglow in which the opened blood vessels are transporting oxygenated blood to the worked muscles."

Weights and Measures

Aerobic exercise is not the only activity that can have a positive effect on blood pressure, says Dr. Effron. In fact, for people with mildly high blood pressure, light weight training in addition to aerobic exercise can reduce systolic pressure by about five points and diastolic pressure by seven. (See "Resistance Training" on page 404.)

Although intense weight lifting has been known to drive blood pressure up to a vein-popping 300/200 reading, based on studies he and his colleagues have performed Dr. Effron feels comfortable prescribing a three-times-a-week regimen of lifting weights at 40 percent of your maximum strength in conjunction with aerobic exercise. "If the maximum you can lift is 100 pounds, for example, you lift 40 pounds for your training routine," he explains.

Lift the weight 10 to 15 times over a 30-second period, then rest for 10 seconds before moving to the next exercise, says Dr. Effron. Proceed through your entire routine twice, raising the load on individual exercises only when you can comfortably lift the weight more than 15 times within a 30-second period.

Be careful, though, that you don't grip the weights too hard during your workouts. A tight grasp creates a demand for more blood flow yet restricts its passage, causing both systolic and diastolic blood pressure

readings to skyrocket. Grasp the weights with enough force to keep them under control, but stay relaxed. If you're lifting a weight that's less than half of what you can really heft, there's no reason to white-knuckle it.

To maximize the pressure-lowering effects of your workout, stretch for 10 minutes or so before every session. And afterward, walk or jog for 20 minutes.

When Pressure Is Not Mild-Mannered

If exercise alone doesn't pull mildly high blood pressure readings down to a normal range or modify moderately or severely high blood pressure after a six-month trial, an approach that combines exercise and medication may prove beneficial, says Dr. Tanji. In fact, he adds, anyone with a diastolic blood pressure reading of 105 and above should probably follow this approach.

Just be sure to work closely with your doctor. Because some high blood pressure drugs are not exercise-friendly, you should make sure your doctor monitors your blood pressure and knows exactly what your exercise program includes. (See "Medications and Exercise" on page 213.)

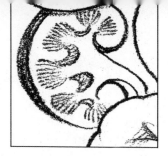

Incontinence

Do you dribble when you giggle? Gush when you guffaw? Leak when you lift? Urinary incontinence—the inability to control a leaky bladder—is coming out of the closet. More people than ever are seeking help for this embarrassing problem. For some surgery shores up a sagging bladder; for others pills help control bladder muscle spasms.

But an increasing number of people, often with their doctor's advice, first try an exercise to strengthen the muscles that control the flow of urine.

They do "Kegels"—pelvic contractions that tighten the muscles around the urethra, vagina, and anus and actually build and strengthen the sling of crisscrossing layers that includes the pubococcygeus (PC) muscles.

Like a sling, these muscles extend from the pubic bone to the tailbone, supporting organs within the pelvis, like the bladder and uterus. If these muscles stretch and sag, the bladder, uterus, or vagina can drop uncomfortably low.

Although Kegels are also known by other names, such as pelvic floor or PC exercises, they can be done correctly only one way. (See "Kegel Exercises" on page 368.) They are the *only* exercise proven to help control urinary incontinence, although overall fitness—and being lean—can also help control incontinence. (Kegels are also used to control fecal incontinence, improve vaginal tone, enhance orgasm, and, in men, help control ejaculation.)

Studies show that one very common type of urinary incontinence is most likely to be helped by Kegel exercises: stress incontinence (leaking urine when you sneeze, cough, laugh, bear down, or lift). This kind of incontinence is related to weak muscles around the neck of the bladder, where a ring of muscles, the external sphincter, helps retain urine.

Expect an Improvement

Studies evaluating the effectiveness of Kegel exercises for urinary incontinence vary tremendously, showing improvement rates in anywhere from 30 to 90 percent of participants. But the studies *do* consistently show improvement, and studies done in the last five or so years support the observation that Kegel exercises can work well for many people—*if* they're properly taught and faithfully done, says Katherine F. Jeter, Ed.D., director of Help for Incontinent People (H.I.P.), a nonprofit patient advocacy organization. If the problem is weak sphincter muscles, the exercises are considered safe and effective and won't do any harm, she says.

A good candidate—one who is motivated and alert—may find that Kegels are all that's needed to get dry and stay dry, says Mimi Gallo, R.N., co-director of the Urodynamics and Incontinence Center at Beth Israel Hospital in Boston. A good candidate should expect to see results in about six weeks, although he or she may not reach peak strength for several months, Gallo says. Someone who is motivated but has very weak muscles may take up to three months to see much improvement.

(Improvement does not necessarily mean cure, therapists point out. But for more serious cases it may mean you are able to switch from adult diapers to panty liners, or go from four accidents a day to one.)

Even people who are overweight, who've had bladder surgery that failed to fix their problem, or who've been incontinent a long time can get some benefit, as long as they are able to properly identify the muscle to exercise, Gallo says.

Those with problems that affect their mind, such as Alzheimer's disease, may have difficulty performing Kegel exercises successfully, says Jeannette Tries, director of the Biofeedback Center at Sacred Heart Rehabilitation Hospital in Milwaukee. Depending on the extent of their mental impairment, people with head injuries, spina bifida, or multiple sclerosis or those who've had a stroke can often successfully use biofeedback with Kegel exercises to improve urinary incontinence. "It's definitely worth an evaluation," she says.

Tuning In to Better Control

Some people have PC muscles that are so weak they can't feel them, or can't tell if they are contracting during exercise. As a result, they can seldom learn to do Kegels on their own. Often, however, they can benefit from a biofeedback-based exercise program, many therapists say. In biofeedback, a person is connected to a machine that helps them recognize their muscle performance.

"People can't see these muscles," says Kathe Wallace, a Seattle physical therapist and H.I.P. advisor who specializes in the treatment of urinary incontinence. "Biofeedback helps the person perform the exercise correctly." Biofeedback can also show small but encouraging improvements in strength, something neither therapist nor patient may be able to detect, Wallace says.

According to the National Institutes of Health, using biofeedback to teach better muscle control results in complete control of incontinence in 20 to 25 percent of people and provides important improvement in another 30 percent.

Good training is important, therapists emphasize. "If you don't learn how to do this exercise right, you can see little benefit," Wallace says.

Some doctors recommend the use of weighted cones, which are inserted into the vagina to train the PC muscles. When cones of the appropriate weight are placed in the vagina, the woman must contract the pelvic floor muscles to keep them from slipping out. Most practice this exercise for two 15-minute sessions each day, with cones weighing from 1 to 2½ ounces. One study, done in Great Britain, shows that using cones may prove effective. Electrical stimulation may also be used as part of a treatment program. Its use helps people become aware of how it feels to activate these muscles.

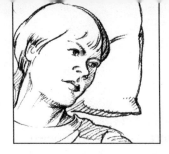

Insomnia

Night falls, but you don't. You're still awake, fantasizing an ancient Aztec kaleidoscope of colors behind restless lids. Sleep extends an open palm, curls a quiet, inviting forefinger, and beckons. You cuddle the covers, punch the pillow, snuggle your head deep in the down. Struggle as you may to will weariness, you cannot heed the beckoner's call.

Every night, millions of people fall short when it comes to falling asleep. Some resort to alcohol or sleeping pills, which may only complicate the problem and increase daytime tiredness.

And they all suffer sleeplessness unnecessarily, because there is an easy, effective answer to sleep's call: Fitness fights fitfulness.

Regular workouts—any exercise, actually—can improve sleep, leaving you feeling more at ease at night and more vigorous during the day. And in the long run, the permanent weight reduction that follows regular exercise may offer relief for those who suffer from the throat-choking, breath-sapping effects of another fairly common sleep disorder—sleep apnea.

As an outlet for reducing muscular tension and stress, exercise "ordinarily will help you fall asleep and sleep better," according to Richard N. Podell, M.D., author of *Doctor, Why Am I So Tired?* and associate clinical professor in the Department of Family Medicine of the University of Medicine and Dentistry at New Jersey, Robert Wood Johnson Medical School.

A Way Out of Insomnia

Virtually everyone has some difficulty getting to sleep at one time or another, and up to a third of Americans complain about what they perceive as a sleeping problem. For some, insomnia is being unable to float off to sleep after shutting off the lights. For others, it's the inability to remain asleep during the night. And for others, insomnia means awakening in the predawn hours and being unable to get that last hour or two of shut-eye.

Needing a half hour or more to fall asleep is considered abnormal. And while most people quite normally wake up anywhere from 15 to 20 times a night, remembering 5 or more of those episodes or being unable to fall back to sleep for 30 minutes or more is also deemed problematic.

Insomnia is not in itself a disease, researchers say; another problem sires the symptom. Sometimes that problem is medical, such as an illness; sometimes it's chemical, such as use of certain prescription drugs or excess consumption of caffeine or alcohol. But more often, insomnia is psychological—the result of stress, tension, or drastic schedule changes.

Move More, Sleep Better

Exercise affects sleep in many ways. It wrestles restlessness to the ground and preps the body for slumber. It elevates the body's levels of epinephrine and endorphins, two chemicals associated with sensations of contentedness and well-being. And it also helps increase the amount of time physically fit people spend in the more restful stages of slow-wave sleep, according to Gary Zammit, Ph.D., director of the Sleep Disorders Institute at St. Luke's/Roosevelt Hospital Center in New York City.

Of the five sleep stages people drift through over the course of the night—stages one through four and the dream state of REM (rapid eye movement)—the slow-brain-wave periods of stages three and four are often considered the soundest, most restful, and most regenerating, explains Dr. Zammit. During these slow-wave stages, body temperature drops, metabolic rate drops, and breathing becomes regular.

It is more difficult to awaken someone from slow-wave sleep than from the other phases, Dr. Zammit says. If aroused during stage three or four, a sleeper likely would report a more placid, more serene mental state than the often surreal dream experiences of the REM phase.

Slow-wave sleep for most people occurs predominantly during the first half of the night. As the sleeper wafts through several sleep cycles over the course of the night, the slow-wave phase tends to fade away, and most of the time is spent in the more easily arousable, less restful states, Dr. Zammit says.

While researchers know exercise improves sleep, they're still trying to figure out how much exercise is enough. "There seems to be a confusion between the effects of exercise and the effects of fitness," says Michael Vitiello, Ph.D., associate director of the Sleep and Aging Research Program at the University of Washington in Seattle. "Anyone can run out and exercise on a given day." And they *will* feel tired and fall asleep more easily, he says. But the evolving pattern in sleep/exercise research favors overall fitness. "Regular, moderate exercise improves general physical fitness," he says, "and with that, there's an improvement in sleep quality."

Fit exercisers with leaner body mass and an improved cardiovascular system do, in fact, seem to rest more easily than out-of-shape, unfit people just beginning an exercise program. People new to exercise may even have some initial disturbance of sleep as they start to work out, particularly if it's later in the evening, says Dr. Zammit.

That's no real cause for concern, he says, and it should not discourage people who already have sleep problems and want to exercise. The sleep disruption "may go away after time," says Dr. Zammit. "If it doesn't after a short period, you can try exercising at an earlier time of day."

To increase your chances of nodding off at night, most sleep experts recommend working out in the afternoon or early evening. "Time your sessions for mid- to late afternoon, maybe between 3:00 and 7:00 P.M. as a general rule," Dr. Vitiello says. People should experiment with different times to decide which is best for them, he advises.

One group of people may want to take special note of the beneficial effects that exercise has on sleep. Sleep for people in their sixties, seventies, and beyond often becomes fragmented, marred by frequent awakenings.

This pattern restricts the amount of time they spend in the deep, restful, rejuvenating slow-wave stages of sleep.

Dr. Vitiello has been studying the effects of two kinds of exercise—aerobics and stretching—on people 60 and older. Although his research is not finished, he believes that both kinds of workouts may affect sleep quality and quantity. Aerobics, particularly, may increase the amount of slow-wave sleep an elderly person gets, he says.

When Snoring Gets Serious

Maybe getting to sleep isn't your problem, but what happens afterward is. Snoring puts the snorer at loggerheads with his or her bed partner at night, and in extreme cases, with his own body. That's because snoring is the chief symptom of obstructive sleep apnea—a severe disruption of nocturnal breathing that leads to a number of health problems and can even prove fatal.

Researchers can't even guess at how many people suffer from sleep apnea, which can affect anyone but seems to occur primarily in middle-aged and overweight men. Fewer women appear to be afflicted, but those who are usually are older and overweight.

Snoring, in which the upper airway is only partly obstructed, "can be benign," Dr. Zammit says. "In and of itself, snoring is not a problem." But when a person has apnea there is so much relaxed tissue in the throat that it mostly or completely

closes off the airway, and the sleeper cannot breathe. People with apnea may stop breathing for several seconds or even minutes before the lack of oxygen arouses them, and they awaken with a sudden jolt and a loud snort. Apnea sufferers choke and arouse themselves repeatedly throughout the night, perhaps as frequently as 400 times, and they may or may not remember the awakenings.

But the disruptions certainly take their toll, for the log-sawer by night just lumbers around by day. "The net result is the person is very, very sleepy during the next day," Dr. Zammit notes. "They may have problems performing in social and occupational settings or just zone out and nap."

Many report a decreased ability to think, concentrate, and remember. Mood changes, headaches, and irritability are common. More serious mental problems, such as psychosis and depression, are also possible. About 42 percent of the apnea patients in one study also complained of impotence or decreased sex drive.

If the apnea is not treated, sufferers are at far greater risk of developing high blood pressure, heart problems, even stroke.

Exercise cannot cure apnea, sleep experts assert, but losing weight may make a significant difference. Because the correlation with obesity is so strong, people who lose weight—through dieting and exercise—often find their apnea has decreased along with their waist size.

While there's "good evidence" to suggest loss of body weight will very often result in an improvement, it is unlikely to make sleep apnea entirely disappear, Dr. Vitiello says. A person who has apnea should be under a physician's care, he emphasizes.

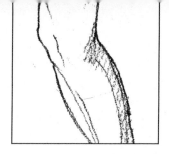

Intermittent Claudication

For years you enjoyed an occasional morning stroll through your neighborhood. But recently you've dreaded walking more than a few yards because of some nasty cramps you've been getting in your calves.

The weird thing is that these cramps occur *only* when you exert yourself. They're so painful that taking another step is unthinkable. If you rest for a few minutes, the pain goes away, and you can resume your stroll. But then, after you've gone a short distance, the cramps strike again.

What's going on here? Well, there's a good probability you're suffering from intermittent claudication, a blockage of the arteries supplying blood and oxygen to the legs. This problem afflicts about 3 of every 100 Americans. It also can strike in the foot, thigh, hip, or buttocks.

"Intermittent claudication is a sign of inadequate blood flow to the lower limbs. As a result, the person gets cramps because their legs aren't getting enough oxygen," says James Skinner, Ph.D., director of the Exercise and Sports Research Institute at Arizona State University in Tempe.

Relief Is Just a Step Away

Fortunately, claudication can be surprisingly simple to treat and in many cases can be relieved without drugs or surgery. In fact, some doctors sum up the cure for claudication in five words: Keep walking and stop smoking.

That's right, walking—the very activity that usually induces the claudication—also is one of the best ways to stop it.

"Exercise has a dramatic effect. If you start someone on a walking program and they stick with it, they can get as good symptomatic relief as they can get from medications," says C. Noel Bairey, M.D., medical director of the Preventive and Cardiac Rehabilitation Center at Cedars-Sinai Medical Center in Los Angeles.

People who have claudication and walk regularly have shown remarkable improvement, says Jay Coffman, M.D., chief of peripheral vascular disease medicine at Boston University Medical Center. In fact, research indicates that if people who suffer claudication do 30 to 60 minutes of walking every other day for several months, they can increase their walking distance, in some cases, from one to ten blocks.

And some doctors say walking therapy can double, triple, or even increase by a factor of ten the distance you can go without leg pain.

Stepping Away from Pain

What is so magical about walking? Why does it have such a powerful impact on claudication? Well, before we can answer those questions, it's important that you understand a little more about claudication.

Intermittent claudication isn't an ailment itself. It's a symptom of peripheral vascular disease (PVD), a malady that blocks circulation in the legs in the same way that coronary artery disease blocks the vessels leading to the heart.

Thirty to 50 percent of people who have claudication probably have coronary artery disease, Dr. Coffman says. So it is important that you seek a physician's care before beginning any exercise program to combat claudication.

High cholesterol levels and diabetes are risk factors for claudication. But smoking is its primary cause—eight out of ten people who suffer from it are puffers. So if you haven't already, you should quit smoking now.

Stop Smoking, Start Walking

"It's extremely important that a person who has claudication stop smoking because the toxins from tobacco produce vascular spasms that reduce circulation of blood," says Richard Hansen, M.D., medical director of the Poland Spring Health Institute in Poland Spring, Maine. "Studies have shown that even one cigarette can drop the circulation 40 percent in the fingers, feet, and toes. It's the nicotine in the cigarette—a potent vasoconstrictor."

In some cases, surgery is necessary to relieve the pain of claudication. But in most cases, walking is your best medicine.

"Combined with a low-fat diet and quitting smoking, walking is a nonsurgical approach that can greatly improve most people. It makes surgery unnecessary 90 percent of the time," Dr. Hansen says.

Walking Opens New Paths

Doctors aren't exactly sure how walking relieves claudication, but some suspect that brisk strolls stimulate the formation of new blood vessels that naturally bypass the blocked portion of the leg artery. It's also likely that regular exercise dilates vessels, increasing blood flow to your legs. Walking also may enhance the ability of your leg muscles to extract oxygen from blood.

But however it works, walking does a better job of relieving claudication than other exercises, says Robert Ginsburg, M.D., professor of medicine at the University of Colorado and director of the Unit for Cardiovascular Intervention at University Hospital, both in Denver.

"Walking is best because you're using the muscles in your calves that are usually affected by claudication," he says. "Swimming is useless because it is primarily an upper-body form of exercise. Bicycling is okay, but not as good as walking."

Other exercise therapies such as dancing, jumping rope, and jogging also are effective, Dr. Coffman says. But few people who have claudication are likely to be able to endure those activities, so walking is prescribed most often.

Easy Does It

Once a physician determines that your claudication is treatable with walking therapy, he or she likely will suggest that you start slowly. When you start feeling the cramps, try to walk a short distance with the pain before you stop to rest, Dr. Ginsburg suggests.

"What I usually tell my patients to do is get up in the morning and go for a walk around the block," he says.

"If you know that you'll start getting leg cramps by the time you get to the third telephone pole away from your house, try walking one telephone pole beyond that, if you can tolerate it. Then stop and rest until the pain is gone, then walk back home.

"The next day, do the same thing, but try to get to the fifth telephone pole. Keep walking like that every day and try to go one more telephone pole every time. You'll find if you do that over a period of months, you'll significantly increase the distance you can walk."

Dr. Hansen advocates a variation of that approach known as terrain therapy. In this form of therapy a person with claudication walks on hillside trails under close medical supervision. The principle is basically the same. The person walks until he feels pain and needs to rest. Then after the pain fades, he begins walking uphill or downhill again.

The method seems to be more effective at relieving claudication than walking on flat surfaces is, Dr. Hansen says.

"It's a special type of interval training that seems to stimulate the formation of new vessels that help blood bypass blockages," he says. "With it, we can take a person who can't walk from one telephone pole to another and possibly have him walking several miles a day before our three-week rehabilitation program is finished."

Your doctor may be able to refer you to someone who conducts sessions in terrain therapy.

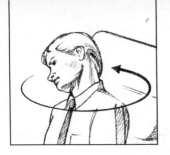

Jet Lag

Young men wait restlessly in a meeting room. An older man bursts in and hastily hands out fat plane-ticket folders. "Time to hit the road," he growls, "and our butts are on the line. We're going head-to-head with Indianapolis, Detroit, Milwaukee, Chicago, Washington, and New York—all by a week from tomorrow—and we've got to bring back nothing but winners."

The basketball team that actually made that trip a few seasons ago didn't do too well on the odyssey. Not many traveling teams would have. Scan the home and away records in the sports section and you'll see how hard it is to maintain an edge during and right after road trips. What with leagues expanding and schedules extending—in duration and in distance—it looks to get tougher. That's why many perfessional sports clubs, not to mention business organizations, are searching for ways to overcome jet lag and other wearying effects of travel.

Stiff, Dry, and Tired

"In a plane, you stiffen up from sitting for extended periods and dehydrate because of the air conditioning, and the effect on physiology from dehydration is severe," says Howie Wenger, Ph.D., an exercise consultant to hockey's Los Angeles Kings and the Canadian Olympic team. This helps explain, he says, why the Kings often play poorly in their first away game or in their first home game after a road trip.

It's worse when flights are 3 hours or longer, or far-flung enough to disrupt the normal rhythms of the nervous system. Those rhythms are sustained by a host of regular environmental cues: eating and sleeping habits, normal exercise patterns, reactions to light and darkness, and so forth. "The problem when you travel," Dr. Wenger says, "is that your baseline rhythm is always under attack." The sum of these factors saps your mental and physical skills. The net effect of jet lag lasts until the body adapts to its new time frame.

West-to-east travel is the toughest because time is lost rather than gained. As a rule of thumb, west-to-east trips require a day of recovery for each time zone crossed; east-to-west journeys require a day after crossing each 1½ time zones. Adjustments get even trickier when altitude and climatic changes are involved.

Alan Coates, assistant to the president of hockey's Calgary Flames, says his team's failure to recapture the Stanley Cup last season was all but guaranteed by a 19-day, five-city, six-game preseason tour of Czechoslovakia and the Soviet Union. "It took us until early January to recover," Coates (continued on page 192)

A NEW SPIN ON RELIEVING JET LAG

Here's a new exercise remedy for jet lag: When you get to your destination, you might want to try "twirling." This unusual technique is recommended by doctors at the Radiant Life Clinic in their book, *Twirling & Jet Lag*.

The doctors are students of Da Avabhasa, a spiritual teacher. Like many such teachers—and many forms of traditional medicine from the East, such as the Chinese and Indian systems of healing—Da Avabhasa says there is an "energy field" surrounding the physical body. "Fast travel," he writes, "sets up a motion in our energy system that takes a little time to return to human speed. Therefore, twirl several times every hour after flying."

Why twirling?

"Through the action or movement of twirling, the physical body and its energy field are equalized or integrated in a mutual harmony, a common speed." In other words, no more jet lag.

One of the Radiant Life doctors, Frans Bakker, M.D., has this to say about his own experience of twirling: "I twirled for the first time about 15 years ago when I went on a lecture tour of Europe. I was in the air for 17 hours straight on my trip across the United States to Holland. As soon as I got to my hotel, I twirled. Because of my lecture schedules, I do a great deal of traveling. Consequently, I have always been troubled by jet lag. This time, I twirled a few times over a period of two days and experienced a gradual lifting of the symptoms. Even while doing the exercise, I could feel the airy feeling I get with jet lag starting to disappear. The pattern of my bowel movements returned to normal quickly. And within two days all the obvious jet lag symptoms were gone. This was quite significant, as they had previously always lasted a week or more. Since then I always twirl after flights and experience the same effects."

Before you attempt this technique, keep in mind that twirling should be approached gradually and with common sense. "Don't try to do too much too soon," warns one of the doctors who wrote the book. "Be particularly careful if you find that you become uncomfortably dizzy while twirling. If you do, slow down your rate of spin and the length of your twirling sessions, and only gradually increase these as your tolerance increases with practice."

You should also be careful of *where* you twirl. "Make sure there are no objects around that you might knock over or that might injure you if you lost your balance and fell into them," he says.

Finally, twirling isn't for everyone. "People who suffer from dizzy spells, physical debilitation, Meniere's disease, or any other inner-ear problems should not try twirling," says the doctor. With that in mind, here's how to twirl.

1. Choose your twirling direction. You want to twirl in the same direction as your flight. If you traveled westward, twirl to the left (counterclockwise). If you traveled eastward, twirl to the right (clockwise). If you travel north or south, choose your direction depending on how you feel: Twirl to the left (counterclockwise) if you feel tired, washed out, or depressed. Twirl to the right (clockwise) if you feel restless, uptight, or irritable.

2. Stand in a relaxed, erect posture with your arms extended straight out to your sides at shoulder level.

3. If you are twirling to the left (counterclockwise), turn your left palm up and keep your right palm down. When twirling to the right (clockwise), turn

your right palm up, keeping your left palm facing down.

4. Keep your eyes open and directed straight ahead as you twirl. Your visual field will blur, but you'll minimize dizziness if you continue to look straight ahead. (Note: First-time twirlers can experience dizziness and even some nausea. You might want to stand near a wall for support. If you feel dizzy, simply do the exercise more slowly. If you're a frequent traveler, you'll adjust to the exercise the more you do it. A few moments of some initial dizziness as you adjust to the exercise are worth it to lose a few days of jet lag every time you travel!)

5. Hold your head, arms, and upper body in the same position throughout the exercise.

6. Don't tighten your muscles. Continue to breathe regularly.

7. Don't skate around the room. Move both feet together in a small circle as your body turns.

8. Twirl 10 to 12 times.

9. Avoid drifting around as you twirl. At first you may find it difficult to maintain your balance. If you do, twirl slowly and gradually increase your speed as you feel more comfortable with the exercise.

10. At the end of twirling, cross your arms over your chest and bend forward from the waist, relaxing your neck and shoulders and letting your head hang down loosely. Stay in this position until all spinning sensations have subsided.

Do not attempt this exercise if you have trouble maintaining your balance.

(For a copy of *Twirling & Jet Lag* call 1-800-524-4941.)

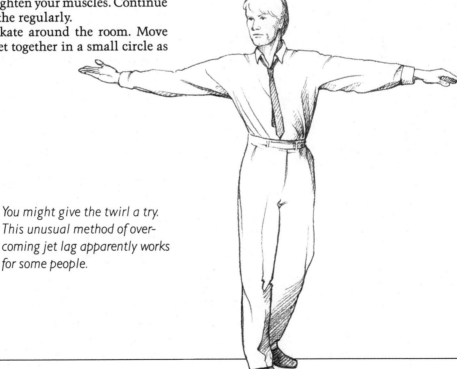

You might give the twirl a try. This unusual method of overcoming jet lag apparently works for some people.

says, adding, "You don't notice the impact of jet lag as much until you become a better team. Then you're trying to win every game, and you realize jet lag can make a difference in your performance."

If jet lag worsens physical performance, could the opposite be true—could exercise help *relieve* jet lag? The pro teams think so—and so do lots of other people.

Head for the Gym, Not the Mattress

Teams feel strongly about the benefits of holding practices and workouts immediately upon arrival, particularly after long flights. "After sitting in the plane for 5 hours, a good aerobic workout gets the metabolism up," says the Seattle Supersonics' trainer, Frank Furtado. Even after returning home, the Calgary Flames have found that a strenuous after-flight practice, followed by a day off (game schedule permitting), is much more productive than allowing the players to "crash" after the flight and stagger in for practice the next day.

But you don't have to be a pro athlete to schedule a workout when you arrive. Greg Finch, a 34-year-old United Airlines pilot who flies from the United States to Europe about four times a month, *always* goes for a run after the plane lands.

"It's well known among flight crews that exercise really helps overcome jet lag. I run," he says, "but others just do push-ups and sit-ups in their rooms.

"We leave the U.S. at 5:00 P.M. and arrive in Europe at 8:00 A.M.—1:00 A.M. body time. Then we return the next day at 9:00 A.M.—2:00 A.M. body time. If I exercise, it makes an enormous difference in how I feel when I'm flying back—if I don't get my workout in, it's extremely hard to stay awake. Here's an example. One week, I flew to London and didn't exercise at all. During the trip home, which lasted about 8½ hours, I felt very tired. A week later I took the same flight, but this time I ran 5 miles when I arrived. The next day on the flight back I felt great the whole way. But I got the same amount of sleep in London on both trips."

Lessening the Lag

A study at the University of Toronto suggests that exercise will actually reduce the number of days jet lag affects you. Researchers exposed golden hamsters (nocturnal animals with stable activity rhythms) to artificial light and advanced the onset of darkness by 8 hours, simulating the conditions of a long flight east.

After dark, one group of hamsters exercised on a running wheel. The other groups mostly slept. While the nonrunning hamsters took 5.4 days to adjust and to resume normal nocturnal activity, the running hamsters adjusted in just 1.6 days.

Exercising *in* the plane can also help you feel refreshed when you reach your destinations. Charles Ehret, Ph.D., the author of *Overcoming Jet Lag,* suggests these exercises for just before you land: squeezing a ball in the palm of your hand for 5 minutes, pressing your hands together in front of your chest, doing deep-knee bends in the back of the plane, and otherwise stretching your body into wakefulness.

Flexible Flyers

Sitting 3 hours or more in the cramped seat of a jetliner can leave a traveler stiff and dehydrated—and both spell trouble if you need to get up and go. The following set of exercises will help the travel-weary flyer loosen up. These movements should be performed in your seat, before the plane begins its descent.

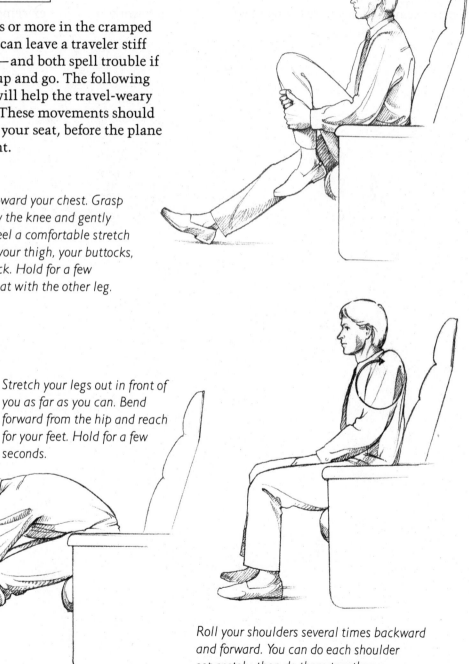

Lift one knee up toward your chest. Grasp your leg just below the knee and gently pull up until you feel a comfortable stretch along the back of your thigh, your buttocks, and your lower back. Hold for a few seconds, then repeat with the other leg.

Stretch your legs out in front of you as far as you can. Bend forward from the hip and reach for your feet. Hold for a few seconds.

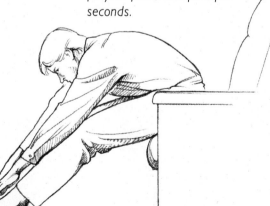

Roll your shoulders several times backward and forward. You can do each shoulder separately, then do them together.

Flexible Flyers—Continued

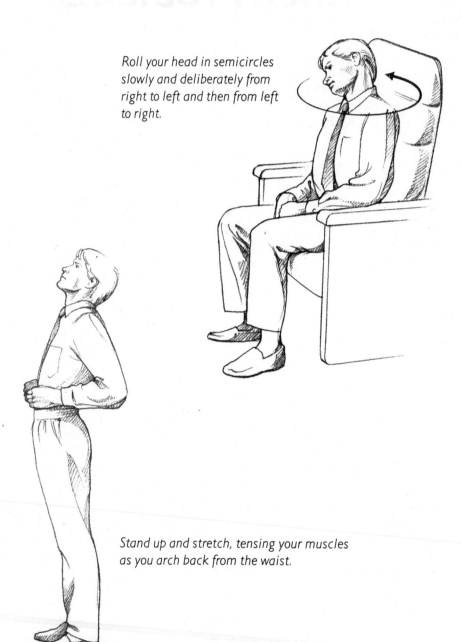

Roll your head in semicircles slowly and deliberately from right to left and then from left to right.

Stand up and stretch, tensing your muscles as you arch back from the waist.

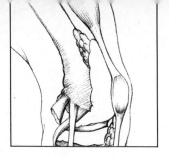

Knee Problems

Who hasn't smashed a knee into the coffee table and cursed the day *Homo erectus* decided to take those first tentative steps?

Knees don't hesitate to let you know you've offended them. They communicate their outrage by swelling up, locking, grinding, buckling, and refusing to go one step farther.

Fortunately, there are ways to coax finicky joints back into service. Rest, ice, anti-inflammatory drugs, and a brace that supports the knee and limits its range of motion may all be helpful. But the backbone of any knee-rehab program consists of exercises that strengthen and stretch joint-stabilizing leg muscles.

Doctors recommend exercises that include range-of-motion and stretching routines to build flexibility; isometrics and weight lifting to strengthen muscles; and biking, walking, and swimming to enhance endurance.

Rubber Bands and Bones

Like a hinge on a wooden chest, the knee opens and closes only within a certain range. Trying to force it further than it's designed to go usually pulls or breaks something—like the ligaments or cartilage that helps hold it together.

A knee joint consists of two bones—the thigh bone (femur) and lower leg bone (tibia)—laced together by thick, rubbery ligaments and encased in a fibrous, fluid-filled capsule.

When you are standing, the femur and tibia fit nicely together, separated only by two crescent-shaped pieces of impact-absorbing cartilage called the meniscus. In front of the joint is the kneecap, a disk made up of cartilage and bone that is connected on either end by tendons. (The thick tendon at the tibia is the one your doctor taps to check your reflexes.)

The kneecap is more than an injury magnet. It acts as a fulcrum for the front muscles of your leg, transferring power from your quadriceps to the rest of your leg, allowing you to kick out, squat, kneel, go up and down stairs, walk, dance—in short, do all the things that you do with your legs. (That's why when the kneecap "pops" out of place, you lose muscle strength in your upper leg, and your leg buckles up.)

All this complicated machinery makes it possible for humans to do marvelously elaborate or challenging things, like figure skating and running 4-minute miles. But it also means lots of things can go wrong with knees. Ligaments can tear; bits of cartilage can break off and make a knee lock; kneecaps can pop off track; tendons can become inflamed.

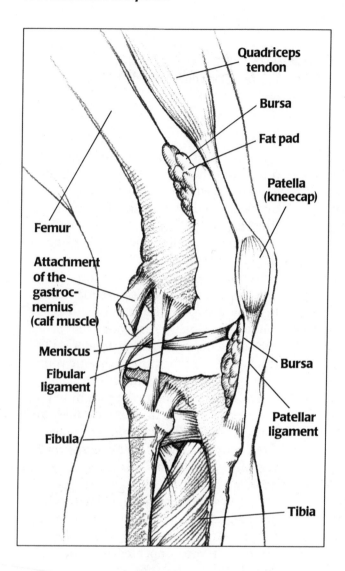

- Quadriceps tendon
- Bursa
- Fat pad
- Patella (kneecap)
- Femur
- Attachment of the gastrocnemius (calf muscle)
- Meniscus
- Fibular ligament
- Fibula
- Bursa
- Patellar ligament
- Tibia

The knee is one of your body's biggest joints. It's also one of the most complex. It's a delicate structure made up of four bones, with more than a half dozen pads (menisci) and cushions (bursae) to help protect it from daily pounding. Nearly a dozen muscles of the thigh and calf all rely upon the knee's ability to turn, twist, and bend, giving you the freedom to dance, twirl, and run. The tough ligaments form protective bands that crisscross to hold the knee intact. Given its complexity and workload, it's no wonder that the knee is a common site of injury and pain.

"Almost everything people do for recreation is tough on their knees—walking, climbing, kneeling. Even being crossed while at rest can stress knees," says James M. Fox, M.D., director of the Southern California Orthopedic Institute in Van Nuys and author of *Save Your Knees*. "Life is tough on your knees."

The knee is so complex, in fact, that when something goes wrong, you need to see a doctor to get it fixed. He or she can diagnose the pain and recommend exercises to get it working again. Far too often, it's some sort of activity that led to a knee injury in the first place. So chances are you could use some help choosing appropriate rehabilitation exercises.

"I don't know of *any* knee problem that

SIDESTEPPING KNEE INJURIES

Most people learn how to avoid knee injuries only after they've had one, says James M. Fox, M.D., director of the Southern California Orthopedic Institute in Van Nuys and author of *Save Your Knees*. Stay ahead of the crowd in the orthopedist's waiting room with these knee-sparing tips.

- If you *must* run downhill, zigzag or adopt a slightly bent-knee stance to reduce pounding on knees.
- If you play football, make it touch. The odds of hurting a knee while playing tackle football are high: about 50-50.
- Cross-train. Never do one exercise exclusively or rely on only one type of exercise machine. Mix aerobic, strengthening, and stretching activities to keep knees in peak shape.
- Always warm up and stretch before any activity.
- If your knees hurt when you bicycle, shift to a lower gear, or reduce the tension on a stationary bike. Make sure the seat is at the proper height. Your knee should be slightly bent when the pedal is at the bottom. Your knees should point straight ahead, not in toward the frame of the bike.
- If you ski, have your bindings adjusted by a pro. Don't do it yourself. Keep bindings clean of dirt and ice. Fatigue figures into ski injuries; take breaks when you get tired. Most ski-related knee injuries occur after 3:00 P.M.
- Know that cross-country skiing can be as risky to knees as downhill skiing. Why? Cross-country ski bindings don't release when you take a tumble. Your knees can get plenty tangled during a fall, even on flat terrain.
- Know whereon you play. Are there woodchuck holes in the meadow where you're playing volleyball? Puddles on the tennis court? Is the soccer field a sheet of icy mud? Serious knee injuries often start with a fall.
- Bare your soles for a stroll through dewy grass, not during running or aerobics. Wear shoes appropriate for your sport, and replace them regularly.
- Stretch to keep your hips and ankles flexible. Hips that can't swing and ankles that can't push off make extra work for knees. (See "Stretching" on page 440.)
- Make fitness a year-round activity. That way you don't have to hustle trying to get into shape for a seasonal sport or special event.

can't be improved by increasing muscle strength," says Dr. Fox. "Even when surgery corrects a problem, it can't rebuild weakened muscles. And with an injury, muscle weakness sets in almost immediately. Each day you rest in bed, you lose about 3 percent of muscle power. It's extremely important to get muscle tissue back to its ultimate level of rehabilitation.

Otherwise, you are at greater risk of reinjuring your knee."

Getting Stronger Safely

For real knee strength and stability, both the quadriceps (the big muscles on the front of the thigh) and the hamstrings (the muscles on the back of the thigh) must be strong, flexible, and balanced. If either is weak or tight, knee strength goes downhill, and injuries are more likely.

"We follow the two-to-one ratio," Dr. Fox says. "If you can lift 20 pounds with your quadriceps (doing a straight-leg, or thigh, extension), you should shoot for 10 pounds with your hamstrings (doing a curl)." To do a straight-leg extension, sit in a chair or on a weight-training machine, bend your knees, and raise your weighted leg straight out in front of you until it is parallel to the floor. To do a curl, simply stand, holding on to a sturdy chair for support, and bend your weighted leg behind you at the knee. Dr. Fox cautions that if these moves cause pain, you should consult your doctor.

Both your legs should be about equally strong, says John A. Feagin, M.D., associate professor of orthopedics at Duke University Medical Center in Durham, North Carolina. "A more than 10 percent difference in strength means the weaker leg has a much higher chance of getting injured."

Strength is easy enough to measure using weight-lifting machines. A doctor can check your flexibility by using instruments that measure the angle of your joint. You can check your own flexibility using the leg-stretching exercise illustrated on page 444. If you can stretch far enough to touch your ankle on one leg but can reach only to midcalf on the other, you can easily figure out which hamstring muscles are tighter.

Agility and endurance are also important, doctors say, to maintain balance and to keep muscles from pooping out before the last dance. (Muscle fatigue is a major cause of knee injuries.) You can help restore agility by dancing or even imitating the fancy floor work that boxers practice to elude each other. Endurance comes simply from sticking to an activity for increasing periods of time—riding your stationary bike not just through the evening news but for the opening scenes of the sitcom that follows, or extending your usual neighborhood stroll to include an occasional jaunt to the other side of town.

Most good knee-rehab programs follow pretty much the same steps, experts say. How quickly you get better depends on the extent of your injury and your willingness to work. The program prescribed by your doctor will probably include the following routines.

Pain-free range-of-motion exercises. These are gentle exercises designed to nudge healing along. That means slowly straightening and bending the knee. This is done with your body weight off the leg, usually while you're sitting or lying down; sometimes a splint that allows you to bend your knee only partway is used. The splint can be adjusted to allow more movement as the knee heals. If your injury involved muscle tears, you may have to work for days or weeks to stretch the scar tissue enough to fully straighten your leg.

Exercises to reestablish strength. Start out with exercises that limit knee motion, such as straight-leg lifts for the quadriceps. (See the bottom illustration on page 201.) Another is the hamstrings exercise: While sitting on the floor, press down with first one heel, then the other, attempting against resistance to pull your leg toward your buttocks. (See the bottom illustration on page 205.) Follow strength building with gentle stretching.

Full range-of-motion exercises. These use your body's own weight, resistance against water, weight-lifting machines, or free weights. "You might use a progressive resistance weight-lifting machine such as Nautilus, for instance, to do straight-leg extensions and hamstring curls, or you might use ankle weights," Dr. Feagin says.

Endurance-building activities. These include exercises that target leg muscles like the quadriceps and hamstrings—bicycling, stair-climbing machines (such as StairMaster), walking, or running.

Exercises that get the rest of your body back into shape. These also provide cardiovascular training. You can do brisk walking, bicycling, swimming, jogging, stair climbing—any activity that makes you huff and puff—as long as your knees enjoy it, too.

A gradual return to normal activities. You should resume walking, going up and down stairs, carrying groceries. If your normal activities have included knee-threatening sports such as break dancing or skateboarding, though, you may be advised to retire while you can still walk.

Snap, Crackle, and Pop

Knees, of course, can do more than open and close. They *can* twist and rock-and-roll—but only within limits. Rotate them or move them sideways more than ¼ inch, and ligaments start to complain. Twist far enough, and you have a partial ligament tear. Twist too far, and you can actually feel—and hear—your ligament pop. Many football players and skiers know that sickening sound all too well.

The ligament on the outward side of your knee, says Dr. Fox, is often damaged—usually a minor injury that does not require medical care.

The ligament that crosses inside the joint itself is often torn in contact sports, during a fall that twists the knee. It's estimated that at least 50,000 ligament tears occur each year in the United States just among skiers. Toss in a few football, basketball, and soccer players, along with a healthy share of out-of-shape "weekend warriors," and you've got a virtual epidemic of popping, flailing knees.

Most partial ligament tears heal well with rest and the kinds of strengthening and stretching exercises described earlier for quadriceps and hamstrings, Dr. Fox says. When done early on, these exercises help a joint heal better, with less constricting scar tissue.

Restoring muscle strength after a ligament tear actually helps to heal partially torn ligaments, says Dr. Feagin. "On a microscopic level, we can see that the diameter of ligaments increases with muscle mass," he says. That means exercise that makes your muscles bigger and stronger is doing the same thing for injured ligaments.

Later, weight-lifting exercises to strengthen leg muscles can partly compensate for weakness and instability caused by the ligament tear. These exercises are done with progressive resistance weight machines, such as Nautilus, and include straight-leg extensions and hamstring curls. Or they can be done with ankle weights. If you're very weak, these movements can be done without weights. The weight of the limb itself provides a certain amount of resistance.

Severe tears are usually repaired surgically, followed by exercises to regain strength, endurance, and flexibility.

Strong quadriceps and hamstrings will help protect knees under normal use and even under some hard use, but don't expect strong muscles to save a knee mangled by a ski that doesn't release during a fall or by a tumble with a 250-pound tight end, Dr. Fox says. The best way to avoid those injuries is to play it safe.

Off-Track Pain

Ligaments are not the only knee parts that cause problems. Kneecaps also take their share of abuse, and often they're first to sound the alarm when something goes wrong, says Dr. Fox. Torn ligaments or damaged cartilage can first appear as kneecap pain.

Deterioration of the cartilage on the undersurface of the kneecap, a condition called chondromalacia (and one of several kinds of knee pain known as "runner's knee"), is also a common cause of kneecap pain.

"Dancers and weight lifters who perform deep knee bends and people whose feet tend to roll toward the inside develop this condition," Dr. Fox says. Arthritis or a long-forgotten injury can also roughen up kneecaps.

Crackling sounds or a grating feeling when you bend your knees may be a tip-off. Pain usually hits both knees, occurring first after running, hiking, or prolonged sitting. Pretty soon you'll be looking for an aisle seat in theaters and airplanes, because you'll have trouble sitting with your knees bent for any length of time.

Tightening and toning your quadriceps can help relieve kneecap pain, Dr. Fox says. Try the straight-leg lift, which strengthens thighs without kneecap stress. The same exercises can help keep a dislocated kneecap on track.

Until the pain subsides, you should steer clear of squats, leg presses, lunges, stair climbing, kneeling, and bent-knee quadriceps stretches.

Inflammation—pain and swelling—hits knees in two common spots, tendons and bursa, and often in tandem. (For information on how to deal with these conditions, see "Bursitis and Tendinitis" on page 92.)

Subject any bone to enough pounding, pumping, or twisting, and it'll crack. Runners, cyclists, and aerobic dance instructors can develop tiny fractures of the femur or kneecap, injuries that produce an intense pain just above or in front of the knee.

"Stress fractures need a very carefully supervised rehabilitation program," Dr. Fox says. He recommends gentle activities that don't force your knees to support your full weight, such as biking and swimming, range-of-motion exercises to keep knees flexible, and strength-maintaining isometrics.

Even when surgery is necessary to correct a knee problem, exercise is always part of the prescription for healing. And when the need for surgery is not clear-cut, as it may be with a partial ligament tear, say, or a wayward kneecap, physical therapy may restore the joint well enough that surgery is permanently sidestepped, says Dr. Fox.

Meeting Your Knees' Needs

Stable, good-for-the-long-haul knees rely on leg muscles, tendons, and ligaments that are strong yet flexible. Like shock absorbers in a car, these support structures help reduce knee joint wear and tear.

The following exercises are designed to strengthen the muscles on the front of the thigh (quadriceps), the muscles on the back of the thigh (hamstrings), and the muscles that help control sideways movement (hip abductors). Since knee pain can be caused by many things, it's best to work with a doctor to determine exactly what kinds of exercises *you* need to do.

Some bent-knee maneuvers put pressure on the knee, causing pain and possible injury. So if it hurts even a little bit, stop!

The exercises included here strengthen muscles without much leg bending. Weight lifting builds muscle quickly—that's why some of the exercises call for ankle weights.

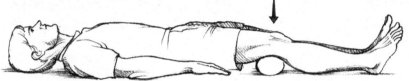

Lie on your back on the floor and place a rolled towel under one knee. Press the back of your knee into the towel without lifting your foot. Work up to ten repetitions. Repeat with the other knee.

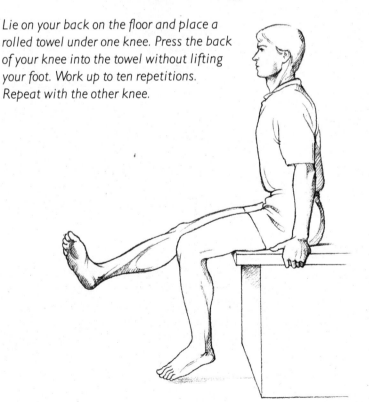

Sit on a chair, a sturdy table, or a kitchen counter. Lift one foot toward the ceiling, first with your foot held straight, then with your foot turned in as shown, then with your foot turned out. Lift, hold, and lower your foot slowly. Work up to ten repetitions in each position. Repeat with the other leg. When you can do this comfortably, use ankle weights to strengthen your knees further.

Meeting Your Knees' Needs—Continued

Sit on the floor with one knee bent and the other leg extended. Tighten the thigh muscles of the extended leg and hold for 2 seconds, then lift your foot about 6 inches and hold a few more seconds. Lower your leg and rest 3 seconds before performing the series once more. Switch legs and repeat.

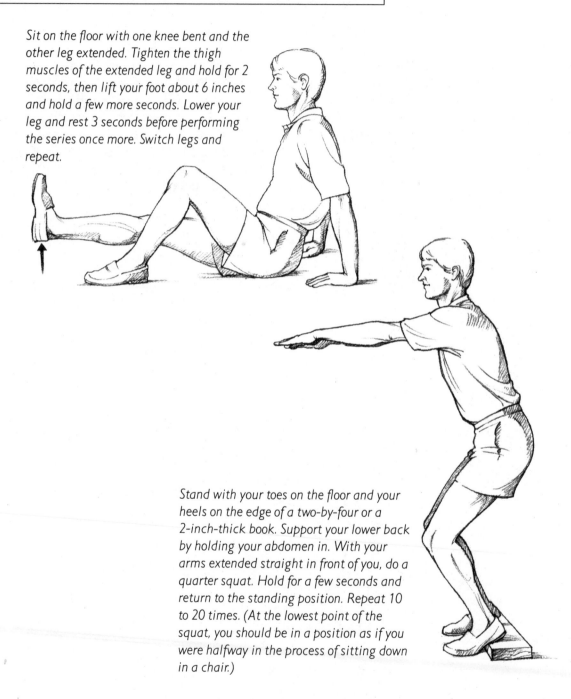

Stand with your toes on the floor and your heels on the edge of a two-by-four or a 2-inch-thick book. Support your lower back by holding your abdomen in. With your arms extended straight in front of you, do a quarter squat. Hold for a few seconds and return to the standing position. Repeat 10 to 20 times. (At the lowest point of the squat, you should be in a position as if you were halfway in the process of sitting down in a chair.)

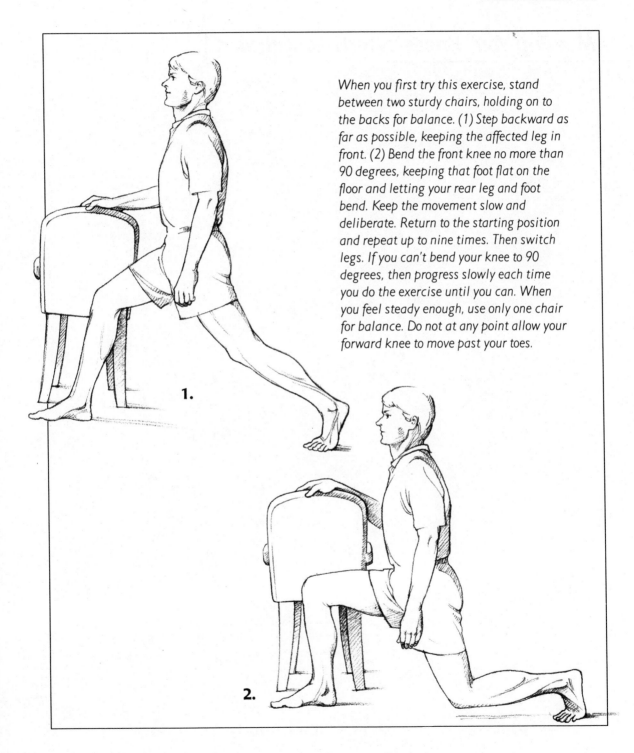

When you first try this exercise, stand between two sturdy chairs, holding on to the backs for balance. (1) Step backward as far as possible, keeping the affected leg in front. (2) Bend the front knee no more than 90 degrees, keeping that foot flat on the floor and letting your rear leg and foot bend. Keep the movement slow and deliberate. Return to the starting position and repeat up to nine times. Then switch legs. If you can't bend your knee to 90 degrees, then progress slowly each time you do the exercise until you can. When you feel steady enough, use only one chair for balance. Do not at any point allow your forward knee to move past your toes.

1.

2.

Meeting Your Knees' Needs—Continued

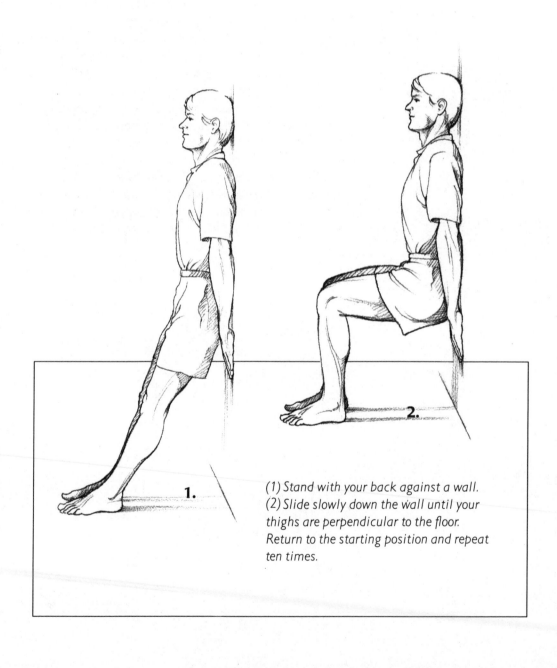

1.

2.

(1) Stand with your back against a wall.
(2) Slide slowly down the wall until your
thighs are perpendicular to the floor.
Return to the starting position and repeat
ten times.

Lie on the floor on your side with your lower leg bent. Slowly lift your upper leg 10 to 14 inches, keeping it as straight as possible. Hold for a few seconds, then slowly lower your leg. Repeat ten times, then switch sides. If the exercise feels easy, you can add ankle weights.

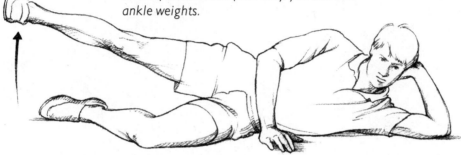

Sit on the floor with one leg extended. Bend your other knee and dig your heel into the floor and pull it slowly toward you. You should feel the muscles in the back of your thigh tighten. Pull for a full 10 seconds, relax for 5, and repeat. Repeat with the other leg.

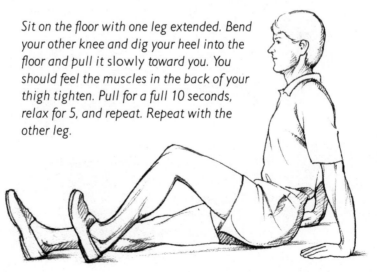

Meeting Your Knees' Needs—Continued

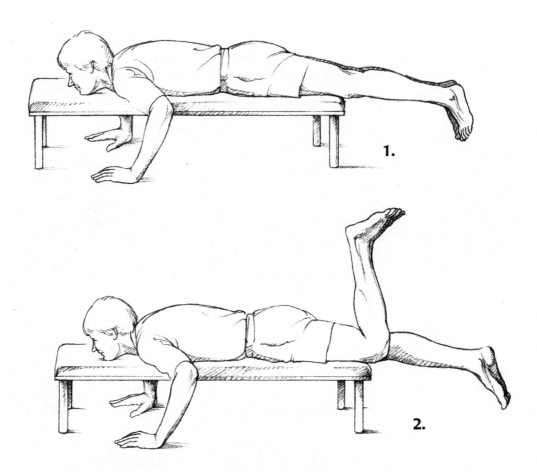

(1) Lie on your stomach on a bed or bench. Be sure your knee is positioned at the edge of the bed or bench as shown. (2) Bend your knee 90 degrees, then lower it slowly. Repeat up to ten times. Repeat with the other leg. Use ankle weights as your knees become stronger.

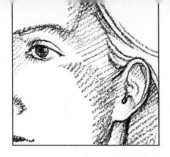

Low Self-Esteem

When you're suffering from low self-esteem, you can easily feel like a bit player in a terrible play, like you're a lousy employee, lousy lover, lousy *everything!*

And no, you don't care to exercise, thank you. "What good would it do *me?*" you ask. No way are you going to join some health club where all the guys resemble decathlon champions, where all the women look like the sun-bronzed creatures you see on the cover of *Shape Magazine.* With your body? Fat chance!

Of course, you may genuinely believe all these things, but experts who've studied low self-esteem insist those kinds of ideas aren't based on reality. "Reality," they say, is a state of mind, and when you've convinced yourself that you just don't cut the mustard, your view of things can truly be distorted.

On the other hand, studies show there's a strong link between physical movement and what goes on in your mind.

The Feel-Good Prescription

When you exercise, it triggers a chemical reaction in the brain that makes you feel good. Even though your body doesn't change immediately, you quickly begin to like yourself. And when that happens, all the worries and fears of inadequacy start peeling off that bruised psyche of yours. You become more confident at work, at home, and in relationships with friends and loved ones.

"I've seen people go from being withdrawn sourpusses to actually having a smile on their face—*after just 10 minutes of exercise!*" says psychologist Tom Collingwood, Ph.D., director of programs at the Institute of Aerobics Research in Dallas. "In fact, I maintain that once you exercise to the point of breaking a sweat, it's impossible to be depressed at the same time."

There's strong evidence that "the more you get involved in physical activity, the more your sense of well-being, value, and self-esteem goes up," says Dr. Collingwood.

"I've worked with some people I'd call real 'ruptured ducks.' They're unfit, obese, uncoordinated, and afraid they'll stumble all over themselves on the gym floor. But once they see even a little improvement, suddenly they're feeling good," he says. "They're saying, 'You know what? I feel good about *me.*' "

Researchers have racked up a body of evidence over the last decade or so that demonstrates a veritable cornucopia of esteem-boosting benefits that exercise offers. Various studies have found that it may help you think more clearly and move more efficiently and energetically. It can increase your sense of power, reduce your anxiety level, make you more creative, and actually increase your mental performance. No wonder it boosts your self-esteem!

So what actually happens inside your body to make all these great things occur? Some researchers have found that exercise causes the brain to manufacture the substance epinephrine, known to be a mood elevator. Others link exercise to higher levels of endorphins, one of the brain's natural opiates associated with pain reduction and increased pleasure.

One study done at the Stanford University School of Medicine measured the effect of aerobic exercise on the sense of well-being in 120 healthy but sedentary middle-aged men and women. After completing a six-month aerobic training program, not only did the participants show a significant increase in confidence and sense of well-being, but their tension and anxiety were also reduced. They even slept more soundly.

In another study, researchers at San Jose State University in California measured the self-concept of students who had jogged regularly for 15 weeks. "We were delighted to find that there was a significant increase in self-worth in about 70 percent of the students, though it was more prevalent with women than men," says psychologist Thomas Tutko, Ph.D., who helped conduct the study. "It was amazing to see how much more students valued themselves after completing the exercise."

Getting Started: One Step at a Time

Because self-esteem is linked to the personal challenges you set for yourself, you should begin an exercise program slowly, advises sports psychologist Bruce Ogilvie, Ph.D., professor emeritus at San Jose State. Stick your toe into the water. Check out the temperature.

"People with low self-esteem don't have confidence," he says. "They're afraid to take something like a Jazzercize class. They'll say, 'People are going to see me trip over my feet. They'll think I'm a fool. They're going to see the folds of skin over my hips.' "

His suggestion? Work with a private training coach three times a week. "Executive women have responded beautifully to this," he says. "It's a warm, supportive situation where someone cares about your progress."

But what if you can't afford the luxury of a private trainer? "Form a walking support group," Dr. Ogilvie suggests. "Get three or four of your friends to meet every morning at 6 o'clock at the bridge, or the grocery store, or the big oak tree on the corner. Make it an opportunity to talk and socialize. For someone with low self-esteem, social support is a very, very powerful tool."

And when you're walking, be sure to take long, healthy strides. Don't slump. Smile. Look straight ahead, not at the ground. Studies show that the *way* you walk can affect how you feel about yourself.

While walking is the best way for physically unfit people to start exercising, Dr. Ogilvie says the biggest danger is that you'll stop because you're bored.

"The best kind of exercise is one that plays on your intrinsic need for something joyful, something aesthetic," he says. "Take my wife and me—we're in our seventies.

We got into mountain biking late. But the visual experiences of going through the mountain trails and coming up on a lake, seeing a magnificent deer or a rabbit thumping along the path are lovely extra rewards that can be a function of the activity itself."

Here are a few more tips.

Says Dr. Tutko: "If you're serious about changing how you feel, make a contract with yourself. Buy an appointment book and schedule three or four 'appointments' a week to walk or jog. It must be a real commitment, because habits take about six months to form."

Reward yourself. "When I first started jogging, it was kind of like, 'What the hell am I doing out here?'" Dr. Tutko laughs. "It didn't make any sense. So I decided to reward myself in two ways. When I got up to the 1-mile mark, I treated myself to a foreign beer I liked, and I set aside a dollar to start saving for a new pair of running shoes. Of course, when I eventually worked up to more miles, I had to limit myself to two beers," he says, "but I then phased that out because I felt so good."

Get creative about keeping track of your progress. Dr. Tutko recalls how every week a friend of his used to tally how many miles he'd run. Above his desk he hung a map of the world. After totaling his mileage, he'd draw a line on the map equal to the distance he'd jogged.

"This guy actually knew how far he'd run around the world. It was a great way of visually presenting what he'd accomplished," says Dr. Tutko.

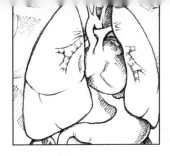

Lung Disease

You've just made a great drive off the 16th tee— 200 yards straight down the center. You drive your cart near the ball and are walking briskly toward it when your chest tightens and you become short of breath. "Oh, no," you moan. "Now I can't even play *golf* any more."

It's an all-too-common scenario. People with lung diseases like emphysema and chronic bronchitis frequently stop doing any activity but those that are absolutely necessary—because exertion leaves them gasping for air. Well, limiting your activities is the *worst* thing you can do, because in the long run, it could make the problem worse.

If you're an exerciser with lung disease, don't stop working out, doctors warn. If you do, within a year you can become so out of shape that a walk to the grocery store will feel like a trek up a mountain.

With continued inactivity you could descend into "the spiral of deconditioning." That means that your breathing muscles become progressively more weakened until you barely have the energy or lung power to drag a comb through your hair.

"The way to break the cycle of deconditioning is through regular exercise," says Donald Mahler, M.D., associate professor of medicine and chief of the Pulmonary Section at Dartmouth-Hitchcock Medical Center in Lebanon, New Hampshire.

Exercising reconditions your breathing muscles so you can take deeper breaths, boosting the oxygen level in your blood. You'll stay healthier and have more pep to garden, drive balls down the fairway, or take a vacation.

"I swear by exercise," says Christena V. Rath of Chicago, whose mix of emphysema, bronchitis, and asthma left her unable to walk across the living room without gasping for air. "Pushing the vacuum cleaner once was a terrible chore," she says. "I stopped visiting my daughter because I felt I was going to pass out climbing up her stairs."

A year in an exercise program that focused on regaining breathing power at the Rehabilitation Institute of Chicago has helped Rath do all the things she thought she would never do again. "Now I walk to the grocery store, carry the bags myself, and climb the stairs to my daughter's without stopping to catch my breath even once," she says.

Breathe with Your Belly

Better breathing starts with toning up the diaphragm, your primary breathing muscle. This dome-shaped muscle, located below your rib cage, moves down when you inhale and up when you exhale. But if you have chronic lung disease, your diaphragm becomes flat and flabby.

Here's why. Lungs damaged by emphysema or bronchitis lose their elasticity; they can no longer deflate fully or push the stale air out completely. The air sacs bulge with trapped air and press down on the diaphragm, preventing it from doing its job. With the diaphragm out of commission, you begin to rely on the less effective upper chest muscles to breathe.

Furthermore, damaged airways can become clogged with mucus and may close down when you exhale. You breathe fast and shallow, trapping even more air.

"Diaphragmatic breathing helps push the stale air out of your lungs so you can take a deeper breath of fresh air," explains Cynthia Kane, R.N., clinical director of the Pulmonary Rehabilitation Program at the Rehabilitation Institute of Chicago. "With enough practice, diaphragmatic breathing could help eliminate shortness of breath entirely."

To do diaphragmatic breathing, lie down (when you get better at it, you can try it sitting up). Place one hand on your abdomen just below your ribs and one on your chest. If you are breathing correctly, the hand on your belly will move out when inhaling, and the hand on your chest will stay still.

As you master diaphragmatic breathing, try this powerful variation: Inhale through your nose, allowing your belly to move out. Now exhale through pursed lips as if you are going to whistle. Taking an extended exhale will further eliminate the trapped air from your lungs. Try breathing in for 2 seconds and out for 4 seconds.

It may feel strange, but this little exercise actually helps you learn to breathe more efficiently, according to Francois Haas, M.D., Ph.D., director of the Pulmonary Function Laboratory at New York University Medical Center in New York City and author of *The Chronic Bronchitis and Emphysema Handbook.* One theory is that the pressure from breathing out against pursed lips opens the airways and helps them release more trapped air.

There are many other methods to help you learn slow, deep breathing, says Dr. Haas. Yoga is one of them. Singing is another. Playing a wind instrument is yet another. "For example, you need a nice, deep breath and long exhale to hold the notes while playing a flute," he says.

However you learn diaphragmatic breathing, practice it until it becomes second nature. (See "Yoga" on page 480 and "Breathing Therapies" on page 333.)

Power Up Your Breathing

It's also helpful to strengthen the other muscles associated with breathing.

"People with lung disease tend to rely on the chest and shoulder muscles to breathe; these muscles become overworked and weak," says Kane. "As a result, they have the most shortness of breath with tasks involving raising their arms."

Studies show that exercising the upper-body muscles can help boost your reaching power and may put more oomph in your breathing.

"I have patients do 15 minutes of arm movements that mimic real-life tasks," says Kane.

Here are two of her recommended exercises.

Stand and hold a broomstick horizontally in front of you, placing one hand at each end of the stick. Slowly raise the stick above your head as you exhale, keeping your arms straight.

Now slowly lower the stick behind your head as far as possible. Reverse the sequence. Repeat eight times.

To strengthen your upper body, use two 1-pound soup cans or plastic detergent bottles, which you can gradually fill with more water or sand as your strength increases. Lie on your back with your arms straight out to the sides in a T position and grasp one weight in each hand. As you exhale, slowly raise the weights straight up over your chest. Gently lower the weights back to your sides, keeping your arms straight. Repeat eight times.

Weight training that concentrates on developing strength in the upper body can also help strengthen these muscles, as can rowing. (See "Resistance Training" on page 404 and "Rowing" on page 418.)

Walking for Endurance

Strengthening your upper body will help you breathe better, but if you want more pep to clean the house, grocery shop, and tend your roses, your best bet is to walk—every day. "Walking builds up the muscles you use to get around," says James Couser, M.D., director of Pulmonary Rehabilitation at the Rehabilitation Institute of Chicago.

Plus, walking is an excellent cardiovascular activity, helping your respiratory muscles become more efficient at using more oxygen. That means your heart and lungs don't have to work as hard.

You can walk indoors at a climate-controlled mall, where frosty air and smog can't further impair your breathing.

Before starting a walking program, get a referral from your doctor or the American Lung Association for a facility offering exercise and pulmonary function tests. These tests tell you how much exercise your heart and lungs can tolerate.

Start by walking as far as you can without getting short-winded. Breathe with your diaphragm. Try to walk every day, increasing your distance a few feet each day until you're up to half-hour walks.

If you get winded, rest and do pursed-lip breathing. Some shortness of breath is fine, says Dr. Mahler, but stop if you experience severe shortness of breath. (For information on how to start a walking program, see "Walking" on page 458.)

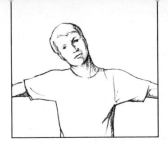

Medications and Exercise

*I*t's seconds before the exciting blast-off of the Top-of-the-Hill Mallwalkers Charity Chase, and you're ready to go. You're wearing your neon crinkle full-split racing shorts, your "Walk Your Buns Off" tank top, your fanny pack and water bottle, your wrap-around shades, your lighter-than-air walking shoes, and your "nitro" patch firmly stuck to your chest. In fact, it's the transdermal drug patch that's allowing you to pace the mall in the first place.

Being on medications for a heart condition, diabetes, or high blood pressure often makes the difference between not being able to exercise at all and leading a normal, active life. But drugs and exercise *do* interact, in ways that can be good or bad. That's because both can affect blood flow, body temperature, and other important functions.

Take blood pressure, for instance. Both drugs and exercise can lower blood pressure, and together they make it drop even lower. That's why people who begin to exercise often can soon reduce their dosage of blood pressure medication. Heart rate, on the other hand, is kept under control by certain medications that can hold it at a fairly constant pace even when *you're* going at full steam. So if you're taking this

type of drug, it wouldn't make any sense for you to try to reach your target heart rate (a measure of exercise intensity often advocated for people participating in aerobic dance and other forms of endurance exercise). In fact, for you to attempt to reach your original target heart rate might be dangerous, explains Douglas McKeag, M.D., professor of family practice and coordinator of sports medicine at Michigan State University's College of Human Medicine in East Lansing.

Knowing how the drugs you're taking interact with exercise can help you get maximum benefit from an exercise program while avoiding dangerous situations.

This chapter examines some potentially troubling drug/exercise interactions and ways to sidestep them. On the plus side, we've also noted when exercise can tame a drug's side effects. (As a general rule, if you are taking any kind of medication, you need to discuss your exercise program with your doctor.)

Stand Up, Black Out

The idea is to anticipate this sort of thing: You've just swum ½ mile in the pool. You climb out, grab your towel, and head for the locker room. Suddenly you're dizzy and weak; your heart starts racing. You feel like you're going to pass out on that cold, wet tile floor.

So you ease yourself down on a nearby bench. In a minute or two, you feel fine again.

So what happened?

Some drugs, especially those that reduce blood pressure, make it harder for your body to maintain normal blood pressure when you're exercising. You may have a sudden drop in blood pressure when you change from a head-down to a head-up position, a response known as orthostatic hypotension. Or you may develop temporary low blood pressure when you stop exercising, a condition called postexercise hypotension, says Dr. McKeag.

With orthostatic hypotension, blood pressure usually returns to normal quickly and remains normal for as long as you are upright. If your pressure doesn't return to normal fast enough, you might experience dizziness or faint.

With postexercise hypotension, blood pressure must adjust to the sudden cessation of activity.

Doing slant-board sit-ups, some kinds of weight lifting, aerobic dancing that involves bends and dips, or any other sport where you quickly change from a head-down to a head-up position can set the stage for orthostatic hypotension. So can simply getting out of bed, which no doubt qualifies as exercise for someone recovering from a lengthy illness. And any kind of vigorous exercise can lead to postexercise hypotension.

Often, diuretics prescribed to lower blood pressure by reducing the volume of fluid in the blood can be a cause of hypotension. Blood pressure drugs that keep blood vessels dilated (beta-blockers and some other new drugs) can also cause

these symptoms. The reason? They slow blood vessels' natural tendency to constrict when you stop exercising, and your heart rate drops.

Antidepressants and some major tranquilizers can also affect blood pressure. So can antiangina drugs, drugs to control chest pain, drugs that control heart rhythm disturbances, antihistamines, and sleeping pills, says Arthur Jacknowitz, Pharm.D., chairman of the Department of Clinical Pharmacy at West Virginia University School of Pharmacy in Morgantown.

If you feel faint when you stand up or right after exercising, see your doctor. Your doctor will take your blood pressure once while you are lying down and then again as soon as you sit up. A significant drop in systolic pressure (the top number in the blood pressure reading) is considered a firm diagnosis of orthostatic hypotension. This means you may need to reduce your dose of a diuretic or change to a different drug, Dr. Jacknowitz says.

To prevent after-exercise wooziness (postexercise hypotension), you've got to decrease your heart rate gradually, Dr. McKeag says. "I have people cool down for at least 5 minutes, at one-half to one-quarter of their peak exertion." If you're running, you may want to switch to a slow jog, then brisk walking for a few minutes before you stop, for example. Your heart rate and breathing should be close to normal before you head for the shower.

Too Hot to Trot

Feeling faint is not the only symptom that exercise can induce when you're on medication. Overheating can also be a problem. Picture this: You're out jogging on an early summer morning. Suddenly, it feels like the Mojave Desert, and you, quite frankly, are beginning to feel like breakfast for a flock of vultures. Your head is pounding, you're weak and nauseated, and your surroundings are taking on a miragelike murkiness. You need an oasis, quick!

Some drugs make it harder for your body to throw off the heat generated by exercise. They slow sweating, which helps you cool down as the moisture evaporates from your skin. Or they interfere with vasodilation, a cooling process wherein blood vessels relax, allowing more blood to flow to the surface of the skin, where heat dissipates into the air. These drug actions can cause heat exhaustion, or even heatstroke—especially if you overdo it on a hot day.

Lots of drugs can turn up the heat. Antidepressants, some tranquilizers, some ulcer drugs, antihistamines, and glaucoma drugs all have what are called anticholinergic properties. That means that they interfere with body secretions, including sweating. (They can also cause a dry mouth, constipation, and difficulty urinating.) Some tranquilizers interfere with the brain's ability to regulate body temperature. This means that they can cause not only heatstroke during hot, dry periods but also frostbite during times of low environmental temperature. Chemotherapy drugs, antibiotics, decongestants, and some cardiac drugs interfere with sweating or vasodilation. Diuretics help the body eliminate excess body fluids and minerals. If you eliminate too much of these essential components because you're taking a diuretic *and* sweating through an

intense workout, you can easily become dehydrated and overheated or chilled. Also take extra precautions whenever the humidity is high during a heat wave. When the relative humidity gets over 60 percent, the air won't absorb as much sweat as your body needs to get rid of, and at 75 percent relative humidity, it won't absorb any. When combined with high temperatures, this can be particularly dangerous.

If your workout makes you feel weak, dizzy, and sick, you should stop exercising, find a cool, shady spot to rest, drink fluids, wet yourself down with cool water, and ideally, catch a breeze. If your body doesn't respond promptly to these measures, you may need to seek emergency medical attention.

It's best to avoid getting overheated in the first place, doctors agree. If you are taking any medications that might turn up your body's thermostat, you should exercise during the coolest part of the day or in an air-conditioned gym. Drink plenty of fluids before, during, and after your workout. And dress in layers you can peel off as you warm up. It might be a good idea to team up with a buddy who can help you stay out of trouble, at least while you're exercising.

If you're taking a diuretic, you have to pay particular attention to mineral loss. Sweating during a workout can deplete your body of four important minerals known as electrolytes—sodium, potassium, magnesium, and calcium. (All can be depleted by sweating, exercise, and diuretic drugs.) Low levels of these minerals can produce muscle cramps, fatigue, and heart irregularities.

"Drinking plain water can just make things worse if electrolyte levels are low," says Maryl Winningham, R.N., Ph.D., an exercise physiologist who works with cancer patients at the University of Utah College of Nursing in Salt Lake City. "I tell my patients to also have V-8 or tomato juice, or chicken soup, which are good sources of sodium and fluids."

People with heart disease, though, should stick with plain water or a potassium-enriched sports drink, Dr. McKeag says. "For safety, make sure the water is tepid and not ice-cold. Ice-cold water can be a stimulus to cardiac arryhthmia in some individuals. Sodium supplementation usually is not considered necessary or advisable in heart patients."

To avoid dehydration, drink 8 fluid ounces (1 cup) of water before exercising, 4 ounces every 15 minutes while exercising, and 4 ounces when you finish, suggests Dr. McKeag.

Pooped Out

Certain medications can also have a strong impact on your endurance. The experience would play out like this: A few weeks ago, you were scaling that big hill behind your house in 30 minutes or less. Now you barely get halfway up, and you're so weak and weary you can hardly drag your tail home. "Hmm," you say to yourself, "could it be that new drug I'm taking?" Yes, it could.

Many things can make you get tired quickly when you exercise—heart or lung disease, diabetes, and just plain sedentary lifestyle for starters. But so can drugs.

If you were exercising for a certain amount of time at a certain level of intensity before you started taking a drug, but find that you now can't go as long or as hard, your new medication may be responsible.

"Just about any drug has the potential to cause fatigue," says Dr. Jacknowitz. Those high on the hit list include chemotherapy drugs, which can cause anemia a few days to a few weeks after therapy, and alpha- and beta-blockers, which blunt the increase in heart rate that normally occurs with exertion. Antidepressants, antibiotics, and anti-inflammatory drugs are also known to drain energy reserves.

Tailor your exercise program during the time you are undergoing chemotherapy or taking an antibiotic, Dr. Jacknowitz says. If you must take a drug long-term, you may find your body adjusts after a few weeks and your energy picks up again. If it doesn't, ask your doctor about adjusting the dosage or trying a different drug that provides the same benefits with fewer tiring effects.

Running on Empty

Some drugs are designed to lower blood sugar. Since exercise can lower blood sugar, too, the combination can lead to hypoglycemia, or too-low blood sugar. The body runs mostly on glucose—sugar broken down from the foods we eat. When blood glucose levels drop too low, we slow down, sometimes very abruptly. (For more information about exercising while taking medication for diabetes, see "Diabetes" on page 138.)

Besides diabetes drugs, beta-blockers can contribute to hypoglycemia, Dr. McKeag says. If you're taking these drugs, your doctor may advise you to have a light snack—such as crackers and orange juice—just before you begin your workout.

You're more likely to develop low blood sugar when you first begin an exercise program, says Tim Rickabaugh, exercise physiologist at the St. Vincent Diabetes Center in Indianapolis. As you become more fit, it's less likely to happen.

Out of Rhythm

Some drugs can contribute to heart arrhythmia, a slower- or faster-than-normal heartbeat during exercise. With these drugs in your system you might pull on your jogging shoes and head out the door only to find your heart pounding even before you break a sweat.

Drugs meant to correct arrhythmia sometimes *cause* the condition when you're exercising, says David Lowenthal, M.D., Ph.D., professor of medicine, pharmacology, and exercise science at the University of Florida College of Medicine and director of the Geriatric Research Center, both in Gainesville.

Antidepressants and some drugs that lower cholesterol can also cause heart irregularities that may worsen with exercise.

Much of the benefit of aerobic exercises such as brisk walking comes from their ability to temporarily increase your heart rate. Medication that you take to maintain your heart rate at an even level—such as beta-blockers—keep your heart rate from rising too much during a workout. That doesn't let you off the hook in terms of exercise, however. You can still benefit, Dr. Lowenthal says. "You'll still develop im-

proved oxygen uptake and gain muscle strength," he says.

People taking beta-blockers need to lower their target heart rate 20 to 30 beats per minute, Dr. McKeag says. (To determine your ideal heart rate—what it should be if you weren't taking medications—see "How Good Is Your Workout?" on page 324.) Dr. Lowenthal prefers his patients who take beta-blockers to simply slow down when they start to feel out of breath.

If you're at risk for heart arrhythmia, you should exercise under medical supervision, Dr. Lowenthal cautions.

Tied Up in Knots

Some drugs can contribute to the development of muscle cramps during or after exercise. You know how it feels when you're breezing along, minding your own business, and your leg suddenly decides it has had enough for the day. Your calf cramps up, and you have no choice but to hobble over to a wall, where you attempt to stretch, rub, and coerce the gnarly muscle into relaxed submission.

If you are taking diuretics, they can lead to dehydration or an electrolyte imbalance, specifically by causing the loss of potassium. Diuretics can cause leg or stomach cramps, or both. If there is a significant loss of potassium, a diet high in this mineral may be helpful. Foods high in potassium include fresh fruits and vegetables, especially oranges, tomato juice, and bananas.

If you experience muscle cramps regularly while you're exercising, see your doctor, Dr. McKeag says. Drinking enough fluids, pacing yourself, doing a warm-up beforehand and a cool-down afterward all

MEDICATIONS AND EXERCISE

Medications affect the body. So does exercise. Taken together, medications and exercise can work together. Exercise enhances the body's ability to use any medication, for example. When you exercise while taking glucocorticoids (powerful anti-inflammatories), the physical activity reduces muscle wasting, and for those receiving chemotherapy, exercise can reduce nausea. But drugs and exercise can also work against each other. This table can help you determine what impact the medication you are taking may have on your body when you're exercising. If side effects are likely, you don't have to stop working out. Just ask your doctor about adjusting your dosage or altering your exercise routine to compensate.

Medication	Possible Side Effects
Alpha-blockers (for heart and high blood pressure)	Fatigue
Antibiotics	Fatigue Tendency to become overheated
Anti-depressants	Fatigue Irregular heartbeat Light-headedness Tendency to become overheated
Antihista-mines	Light-headedness Tendency to become overheated
Anti-inflam-matories	Fatigue
Beta-blockers (for heart and high blood pressure)	Fatigue Irregular heartbeat Light-headedness

Medication	Possible Side Effects
Chemotherapy	Fatigue Tendency to become overheated
Decongestants	Tendency to become overheated
Diabetes medications	Fatigue
Diuretics	Light-headedness Muscle cramps Tendency to become overheated
Glaucoma medications	Tendency to become overheated
Heart medications	Tendency to become overheated
Sleep aids	Light-headedness
Tranquilizers	Light-headedness Tendency to become overheated
Ulcer medications	Tendency to become overheated

make muscle cramps less likely to occur. A condition called intermittent claudication can also cause what feels like a muscle cramp. (See "Intermittent Claudication" on page 186.)

Sidestepping Side Effects

A number of medications, it seems, have the ability to complicate your best-laid exercise plans. Sometimes, however, exercise helps banish uncomfortable side effects.

Chemotherapy is notorious for its side effects, including hard-to-control nausea. So in a recent study, researchers were pleased and surprised when women with breast cancer reported that riding a stationary bicycle relieved their nausea. The effect started within a few minutes of beginning the exercise and lasted most of the day, says Dr. Winningham.

Exercise can also circumvent two nasty side effects of a drug sometimes used for arthritis or severe allergies—glucocorticoids (cortisol). Research suggests that either aerobic exercise or strength training reduces the muscle wasting and weight loss that occur with the use of this drug.

Banishing certain side effects is not the only payoff for exercising, however. Medications sometimes work better if you exercise regularly, says Dr. McKeag. The increased blood flow that exercise produces helps speed delivery of a drug to every part of your body, he says.

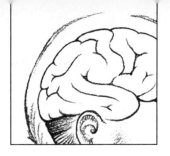

Memory Problems

You might remember your first kiss but not have a clue where you parked your car when you came to work this morning. You can rattle off the names of the entire cast of *Gone with the Wind*, but you don't remember the name of the movie you watched last night. The image of a childhood friend easily flashes into your mind, but you can't recall her name.

Yes, our memory lets us down at the most inopportune times—and more often than we'd like to admit.

"There isn't anyone who can remember everything," says Pierre Haber, Ph.D., director of the Psychology Society in New York City. "The amount of material that we forget is very large because the brain can't store everything that we see, hear, or touch every day."

Remembering absolutely everything is not a realistic goal, but some researchers believe that you're less likely to forget if you remember to get out there and exercise. This doesn't mean your memory is at its best *while* you're exercising.

"If anything, it becomes harder and harder to remember things while exercising because you're depleting your oxygen supply," says Bruce W. Tuckman, Ph.D., professor of educational research at Florida State University in Tallahassee.

Exercise can do for the mind what it does for the body—that is, energize and revitalize.

"Some time after you're done with your workout, you can suddenly think of those things you've been trying to remember," says Dr. Tuckman. Exercise, it seems, has the ability to clear the blocks that are preventing you from accessing your memory. "There is some sort of reorganization going on in the mind during exercise," he suggests.

"Exercise does appear to have an effect on cognitive [thinking] ability," says Louise Clarkson-Smith, Ph.D., of Scripps College in Claremont, California.

In a pair of studies, Dr. Clarkson-Smith and Alan A. Hartley, Ph.D., compared 62 physically active adults aged 55 to 91 with an equal number of sedentary people in the same age group. The active group included walkers, weight lifters, and marathon runners. Both the active and inactive participants were evaluated in a series of tests that measured reasoning, reaction time, and memory.

The researchers found that the exercisers did significantly better on all of the reasoning and reaction-time tests. They also outperformed the sedentary group on two of the three memory tests.

"I think this study strongly suggests that exercise may be important in preserving our mental abilities as we get older," says Dr. Clarkson-Smith.

Holding On to What You Have

Scientific studies leave little doubt that our short-term memory—the ability to recall new information—erodes as we age, particularly after age 50. But scientific studies also demonstrate that exercise can help improve short-term memory in older people.

One study, done at Ohio State University in Columbus, looked at 72 people who rode stationary bicycles three times a week for nine months. People participating in the study (average age 63) were divided into two groups. The first did moderate exercise, which elevated their heart rate to 75 percent of their maximum capacity. The second group did light exercise, which raised their heart rate to about 50 percent of maximum capacity.

Surprisingly, *both* groups showed significant improvement in mental abilities, says researcher Joanne Stevenson, R.N., Ph.D., professor in the College of Nursing at Ohio State University. The researchers found that exercise substantially improved attention span, concentration, short-term memory, and other measures of higher brain function.

In another study, researchers at the Veterans Affairs Medical Center in Salt Lake City found that brisk walking seems to jog the memory of forgetful adults. Over a four-month period, sedentary people aged 55 to 70 were randomly assigned to groups that did fast walking, strength and flexibility training, or no exercise at all.

"We found memory and other cognitive measures from the walkers improved significantly," says Robert Dustman, Ph.D., author of the study. "There was a bit of improvement for the strength and flexibility group, but not nearly as much as for the walkers."

In contrast, the nonexercisers showed no improvement at all, Dr. Dustman says.

Another study looked at memory in 20 older men, aged 50 to 70. Some of the men had run at least 25 miles a week for the previous five years. The rest didn't exercise regularly. To measure their short-term memory, researchers asked the men to listen to two sequences of numbers that were broadcast simultaneously through headphones. For example, a subject might have heard "1-3-9" in his left ear and "2-7-8" in his right. His task was to recall both sets of numbers. The runners more accurately remembered the numbers than the nonexercisers.

Sharpen Your Powers of Observation

There also is evidence that physically active people may have better visual recall than nonexercisers. Researchers at the University of Alabama in Birmingham studied 105 sedentary and active men aged 18 to 73. The active group included several marathoners, triathletes, and a world champion long-jumper. The men were asked to examine three cards with printed designs for 10 seconds and then to draw the designs from memory. Then 30 minutes later, they were asked to draw the designs from memory again.

The physically active participants were better able to recall the designs than their inactive counterparts.

"Quite honestly, part of the difference may be because the active people have to use their mental apparatus more," says David Roth, Ph.D., associate professor of psychology at the University of Alabama. "They have to use their visual memory to remember such things as their running routes. So it may be they're using those skills a lot more often than the people who aren't running around town."

Another factor is that exercise may increase blood and oxygen flow to the brain.

"As you become more aerobically trained, the body becomes more efficient at transporting and utilizing oxygen, so you're getting more oxygen to the neurotransmitters in your brain," says Dr. Dustman.

Put Balance in Your Life

So what types of physical activity might improve your memory and provide some mental health benefits as well? Some researchers believe that aerobic exercise—the kind that gets your blood pumping—is the best. Biking, walking, and running are at the top of the list. (To find out how to participate in any of these exercises, see the appropriate chapters in part 2.)

Even a modest walking program— 20 minutes a day, three times a week—can be beneficial, says Dr. Tuckman.

"You don't have to walk fast, but you should feel like you're exercising," he says.

Aerobic workouts, however, aren't the only type of exercise that leads to better memory and mental health in general. Exercise such as weight lifting may have some beneficial effects on emotions, too, says Dr. Roth.

"The main requirement of exercise for promoting psychological well-being is that it's healthy for you and leads to noticeable changes," according to Dr. Roth.

"It used to be thought that you needed a high level of aerobic fitness to get mental health benefits from exercise," Dr. Stevenson adds. "What we've learned over the past five years is that you don't have to kill yourself with exercise to get the benefits. There are beneficial effects from low levels of exercise," says Dr. Stevenson.

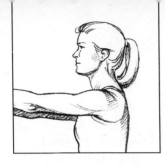

Menstrual Problems and PMS

Month after month, year after year, it was always the same. The week before she began menstruating, Gail Schlack's mind and body went into what she remembers as "utter chaos."

"I'd dissolve into tears over nothing, fly into a rage if somebody so much as looked at me cross-eyed," she recalls. "For a solid week, I was puffy and bloated and miserable. If I'd been a horse instead of a woman, they would have shot me out of pity!"

Gail, a Rochester, New York, business-woman, finally realized her "premenstrual jitters" were out of control the day she wrestled the last box of Pampers on the supermarket shelf out of another customer's grip.

"I had a wet kid at home and needed them badly. I yelled, 'Okay, buddy, this is it. Gimme those Pampers.' Then I rushed out of the aisle thinking, 'You're going crazy.' "

A consultation with her physician amounted to this advice: "Take some Midol. You're getting your period."

"The Best Medicine We Know"

Years later, Gail enrolled in a judo class "just for fun." Before each session, the class did warm-up exercises, stretches, and jumping jacks. Within a week, she says,

she felt great. And she noticed she was less irritable the week before her period. And within four months, her premenstrual symptoms and cramps were dramatically reduced.

"I think of all those times I felt like Beulah the Witch," she says, only half-jokingly. "How come doctors know how to transplant hearts but couldn't figure out that exercise could help me?"

Well, medical researchers are still figuring out how to relieve the symptoms of both PMS (premenstrual syndrome) and menstrual problems. But experts now agree that exercise is one way to deal with both.

"Without any question, regular exercise plays a major role in improving certain menstrual symptoms," says Joseph Mortola, M.D., a psychiatrist at Beth Israel Hospital in Boston. "It's the best nonpharmacological medicine we know of."

Do You Have PMS?

You've no doubt heard PMS mentioned a lot—in newspapers, on television, in off-color jokes—giving the idea that every woman in America has "it." But if you're a tad touchier than normal, or even cry during the week before your period, does that mean you suffer from PMS?

Absolutely not, says Jerilynn C. Prior, M.D., associate professor of endocrinology at the University of British Columbia Faculty of Medicine in Vancouver.

"These 'symptoms' are simply a natural physiological result of ovulation," she says. "In fact, if you *didn't* experience some changes, you'd have a problem. PMS has become a convenient label that reflects the tendency of our culture, and the male-dominated technology of medicine, to make diseases out of anything that relates to women's reproduction."

In fact, one doctor says, only two out of ten women who think they have PMS actually do.

The difference between normal premenstrual changes and PMS is intensity, says Dr. Prior. Also, to be diagnosed with PMS, your symptoms must occur before *every* period and be totally absent the remainder of the month. These symptoms include water retention, irritability, mood swings, cravings for high-carbohydrate foods, headaches, backache, abdominal bloating, and breast tenderness.

Stopping Your Body's "Mini-Heroin Withdrawal"

There are conflicting theories about what causes PMS. Experts have blamed the monthly roster of unpleasant symptoms on hormonal imbalance, vitamin B deficiency, or low levels of certain neurotransmitters (the chemicals that carry messenges from brain cell to brain cell). But one of the most widely accepted theories may also explain why exercise can help relieve the symptoms. One particular kind of neurotransmitter—the beta-endorphins—is chemically related to opium.

Our body's own beta-endorphins can supply us with a natural "high" that suppresses pain and generally makes us feel good.

About a week prior to menstruation, beta-endorphin levels naturally decrease. We experience a kind of "mini-heroin withdrawal," says Dr. Mortola. "The withdrawal symptoms from opium and PMS symptoms are very similar—irritability, anger, depression."

So what's this got to do with exercise? Plenty. Researchers have shown that after 20 minutes of exercise, beta-endorphin levels increase dramatically. This natural "fix" wipes out the withdrawal symptoms associated with PMS. With regular exercise over time, these endorphins build up, and your PMS symptoms go down.

But whether it's extra endorphins or some other factor that's ultimately proven to be behind exercise's effectiveness, the fact that it *is* effective is scientifically indisputable.

In a study at the University of British Columbia, for example, Dr. Prior and her associates asked nonexercising women to begin a running program. After six months, the women were running 1 mile a day. Not only did these women experience significant decreases in water retention and breast tenderness, but they also reported fewer premenstrual symptoms overall.

Symptom-Specific Exercise Routines

So what are the most effective exercises if you have premenstrual symptoms?

"Any aerobic exercise," says Susan Lark, M.D., author of *Premenstrual Syndrome*

Self-Help Book. "Walking, jogging, tennis, and aerobic dancing are particularly effective in helping you avoid fluid congestion in the breasts and abdomen. Aerobic exercise definitely stabilizes mood swings and decreases irritability and anxiety." Dr. Lark recommends that these be done *in moderation,* no more than three or four times a week, for about 30 minutes each time. She also recommends the two "extremely useful" yoga positions described below in the section on cramps.

Stair climbing, bicycling, swimming, and using a rowing machine are also effective, says Dr. Prior. But if you're not a big exerciser, she advises starting out with a program that lasts no longer than 15 minutes daily. Be sure to check your heart rate, though. The exercise won't be terribly effective if you don't get it above 130. (To determine your maxiumum heart rate, see "How Good Is Your Workout?" on page 324.)

Putting the Crimp on Cramps

There was a time, not that long ago, when one of the "cures" for painful cramps was to wipe out your reproductive system altogether—130,000 complete hysterectomies were performed on women *solely* to eliminate menstrual cramps.

While this procedure was no doubt effective in eliminating women's complaints about cramps—they're caused by contractions in the uterus—medical science offers a less drastic form of relief these days. Because uterine contractions are triggered by the chemical prostaglandin, there are antiprostaglandin drugs on the market that usually can treat the problem with few side effects.

But what about natural remedies? The answer, some experts believe, may be gentle exercise. (Just make sure the cramps are caused by menstruation, not some serious underlying disorder such as endometriosis. See your physician if debilitating cramps continue month after month.)

"To relieve the pain of cramps, do exercises that encourage gentle stretching," says Dr. Lark. The most effective exercises for cramps and related symptoms such as stomachaches and backaches are those that relax you *and* your muscles, she says.

"Yoga positions are wonderful for cramps," she says. "Any easy movement that stretches the spine and the pelvis is good."

Here are the yoga postures that Dr. Lark prescribes to relieve menstrual discomfort.

The child pose. "This is one of the best exercises for cramps," says Dr. Lark. "I have patients who absolutely swear by it."

To get into this posture, sit on your heels with your arms relaxed at your sides. Bend over until your forehead touches the floor. Make sure your spine is stretched and your body is totally relaxed. Close your eyes while breathing slowly and deeply. Do this for about a minute or for as long as you're comfortable.

The sponge. "This is a really simple exercise that helps not only cramps but also premenstrual irritability and anxiety," says Dr. Lark. To soak up the relaxing benefits of this posture, lie on your back with your arms and legs spread-eagled. Relax your body and close your eyes. Very slowly inhale and exhale. Do this for as long as you're comfortable.

Cramp Chaser

The emotional side of premenstrual syndrome (PMS) is tough enough to contend with without having to deal with cramps and abdominal discomfort as well. Here are a few moves to help you ease the cramping and get through that difficult time of the month.

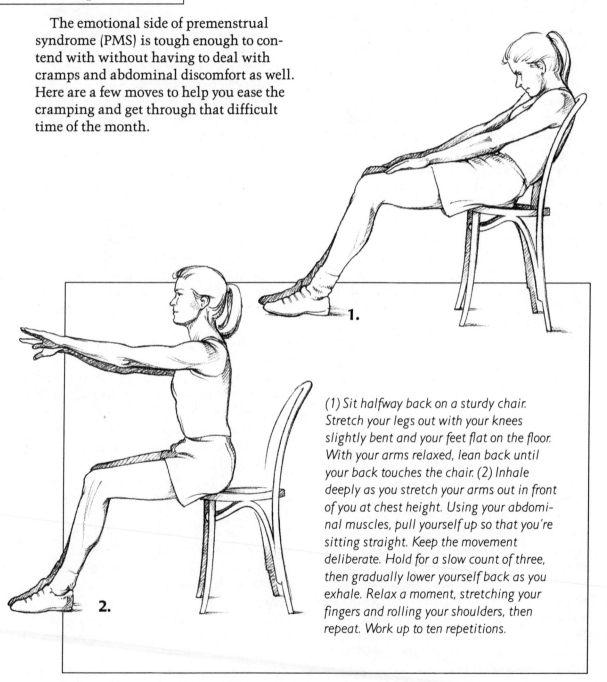

(1) Sit halfway back on a sturdy chair. Stretch your legs out with your knees slightly bent and your feet flat on the floor. With your arms relaxed, lean back until your back touches the chair. (2) Inhale deeply as you stretch your arms out in front of you at chest height. Using your abdominal muscles, pull yourself up so that you're sitting straight. Keep the movement deliberate. Hold for a slow count of three, then gradually lower yourself back as you exhale. Relax a moment, stretching your fingers and rolling your shoulders, then repeat. Work up to ten repetitions.

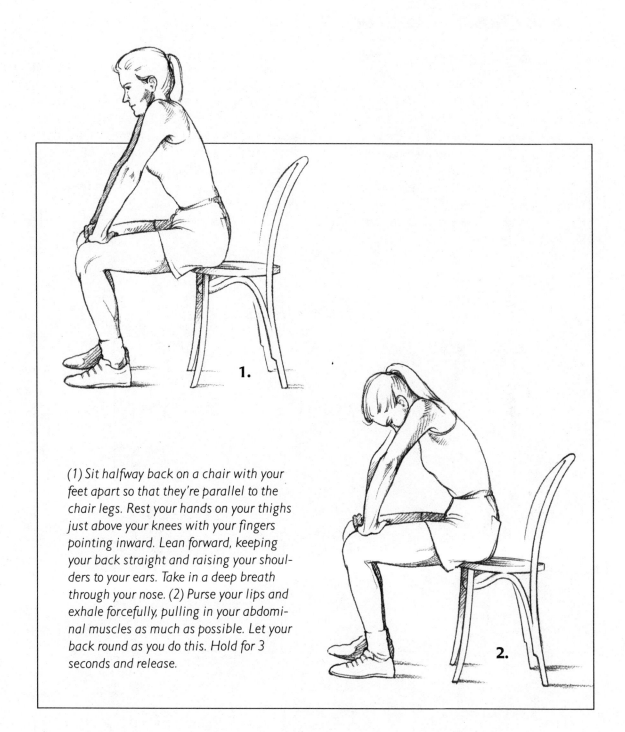

(1) Sit halfway back on a chair with your feet apart so that they're parallel to the chair legs. Rest your hands on your thighs just above your knees with your fingers pointing inward. Lean forward, keeping your back straight and raising your shoulders to your ears. Take in a deep breath through your nose. (2) Purse your lips and exhale forcefully, pulling in your abdominal muscles as much as possible. Let your back round as you do this. Hold for 3 seconds and release.

Cramp Chaser—Continued

(1) Stand with your back and heels against a wall. (2) Inhale and bend your knees, tuck in your buttocks, and pull in your abdominal muscles to flatten your lower back against the wall. You will need to contract your muscles strongly. Hold this position for a count of five as you exhale, then hold a few more seconds. Increase your holding time as you are able.
(3) Inhale as you straighten your knees and arch your back. Alternate from the flat-back to the arched-back position, beginning with five repetitions and working up to ten. (Do not do this exercise if it causes back pain.)

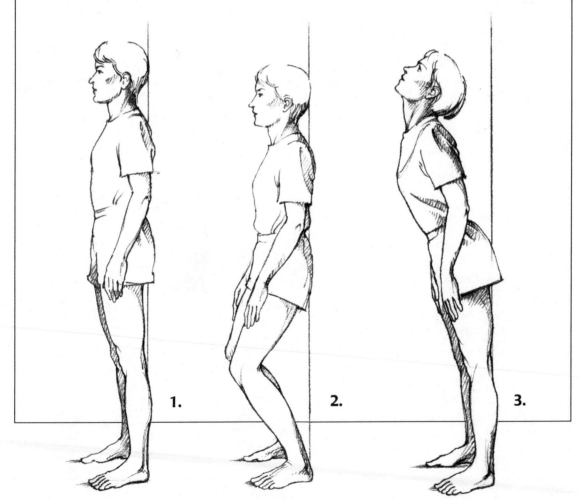

1.   2.   3.

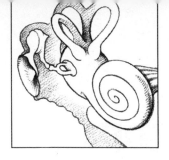

Motion Sickness

Look up, then down—at first slowly, then quickly, 20 times. Then look from side to side—at first slowly, then quickly, 20 times.

Gentle exercises like these may be one way you can prevent seasickness when you can't take medication or it isn't available. Called Cawthorne's Head Exercises (named after the 1930s British surgeon who devised them), they're designed for people who are prone to dizziness.

Cruise Control

"If you practice them before a cruise, you may help train your body and your brain not to become dizzy," says Christopher Linstrom, M.D., assistant director of otology at the New York Eye and Ear Infirmary. "If you do them during or after the cruise, they may help reestablish your sense of balance."

According to the doctor, since the nausea of seasickness is often closely related to dizziness, preventing the dizziness may help prevent the churning stomach for many people.

"I'm not aware of any studies that prove these exercises work for seasickness, but many specialists in the field prescribe them and report success," says Dr. Linstrom. The exercises aren't meant to be a substitute for medication but may be worth a try when medication isn't an option.

You can do these exercises anytime, except when you're already dizzy or seasick. In that case, just lie down. If you feel motion sick without feeling dizzy, these exercises will probably not help you. Here are a few more of them.

Nodding the head. Slowly, then quickly, bend your head forward, then backward, with your eyes open, 20 times. Turn your head from one side to the other slowly, then quickly, 20 times. Repeat with your eyes closed.

Shrugging it off. While sitting, shrug your shoulders 20 times. Turn both shoulders to the right, then to the left, 20 times. Now bend forward and pick up objects from the ground and sit back up 20 times.

Up, down, up, down. Change from sitting to standing and back again, 20 times. Do this with your eyes open, then repeat the routine with your eyes closed. (It's okay to open your eyes if you feel yourself losing your balance.) Now throw a small ball from hand to hand above eye level.

Keep on moving. Walk across the room with your eyes open, then closed, 10 times. Walk up and down a slope with your eyes open, then closed, 20 times. Repeat this on steps. (Hold on to a railing for the shut-eyed portion of this exercise.)

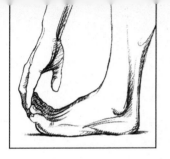

Muscle Cramps

*I*t felt as if someone had shoved a hot harpoon up the back of my calf," says dancer and dance instructor Karen Carlson, recalling a particularly bad muscle cramp suffered during a dress rehearsal. She blames the cramp on fatigue and stress coupled with a failure to warm up properly. The result: pain so severe it affected her dancing for the next three nights.

What's a Cramp?

If you have ever been yanked from sound sleep by a charley horse in your calf, you know about Karen's distress: Sudden muscle cramps, such as the ones that clamp on to your leg in the middle of the night, are usually excruciating (if short-lived).

These painful, involuntary muscle contractions can occur in almost any muscle at almost any time. The most common form attacks unsuspecting muscles at rest or between bouts of exertion.

Why do cramps often wait until you're sleeping to ambush you? It's not because they're sneaky. "When you're up all day, walking around, your ankle is at least a 90-degree angle," says Charles Norelli, M.D., physiatrist at Good Shepherd Rehabilitation Hospital in Allentown, Penn-

sylvania. "When you lie down, your toes point, your calf muscle shortens, and—boom—you cramp. The same thing happens when you're running around playing tennis, or you're in the pool. You step up, your toes point down, the calf muscle shortens, and—whammo—it cramps."

Ordinary cramps affect up to 95 percent of the population at some time. Fortunately, most ordinary cramps can be treated—and frequently prevented—through exercise.

How to Stay Cramp-Free

One of the first steps toward staying free of cramps (and injuries) is to add a warm-up routine to any new fitness program.

Warming up means gradually increasing your muscle temperature, breathing rate, and blood flow through controlled, easy motions. This readies the muscles for more aggressive stretching, working, or exercising, and it also aids flexibility, which many experts believe helps prevent injuries.

Any basic warm-up includes gently and gradually moving your spine, shoulders, and hips through their ranges of motion, without straining. The usual recommendation is to warm up until you feel loose and break a light sweat. This will take from 2 to 15 minutes, depending on your overall fitness, says Ronald Lawrence,

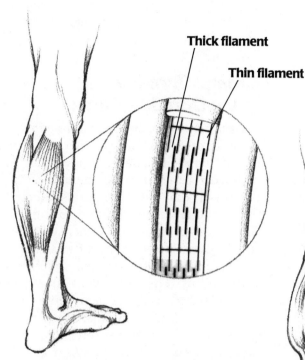

Thick filament

Thin filament

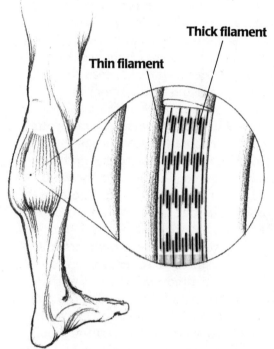

Thin filament

Thick filament

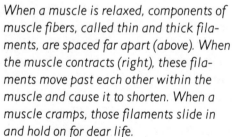

When a muscle is relaxed, components of muscle fibers, called thin and thick filaments, are spaced far apart (above). When the muscle contracts (right), these filaments move past each other within the muscle and cause it to shorten. When a muscle cramps, those filaments slide in and hold on for dear life.

M.D., founder of the American Medical Athletic Association and clinical professor at the UCLA School of Medicine.

Warm-up routines and subsequent stretching exercises are numerous and varied and should be geared to the type of sport or activity you intend to perform. (See the appropriate chapters in part 2.) One example of a very sport-specific warm-up is pedaling your bicycle with as

little resistance as possible (low tension if you use a stationary exercise bike) for a few minutes or miles before taking off on a trip or a race.

Don't Cramp Your Style

What if you're good and warmed up and you suddenly find yourself clamped by a cramp anyway? If the cramp affects your calf, the prescription for relief is to stay calm and encourage the muscle to do the same by gently stretching it into a relaxed state. "Walk gently," advises Colorado physical therapist David Balsley. Other experts call for gently stretching your toes toward your shin to lengthen the cramped calf muscle.

Stretches can serve as preventive medicine, as well as a treatment. "I recommend 'foot drop' exercises," says Leon J. Weiner, M.D., staff member of Holy Redeemer Hospital, Meadowbrook, Pennsylvania, and the Pain and Stress Center in Philadelphia. "While sitting, raise your toes so the weight of your feet is on your heels. After about 5 seconds, you'll feel a little discomfort in your ankle and calf. Lower your foot. Rest for 3 or 4 seconds, and repeat. Next, lift your heels off the floor while your toes stay planted. Hold for 3 or 4 seconds, then relax for 3 or 4 seconds." If you are prone to night cramps, you can do these exercises any time during the day, and almost anywhere. "With regular practice of this exercise, the muscle cramps will go away," says Dr. Weiner.

In fact, one group of 44 crampy people studied by Harry W. Daniell, M.D., clinical professor of family practice at the University of California, Davis, Medical School, became free from night cramps after one week of performing these simple calf stretches: Stand barefoot facing a wall, 2 to 3 feet away from it. With your palms against the wall, bend your arms and lean forward, keeping your heels flat on the floor, until you feel a "pulling sensation" in your calf muscles. Hold the stretch for 10 seconds, relax for 5 seconds, and repeat once. Do this gentle stretch three times a day, says Dr. Daniell, and if your cramps are the ordinary type, this practice should quickly relieve them.

Cramps Turn Up in the Darndest Places

Occasionally, ordinary cramps pay a visit to muscles around the rib cage, arms, or shoulders. The familiar "side stitch" is believed to be a cramped diaphragm—that's the muscle that helps the lungs do their job. For both preventing and treating upper-body cramps, Dr. Weiner suggests these moves: "Lie down on a flat, firm surface, such as the floor. Look straight up at the ceiling. Then move your arms out to your sides and over your head while still touching the floor." This maneuver can serve both as a warm-up exercise and for preventing and treating cramps in home exercisers at all levels of fitness. Gently stretching the areas where cramps might occur is the key, says Dr. Weiner.

If any cramps occur more than occasionally, it's time to enlist your physician's help to explore the possible causes.

"Muscle cramps should not keep people from exercise," asserts Marjorie Albohm, certified athletic trainer and director of sports medicine at the Center for Hip and Knee Surgery in Mooresville, Indiana. "For the most part, they can be prevented, are not that common, and should not be a detriment to good, sound physical exercise."

The Right Fuel

Other types of cramps, such as heat cramps and those caused by dehydration or overexertion, are sometimes exercise-related. They may also be prevented or treated with good exercise-related practices. Exercise, however, is not the only factor. Preventing cramps also entails proper diet, says Dr. Daniell. You must eat a balanced diet that provides protein, carbohydrates, vitamins, minerals, and other vital nutrients, he says.

"Work with your physician to design a diet that will fulfill your personal nutrient needs and to deduce other possible underlying diseases or conditions that are causing cramps," suggests Albohm.

"Some medications, such as diuretics, upset electrolyte [mineral] balance, and some people who take them are more likely to have leg cramps unless they take potassium or calcium supplements, but nobody has worked out the details of why that is so," says Dr. Daniell. "Certainly, a person taking a diuretic of any kind should make sure they get a lot of fruits and vegetables in their diet, because that's where they get their potassium. That's good advice for anyone."

A clear complement to healthy eating is getting enough fluids, especially when you're working out. Sweat is more than 99 percent water; when it flows freely, during exercise or work, it's important to refill your tank of vital fluids. This will prevent dehydration, heat exhaustion, and mineral imbalances in the blood—all of which may lead to cramping and other problems.

"Drink water to rehydrate and rebalance mineral concentrations in the body," Albohm says. Most experts agree, adding that sport and energy drinks are usually not necessary, because the minerals and other nutrients they contain can come from a balanced diet.

Gearing Up

Is there anything else you can do to prevent an onslaught of painful cramps? "One thing is to train adequately," says physical therapist Balsley.

"In other words, if you're going to run a marathon in hot weather, and you've only trained in cold weather, there's a good chance you'll get a cramp. If you want to run in the heat, you've got to train in the heat."

Exercise experts say that gradually adapting to and preparing for whatever conditions you are going to exercise in—heat, cold, rain, high humidity—will help stave off both injuries and cramps.

Unclench Those Cramps

Surely you've had your share of memorable muscle cramps. There's the foot cramp that sidelined you during your first college soccer game, the cramp in your buttock that almost crippled you during the charity dance marathon, a nasty hamstring cramp that spoiled the second day of your long-awaited ski vacation, and one doozy of a calf cramp that hits you every time you take off your dancing shoes.

Muscle cramps are always a shock, aren't they? You're busy pursuing fun that you waited for all week—or all year—and the next thing you know, your body turns on you with a vengeance. There is blessed relief from muscle cramps, however, and it's as easy as one-two-three. One: Let out a yelp. (It's good for the soul.) Two: Grab the offending body part. And three: Keep these stretches in mind.

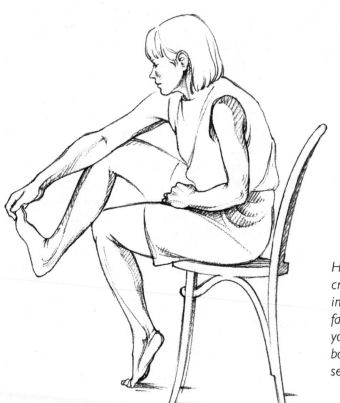

Here's stretch for quick relief of calf cramps. You'll probably already be kneading that calf, so just reach down a little farther and grasp the ball of your foot and your toes. Pull your foot up toward your body in an easy stretch. Hold for up to 25 seconds; you should feel the muscles relax.

To work out a foot cramp, place the tips of
your fingers under the tips of your toes and
pull back until you feel the stretch in the
foot muscles. Hold for a few seconds.

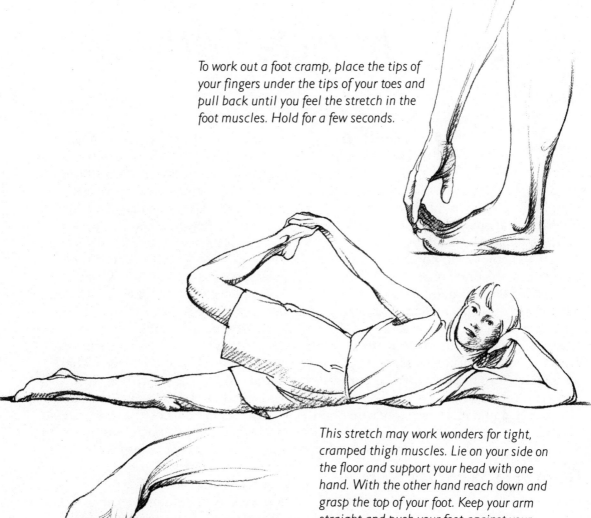

This stretch may work wonders for tight,
cramped thigh muscles. Lie on your side on
the floor and support your head with one
hand. With the other hand reach down and
grasp the top of your foot. Keep your arm
straight and push your foot against your
hand, while at the same time contracting
your buttocks muscles so that your hip
moves forward. Hold for 10 seconds.

To take the ache out of cramped
fingers, simply use the fingers
of one hand to push apart and
stretch the fingers of the other.

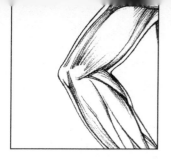

Muscle Pain

*I*t's a pain in the neck. It's a pain in the ankle. Sometimes it's a pain in the face, or in the thigh, or everywhere at once. It's chronic muscle pain, and it goes by the name myalgia, or myositis, rheumatism, fibrositis, fibromyositis . . . the roster of possible IDs is long. Many doctors prefer the term *fibromyalgia.* Medical scientists aren't quite sure what causes it. In some people, fibromyalgia is a condition unto itself; in others, it heralds future neural or muscular diseases. Two things about this curious syndrome are certain, however: The pain is very real, and it is relieved somewhat by exercise.

What It Is, What It's Not

Fibromyalgia is an as-yet mysterious affliction loosely characterized by pain or tenderness in one or more (usually more) groups of muscles or joints, along with stiffness and fatigue. "Fibromyalgia is muscle pain without any evidence of cause," explains Leon J. Weiner, M.D., staff member of Holy Redeemer Hospital, Meadowbrook, Pennsylvania, and the Pain and Stress Center in Philadelphia. In other words, fibromyalgia is *not* a sore shoulder that begins hurting after you paint the ceiling.

The pain of fibromyalgia—sometimes dull and achy, sometimes numb or tingling, sometimes so intense it is debilitating—is chronic, meaning it lasts for at least six months. It may mimic nerve damage at one time, a digestive disorder at another.

"A person with fibromyalgia may complain initially of a neck ache. Then I start poking around and their forearms ache. Then they're tender in the buttock, then in the back, then in the calf. Then all the areas are tender, and they tell me they can't sleep very well. Then they may have irritable bowel syndrome," says Charles Norelli, M.D., a physiatrist at Good Shepherd Rehabilitation Hospital in Allentown, Pennsylvania. It is not just lucky guesswork when a doctor knows just where to touch a patient to get a response like, "Ouch! That hurts." Doctors have a pretty good idea where a person with this condition is likely to harbor the pain.

Doctors also know that fibromyalgia is frequently accompanied by depression, yet they are uncertain whether depression precedes the pain or is caused by pain, Dr. Weiner says.

Gathering the Puzzle Pieces

Unfortunately, many fibromyalgia sufferers go from one doctor to another for a year or more before being diagnosed. So how do you know you have fibromyalgia?

You should see your doctor for any ongoing unexplained muscle pain. "The diagnosis is one of exclusion," says Dr. Weiner. "Begin with your family doctor and get a thorough medical 'workup.' If the x-rays, nerve tests, and blood tests are normal, and the behavior pattern is a certain way, it's fibromyalgia."

Treatment after these rigorous diagnostic tests may include heat therapy, massage, acupuncture, nerve stimulation, and injection of tender points with local anesthetic. All of these treatments may bring some temporary relief, but every one of them is said to be ineffective in the long run. So what really works? The answer: You do.

Exercise is one of the universal recommendations for people with fibromyalgia, whether their pain is mild or severe. And exercise can often stop mild pain from *becoming* severe, says Dr. Weiner.

Now many people with fibromyalgia may have poorly developed muscles and feel they're not equipped for exercise (as with depression, the experts don't know if weak muscle systems are a cause or effect of fibromyalgia). But poor muscle tone shouldn't stop them from exercising: People who exercise regularly—no matter what their muscle tone—usually experience the most improvement.

Regular aerobic exercise can also bring blessed relief from the restless sleep that is so common in fibromyalgia sufferers. Sound sleep, in turn, can reduce fatigue and can further break the pain/sleeplessness/fatigue/weakness cycle of fibromyalgia.

You'll have to work closely with your doctor or physical therapist to design a program of aerobic activity that will gradually create overall fitness. Brisk walking, swimming, and cycling are some of the low- or no-impact aerobic sports your doctor may recommend as part of your exercise regimen.

Stretch It Out, Too

Your program will undoubtedly include a stretching routine as well.

A daily, or several-times-daily, stretching routine is an important part of the path to living with and controlling the pain, says Dr. Weiner. Stretching feels good and can also help you avoid muscle injuries.

Your doctor or therapist will work closely with you to create a series of stretches designed to relieve your specific fibromyalgia pains.

Here are some examples of stretches you can do on your own. Before stretching, you may find it helpful to apply a hot compress to the area to be stretched to warm the area and make it more flexible, says Dr. Weiner.

To stretch a sore neck, begin by lying flat on your back on a firm surface. Place your right hand under your right buttock. With your left hand, reach across the top of your head to your right ear, then smoothly pull your head and neck to the left. Concentrate on stretching and relaxing the tight neck muscles as you do this. Hold for 6 seconds before allowing your head to return to the center position. Reverse arms and repeat the stretch on the other side of your neck. Breathe deeply between stretches to complete the muscular relaxation. Always stretch both sides of the neck equally.

To relieve pain in your hands caused by holding them in tense positions or by performing repetitive finger movements, practice the "artisan's finger-stretch exercise": First hold your hands at a comfortable distance in front of your face, with your palms away from you. Slowly form two fists by curling each finger, beginning with the pinkies, into position, ending with the thumbs folded over the index fingers. Complete the stretch by flexing your wrists and drawing your fists toward the insides of your elbows.

To stretch the muscles over the front of your rib cage, first stand in a narrow doorway. Raise your arms to a comfortable height and rest your forearms against the left and right doorjambs, palms facing forward. Place one leg in front of the other, bending that knee. Look straight ahead, keeping your head erect, and slowly and gently lean forward through the doorway, bending the forward knee further. Hold for only a few seconds. Relax and breathe deeply between repetitions. Raising or lowering the arms to various positions will stretch different sections of this vast sheath of muscles. With a little experimenting you should be able to home in on the painful area and give it a deep, relaxing stretch. (For additional stretches, see "Neck and Shoulder Pain" on the opposite page and "Stretching" on page 440.)

Pain, Pain, Go Away

Some people with fibromyalgia are in such pain by the time the syndrome is diagnosed that they cannot even raise their arms over their head. When a person is in this much pain, Dr. Weiner sends him or her to the kitchen as the first line of treatment. He has his patients begin cooking fresh foods at home and stop eating "junk foods" (which people in severe pain often rely on to avoid moving about a kitchen). He may also prescribe low-dosage antidepressants in some cases as sleep aids and to give the person's feelings a slight shove in a positive direction.

"Once the patients start feeling a little better, they can begin the exercises," says Dr. Weiner. For people in extreme pain, he recommends taking a hot shower or applying hot compresses to warm up the muscles and improve their diminished flexibility. He has them begin their exercise program by sitting in a chair and getting used to moving and stretching very gradually. "I ask them to do the simplest possible exercises first: Move your head from side to side; lift your arms over your head; bend forward, backward," Dr. Weiner explains. "Then I try to get them to walk. If they can't walk outside, they can walk in their house or apartment. Next, I encourage them to do measured walks around their neighborhood, gradually increasing their speed." It may take many months of work to rebound to this basic level of fitness.

What motivates people to work through such pain to get there? "It's fear," says Dr. Weiner. "I just tell them quietly, softly, 'If you don't keep doing these things, you're going to get worse.' If they listen to me, they get better."

Some physicians and physical therapists also recommend Eastern exercises, such as yoga or t'ai chi. (See "Yoga" on page 480 and "Martial Arts" on page 370.) Whatever routine you and your physician choose, remember that a more comfortable world awaits you on the other side of exercise.

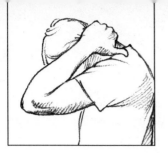

Neck and Shoulder Pain

Remember the kid in grade school who could never sit still? The one who wriggled and cavorted and always found some excuse to leave his desk?

Chances are *he's* not going home from work every day with an aching neck and sore shoulders (assuming he's still a fidgeter). Health-care professionals agree that sitting still or working in one position all day is a major cause of neck and shoulder pain.

"One of the biggest problems is that we're trained as children that the proper thing to do is sit still," says physical therapist Philip Tygiel of Tygiel Physical Therapy in Tucson, Arizona. "We train people to deny the natural urge to move around."

From keyboard operator to draftsman to truck driver, many of us are guilty of blithely carrying out those lessons we learned too well as schoolchildren. We sit or stand in one position all day—restricting our movements and wreaking havoc with our muscles, joints, and ligaments.

The result is often a stiff, sore neck and aching shoulders.

Many people suffer neck pain simply because they hold their neck in one position all day, says James Richards, M.D., an orthopedic surgeon at Matthews Orthopedic Clinic in Orlando, Florida. "As you go through the day those neck muscles don't relax, and that means they're going to get sore and stay sore," he says.

Muscles that aren't regularly moved tighten and shorten, and they also become tired under the constant strain. The muscles of your neck and shoulders are particularly vulnerable because they're hard at work holding up your head all day (unless you have the habit of nodding off at your desk). "They're not like the muscles of the arms and legs that are resting when you're not using them; they're continuously being used," says Edward A. Rankin, M.D., professor of orthopedic surgery at Howard University and chief of orthopedic surgery at Providence Hospital, both in Washington, D.C.

There are several things you can do to avoid those pains in your neck. First, take a close look at how you use your body in your day-to-day routines; you can probably make a number of small adjustments in how you move and work that will ease the strain on your neck and shoulder muscles.

Also, take care of your muscles and joints by taking frequent stretch breaks and by exercising regularly to maintain flexibility and strength.

De-stressing Your Routines

Stress on the neck starts early in the day, according to David F. Fardon, M.D., an orthopedic surgeon at Knoxville Orthopedic Clinic in Knoxville, Tennessee, and author of *Free Yourself from Neck Pain and Headache.*

To spare yourself the strain of leaning over the sink to shave or apply makeup, use a hand-held mirror or one that extends out from the wall. When you shave, don't throw your neck back; instead, use your fingers to pull your skin taut.

Okay, now you're in your car driving to work. While you may not think of driving as a neck-straining activity, it is. You have to hold your head erect and fairly rigid— there's a limit to how much you can waggle your head while driving. What you *can* do is make sure you don't lean forward excessively. Dr. Fardon recommends moving your seat forward so your knees are bent and your shoulder blades touch the seat back. If your steering wheel is adjustable, move it low and close to your body.

Work, however, is the real danger zone for many of us. People who work at video display terminals (VDTs) are at high risk for neck and shoulder pain because they hold their head and neck in precise positions for long periods of time. Altering your desk setup may help: You can move your keyboard so you don't have to lean forward, and elevate one foot on the rung of your chair or other object. Using arm supports may also help reduce muscle strain.

But it's not just VDT operators who suffer neck and shoulder pain. Anyone who sits or stands in one position can suffer, whether barber, writer, dog groomer, or nurse. Incorrect posture takes its toll, because standing or sitting incorrectly

puts a lot of stress on your neck and shoulders. (See "Posture Training" on page 387.)

Holding a phone receiver cradled against your shoulder so you have both arms free also strains the neck. Use a headset, or hold the receiver in your hand. You should also avoid stooping or bending, which can be tough on your back and neck.

Keep It Moving

Although eliminating undue stress and strain in your daily routine helps, what's crucial in maintaining healthy muscles and joints is *motion.* "Joints require movement for life; muscles require activity to remain viable," says Tygiel. Studies have shown that VDT operators experience fewer problems when they take exercise or stretch breaks, and experts agree that we're *all* better off moving around.

You say you're at a high-pressure job with no time to walk around or take exercise breaks? Tygiel recommends these easy exercises to prevent neck and shoulder pain—and you can do all of them sitting right at your desk. (For more exercises, see the illustrations on page 242.)

While sitting with your chin in and your neck straight, take a deep breath and drop your chin to your chest. Breathe out, and bring your head back to the starting position. Repeat ten times.

With your chin in and your neck straight, take a deep breath and bend your head as far as you can to the left (moving your ear toward your shoulder). Breathe out and bring your head back to the starting position. Repeat ten times on each side.

With your chin in and your neck straight, breathe in and turn your head as far to the left as you can. Breathe out and turn your head back to the starting position. Breathe in and turn your head to the right as far as you can. Breathe out and return your head to the starting position. Repeat ten times on each side.

To exercise and free your shoulders from tension, clasp your hands and raise them over your head with your arms straight. Repeat ten times. Another simple exercise—don't laugh—is to reach up and scratch the back of your head with one arm. Now lower your arm, reach behind you, and scratch the small of your back. Do this exercise ten times, then repeat with the other arm. These will take your shoulders through most of their normal range of motions.

You should do these at least once a day, and up to three times a day if you've been experiencing stiffness, says Tygiel.

Dr. Fardon recommends a simple "chin wipe" exercise: Rub your chin along your chest from one shoulder to the other, as if there were something under your chin that you wanted to wipe off.

While flexibility is more crucial than muscle strength in avoiding neck and shoulder pain, well-conditioned muscles may help you resist injury. To strengthen shoulder muscles, you can do "shoulder shrugs" against resistance: While seated with your feet flat, hold approximately equal weights in each hand (a couple of books will do) and slowly lift the weights by shrugging your shoulders.

What to Avoid

If you have seriously limited shoulder motion (say you can't raise your arm up past your shoulder) or are in pain, you shouldn't try exercises on your own, Tygiel warns. "If you use the wrong exercise, it can aggravate the condition," he says. What you need are specific exercises prescribed by your doctor or physical therapist.

And stop if you experience dizziness while doing exercises, Tygiel advises.

Realize that sharp pains or severe stiffness in your shoulders may result from other problems, such as tendinitis, bursitis, or arthritis. (See "Bursitis and Tendinitis" on page 92 and "Arthritis" on page 18.) In general, if your problems persist past a week or ten days, seek professional advice.

One symptom you should always get checked out immediately, however, is pain in your left shoulder that appears for no discernible reason. Some heart problems refer pain to the left shoulder. "It's worthwhile to have a doctor check it out," says Tygiel.

Most of your day-to-day neck and shoulder aches and pains, however, have a simpler origin and can be prevented—if you'll forget those childhood "sit still" lessons and just keep moving around.

Stretch into the Comfort Zone

Stiff neck and shoulders? Whether your problem stems from sitting too long in one position, an overdose of tension, or a combination of the two, you can avoid this painful condition by remembering to break your daily routine with stretching. Stretching not only helps prevent the stiffness that results from lack of motion, it also improves the flexibility of your muscles and tendons and your range of motion.

Experts recommend doing stretching exercises at least twice a day, and more often if possible.

If you're troubled by dizziness, however, or have severe pain (rather than just stiffness), consult your doctor before trying any of these exercises.

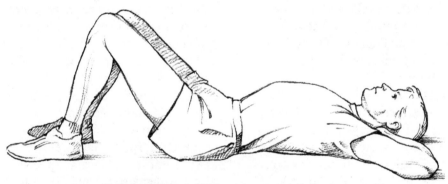

To help loosen tight shoulder muscles, lie on the floor with your hands clasped behind your head and your elbows touching the floor. Slowly try to bring your elbows together above your head. Hold for 6 seconds and return to starting position. Repeat three times.

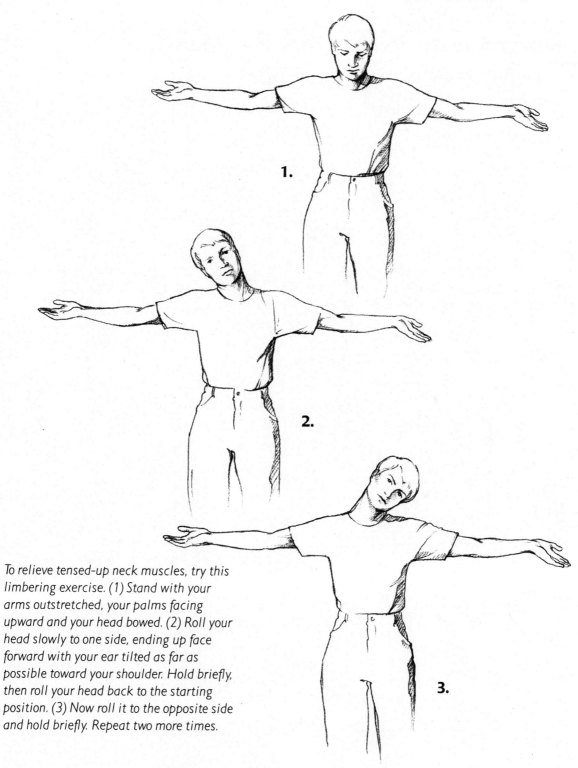

To relieve tensed-up neck muscles, try this limbering exercise. (1) Stand with your arms outstretched, your palms facing upward and your head bowed. (2) Roll your head slowly to one side, ending up face forward with your ear tilted as far as possible toward your shoulder. Hold briefly, then roll your head back to the starting position. (3) Now roll it to the opposite side and hold briefly. Repeat two more times.

Stretch into the Comfort Zone—Continued

(1) Sit in a straight-backed chair and clasp your hands behind your head. Stretch your elbows back, pressing on your hands slightly with your head. Hold for 6 seconds. (2) Now bring your elbows forward and down and bend your head forward. Hold for 6 seconds before returning to the starting position. Be careful not to stretch too far in either direction—just enough to feel the muscles relaxing. Repeat three times.

1.

2.

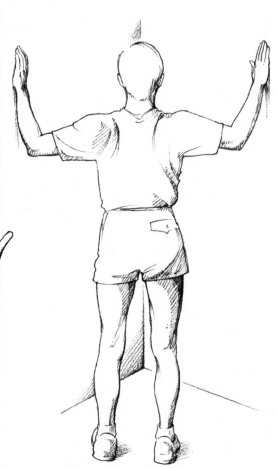

Stand in a corner of a room or facing an open doorway, with your elbows bent and your hands on the wall on each side of the corner or doorway. Bend your knees slightly and lean forward with your whole body, feeling the stretch in your shoulder area. Hold for 6 seconds and return to starting position. Repeat three times.

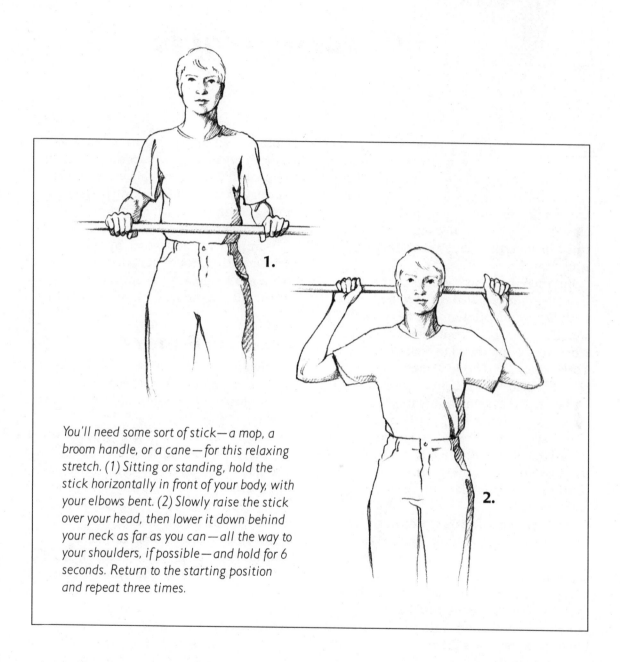

1.

2.

You'll need some sort of stick—a mop, a broom handle, or a cane—for this relaxing stretch. (1) Sitting or standing, hold the stick horizontally in front of your body, with your elbows bent. (2) Slowly raise the stick over your head, then lower it down behind your neck as far as you can—all the way to your shoulders, if possible—and hold for 6 seconds. Return to the starting position and repeat three times.

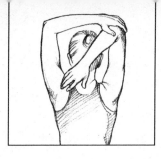

Osteoporosis

At age 69, Baltimore real estate agent and artist Baylis Love was an ad man's dream . . . the kind of svelte, classy, model-beautiful woman who's featured in advertisements geared to older Americans.

But then the bone fractures began. The first when she tumbled while roller-skating with her grandchildren. The next when she slid on her bathroom tiles. And again when she bent forward to pick up the *New York Times.* Finally, doctors confirmed her fears: She had "brittle bones"—osteoporosis.

"I'd been confident all my life," says Baylis, now 78, in a soft, southern drawl. "Then suddenly, I found myself terrified I'd fall out of my half-inch heels. And terrified to cook Thanksgiving dinner because lifting that darn turkey could crack my ribs!"

She experienced years of excruciating bone breaks—and years of ineffective treatments. "I felt like Alice in Wonderland, just running in place to stay the same." Exasperated but determined, she decided to enroll in a treatment program at Baltimore's Union Memorial Hospital. And that's when her life started to turn around.

Slowly, the number of fractures diminished. And today, she says, "Eureka! They've stopped altogether!"

Baylis and her physicians attribute her improvement, in part, to an important factor in preventing osteoporosis: exercise. Coupled with estrogen replacement therapy, her treatment includes taking brisk walks of up to 2 miles a day at a local mall. She feels stronger. More confident. *Elated.*

"I simply can't believe it; my bones aren't cracking any more," she laughs. "Alice in Wonderland is finally moving, or I should say, she's very happily *walking!*"

Some Face Greater Risk

Times have changed since the days when thinning bones were considered an inevitable part of growing old—particularly for women.

"Today, women have a marvelous advantage that their mothers and their grandmothers did not have," says Sydney Bonnick, M.D., director of osteoporosis services at the Cooper Clinic in Dallas. Special diagnostic equipment can detect the first hint of thinning bones. And research has shown that exercise (among other things) is an excellent way to help prevent osteoporosis, stop its progression, and even, in many cases, actually partially reverse it.

About 25 million Americans, mostly women, have osteoporosis. In a person who has this all-too-common condition, the bones gradually lose substance and grow weak and brittle. Over time, the strength and density that calcium and exercise pack into the bones can be leeched from the spine, hips, and essentially every part of the skeleton. The bones necessary to support the body's weight begin to fracture and cave in on each other—even from something like bending to lift groceries—eventually compressing the back into a disfiguring, painful slump.

Who's at risk for the disease? Women are five times more likely to have the disorder than men, whose bones are naturally denser and less likely to erode. Particularly at risk are women who are white or Oriental, are small-boned and thin, and whose families have a history of osteoporosis. Other factors found to increase the risk include a high-protein diet, low calcium intake, smoking, and high alcohol and caffeine consumption.

By age 65, the average woman can lose one-quarter of her bone mass. In fact, over the course of her lifetime, she can lose from 35 percent to 60 percent of her bone. But that's only if she doesn't take precautions.

Adolescence to 35: The Skeleton Crew

The body builds most of its bone during the first 35 years of life, 45 percent of it during adolescence. A number of factors play a role in bone formation—genetics, nutrition, calcium intake, hormones, and exercise.

Experts agree that exercise—particularly exercise such as walking, running, stair climbing, and weight lifting—is one of the essential elements for growing strong bones. Such exercises are known as weight-bearing exercises because they force the skeleton to support the weight of the body as you move. Bones are composed chiefly of calcium. The more you engage in this kind of exercise, the more calcium you deposit in your bones, making them stronger and thicker. And the thicker your bones are when you're young, the stronger your reserves will be when aging begins to erode them.

"Think of your skeleton as a bank of calcium," says Kathleen Little, Ph.D., exercise physiologist with the MetroHealth Medical Center in Cleveland. "The more calcium you put in your account, the more you'll have to draw upon as you get older."

Exactly what *is* the physiological link between bones and exercise? "Bone is not static, not inanimate," Dr. Little explains. "People think of the skeleton as inert, but it's really a living tissue that responds, moves, bends."

When bone has pressure applied to it through weight-bearing exercise, after an extended period of time its density will have increased. The pressure placed on the bone from gravity, muscle contractions, and the demands of exercise not only discourages calcium from leaving that area being stressed but actually stimulates its deposit, explains Dr. Little.

No Bones about It

Of course, intuitively, we've always known there is a connection between strong muscles, strong bones, and certain types of exercise. Not surprisingly, studies have found that the bones in the forearms of tennis and baseball players, weight lifters, and even lumberjacks are thicker.

Scientists have shown that there's a relationship between the strength of the muscle and the density of the bone to which it is attached.

There's also evidence suggesting that people in sedentary occupations are far more likely to have bone fractures later in life than those who work at jobs requiring weight-bearing activities. The epitome of what can happen to your bones if you're inactive was exemplified in another study of people who were totally bedridden. After two weeks, their calcium loss because of immobility had aged their bones by a full year.

"The bottom line is use it or lose it," says Miriam Nelson, Ph.D., researcher at the U.S. Department of Agriculture's Human Nutrition Research Center on Aging at Tufts University in Boston. "It is very, very clear that exercise is an excellent way to build strong bones."

All exercise may, to a degree, help build bone mass. But Dr. Nelson emphasizes that to protect your bones you must engage in weight-bearing activity. "Brisk walking is excellent for the hips and spine. Stair climbing and aerobic dancing are wonderful for the entire skeleton," she says. "Strength training probably is most important for muscle and bone, provided the intensity is high enough. All the muscle groups should be worked on."

35 to Menopause: Hold On to What You've Got

By the time you've reached 35, you've most likely developed your peak bone mass. This represents the point in life when your bones have reached their maxi-

mum density and toughness. From now on, calcium from your diet is no longer deposited in your bones as quickly as it is removed.

Although bone loss is minimal until menopause (only about 0.5 percent annually), doing weight-bearing exercise during this period of life becomes even *more* important. It helps retard bone loss.

At this point, the best route is a vigorous one—filled with the same exercises that helped you stockpile calcium in your earlier years: walking, running, cycling, aerobic dancing, and so on.

Menopause: Bones of Contention

After menopause, a woman's ovaries stop producing estrogen, a hormone that plays a major, though indirect, role in depositing and maintaining calcium in the bones. For the next five years, there is a dramatic loss in bone mass—generally from 3 percent to 5 percent annually— with a leveling off after 10 to 12 years.

As a result, your bones are far more susceptible to fractures. Most occur in those spots where the spongy, meshlike bone (trabecular) most susceptible to osteoporosis is heavily concentrated: the spine, hips, and forearms close to the wrists.

Would increasing calcium in your diet prevent osteoporosis at this point? Although pharmaceutical companies have for years bombarded consumers with ads suggesting calcium supplements are a cure-all for osteoporosis, many experts say it's not the only answer. Study after study shows little evidence that calcium supplementation alone will stop the rapid erosion of bone mineral density in the postmenopausal woman.

Physicians do prescribe a variety of drugs to treat osteoporosis, but many are fraught with problems. Take fluoride, for example. Although it's been used to increase bone mass by up to 10 percent, new evidence shows that bone treated with fluoride may be inferior. While fluoride does increase bone mass in certain kinds of bone, it apparently doesn't stop fractures.

And while many women benefit from estrogen replacement therapy (according to studies, the incidence of bone fracture drops by as much as 70 percent), estrogen isn't a panacea for everybody. For many women, it causes negative side effects. When taken alone it increases the risk of uterine cancer (when it is combined with the hormone progesterone, however, the risk of uterine cancer is reduced).

Accentuate the Positive

There is, however, a proven bone builder that carries only positive side effects: exercise.

"Physical activity promotes bone density," answers Myroslaw M. Hreshchyshyn, M.D., professor and chairman of the departments of gynecology and obstetrics, State University of New York at Buffalo, School of Medicine. "It's good for the bone, any bone, at any age."

In one study, Dr. Hreshchyshyn and his associates found that postmenopausal women who in the course of a normal day walked 1 hour more than other women had thicker, stronger bones in their hips. In fact, they concluded that the bone mass in the hips of the more active women was comparable to that of women four years younger.

In another study, researchers at the Washington University School of Medicine, in St. Louis, examined the bone mass of postmenopausal women before and after an exercise program to determine what impact exercise might have. One part of the group, healthy but previously sedentary women aged 55 to 70, underwent a 22-month regimen of weight-bearing exercises: walking, jogging, and stair climbing. Exercise sessions also included cycling, rowing, and bench pressing.

Another group of women with similar characteristics did no exercise. The result? The exercisers increased their bone mass by about 6 percent; the inactive women experienced no significant change in their bone mass.

But suppose you don't want to do all that exercise? Just take a brisk walk every day. Researchers at the Tufts Human Nutrition Research Center examined the bone density of postmenopausal women before and after a year-long program of brisk walking—just 45 minutes a day four times a week. Their findings were similar to those of numerous other studies: All other factors being equal, women who are active (versus those who aren't) increase their bone mineral content.

A Word of Warning

Once you begin any exercise program, be sure to stick with it. Repeated studies show that people who've increased their bone mass through exercise lost bone density if they stopped exercising.

And remember, it's not just for preventing or treating osteoporosis. Exercise is an excellent way to become healthier—it benefits the entire body, including the nervous system, which can help people who have osteoporosis keep their balance and help prevent those falls that cause fractures.

If you have osteoporosis, cautions Dr. Little, you should consult with a health professional with expertise in exercise physiology before starting an exercise program. And, she urges, "proceed with caution. You should begin with moderate exercise, which is best for women with thinner bones. Sudden movement, too much strain, or pounding could cause fractures."

Firming the Foundation

Just what kinds of exercise are best for women who are most at risk?

For women past menopause, "we want to work on those parts of the skeleton most at risk for fracture, those predominantly weight-bearing portions of the skeleton—the spine and the hip joint," says Dr. Bonnick. "And also we work on the wrist, because that's usually what breaks when someone tries to stop a fall."

In general, bone-strengthening exercises are basically the same for all women, before or after menopause, but they should vary in intensity, frequency, and duration depending on age, health, and degree of bone loss, says Dr. Bonnick.

First, warm-up exercises are important to reduce the risk that you'll pull a muscle, says Dr. Little. A few slow stretching activities done for about 5 minutes will do the trick: Stand and touch your toes, bend

to both sides from the waist, clench your hands into fists, then release.

"Walking is an excellent weight-bearing exercise, but start out slowly," says Dr. Little. "If you're older and haven't exercised regularly, maybe take a walk to the mailbox or the grocery store, working up to a minimum of 20 minutes a day three times a week." Eventually, Dr. Little suggests, increase the pace so that you're walking briskly—about 45 minutes daily for 1½ miles, three to five times a week.

"You'd be amazed how good stair climbing can be for your bones," particularly the spine and the hip, says Dr. Little. She recommends starting out slowly, making about five round trips on a flight of ten steps. Do this about three times a week, eventually increasing the climbing to an 18-minute session.

Also, warns Dr. Little, don't forget to breathe when lifting weights. "Although the tendency when exerting your muscles may be to hold your breath, your muscles need the oxygen that natural inhaling and exhaling provides.

"If you find yourself suddenly breathless, stop and rest. If you experience more severe symptoms, like chest pain, see a physician," advises Dr. Little. You may have exceeded your maximum heart rate for your age level.

Harden Your Hips

In addition to exercises that strengthen your entire skeleton, a routine to tone and strengthen areas that are especially vulnerable to fracture may also prove useful.

Hip-kick exercises are excellent for

strengthening hip bones, Dr. Little says. For beginners, start out using your own body weight and gradually progress to working with resistance bands. You can purchase them in any sporting goods store—just look for the exercise aids resembling big rubber bands. For this exercise, place the band around both ankles.

With or without the band, here's what you do. Stand with one hand against the wall for support and raise your leg—making sure it's straight—out to the side as far as you can go. Return your foot to the floor, then extend your leg behind you, again as far as you can go. Return your leg to the floor and then extend it in front of you in the same manner. Do this routine about eight times. Repeat with the other leg.

Dr. Little notes that you can achieve a similar effect if you lie on your side—be sure you have a soft but firm mat—and lift your leg up and down, scissors-style, about ten times. Repeat with the other leg.

Strengthen Your Spine

An exercise that will help firm up the spine and the muscles surrounding it is the back extension, according to Dr. Bonnick. Lie on your stomach with your arms at your sides, palms facing up, with a pillow beneath your pelvis. Have someone hold your feet, or anchor them under the sofa. Using just the muscles in your back (not your hands or arms), very slowly and gently try to raise your head and shoulders, keeping the rest of your body on the floor. Lower your head and shoulders just as

cautiously, and repeat several times, always remembering to stop the movement if you feel actual pain, not just muscle tension.

Don't Risk Your Wrists

To strengthen the bone in your wrists, support your forearms on a table or your thighs. Holding a very light weight—1- to 2-pound dumbbells or even soup cans—slowly curl your wrists toward you, then return to the original position. Repeat about ten times.

In a variation of this exercise, hold the weights with your forearms resting on your thighs and your wrists slightly dangling over your knees. Your palms should be facing the floor. Do the same curling motion described above.

Dr. Bonnick also recommends the wall push for strengthening bone in the wrist. Stand about 20 inches from a wall, with your legs about 10 inches apart. Place your palms on the wall at about shoulder level. Slowly move your body toward the wall, then push away from it to your original position. Repeat this about ten times. Rest a minute or so before doing more exercise.

All experts agree that given the potential risks of injury, anyone with osteoporosis should not do intense exercise without first consulting a professional with expertise in the area. They also agree that exercise is necessary to prevent and even reverse osteoporosis.

The right moves today will build a strong base that can protect you in the years to come.

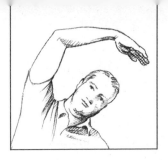

Overweight

Have you noticed they're cutting clothes smaller this year? Or maybe that your bathroom scale is broken? Or perhaps your weight hasn't changed, but they're not making mirrors like they used to? Well, the problem may not be shoddy clothes, faulty scales, or inept glassmaking. More likely, your body is taking advantage of its modern, easygoing lifestyle. And it's thanking you for making life easy by padding your flanks with unwanted pounds of fat and by losing underused muscle.

In fact, an inactive lifestyle is one of the biggest weight-gain villains. It may be, say weight-loss experts, an even greater cause of excess fat than overeating. Not only that, lack of exercise plays a major role in weight gain in people whose genes predispose them to heaviness.

Inactivity does not necessarily mean lying in bed all day. The types of inactivity that allow fat cells to grow and flourish include things like finding the parking space closest to a store's entrance, watching TV after dinner rather than walking around the neighborhood, lying on the beach instead of exploring it, driving a golf cart instead of walking the links, being a sports fan but not a player, and taking the elevator and avoiding stairs that don't move.

Get the picture? Are you in it? Then count yourself among the inactive, but brace yourself for the good news: You can reverse the inactivity/fat-gain spiral and lose unwanted weight through exercise.

Why Exercise?

Notice we said "exercise," not "diet." Studies show that weight lost only through dieting—as in counting and drastically cutting calories in order to shed pounds quickly—is almost inevitably regained. You may be all too familiar with this scenario: You diet and lose weight, then stop dieting and gain weight. It's called the yo-yo syndrome. Not only is yo-yo dieting disheartening, it's unhealthy. That's because some of the weight lost through dieting without exercising comes from valuable muscle tissue, not just fat. Furthermore, when your weight goes back up, you gain fat, not muscle. So if you feel as if you get flabbier every time you gain weight back, you now know it's not just your imagination. You *are* getting flabbier.

"The only way to lose fat forever is through regular aerobic exercise," says exercise physiologist Barbara Frey-Hewitt, Ph.D., of Diablo Valley College in Pleasant Hill, California. And many other experts agree. In fact, they would like to have the concept of *dieting* eliminated from our culture altogether. That is not to say that adopting and conscientiously maintaining healthful *eating habits* can be ignored. A nutritious and healthful diet, followed on a permanent basis as part of a healthy lifestyle that includes regular exercise, is the *best* way to get those excess pounds off and keep them off.

Research suggests that exercise is a boon to weight loss for several reasons. According to Kelly Brownell, Ph.D., professor of psychology at Yale University, exercise does the following:

- Boosts your metabolic rate
- Builds nice, firm muscle
- Suppresses your appetite
- Provides important psychological benefits that spill over into your attitudes about yourself and about eating (see "Low Self-Esteem" on page 207)

Let's look at these powerful benefits of exercise one by one.

Metabolism: Your Fat Burner

You've probably heard that working out revs up your metabolism, but what exactly does that mean? Metabolism is your body's system for converting food into new cells and energy (calories). When you eat more food than you use as energy, the excess food is converted to fat for storage. It's like keeping butter in the refrigerator . . . except it's on your hips, belly, and . . . well, you know where your butterballs are. Increasing the rate at which your metabolism works lets you burn more stored food, and a great way to increase your metabolic rate is through regular—repeat, *regular*—exercise.

The metabolic boost from exercise does not shut off when your exercise session ends, either. "When you exercise, your body temperature [a gauge of metabolic rate] rises and can remain elevated for 6 to 18 hours, resulting in increased calories burned while you're sleeping that night," explains Gabe Mirkin, M.D., associate clinical professor at the Sportsmedicine Institute of Georgetown University School of Medicine in Silver Spring, Maryland.

Many recent studies confirm that sustained exercise speeds up metabolism, burns up more fat stores in overfat people, and leads to weight loss. On the flip side, inactivity during quick weight-loss schemes can depress your metabolism, making it harder than ever for your body to lose fat.

Also, the more fat (and less lean muscle) you have, the slower your metabolism will be. That's because muscle is metabolically active: It "works," uses energy, and gives off heat when your metabolism is cranking. Fat (you might expect this) just sort of sits there like a blob. It can't do much work. Remember, it's in storage, waiting to be used. When working muscles need extra energy to keep on working, they tap into those stored fat reserves and start to use them up. So the more muscle you build up, the more energy that muscle needs to work, and the more stored fat it uses as fuel.

How do you know your muscle is gaining ground over fat? "Get a tape measure and throw away your scale," Dr. Mirkin suggests. The reasoning behind this drastic suggestion is that muscle is denser than fat. In other words, a pound of fat takes up more space than a pound of muscle, and a 150-pound fat-laden person takes up more space than a 150-pound muscular person. As your exercise program progresses, some of your fat weight will be converted to muscle weight. Your scale cannot reveal this change, but a tape measure and your clothes can, says Dr. Mirkin.

Exercise as an Appetite Suppressant

You might think all that exercise is going to make you ravenous. Not necessarily.

Oddly enough, regular exercise often helps to curb an overactive appetite in overweight people. The scientific explanations for this are complex, and unfortunately, the studies that examine this phenomenon often say more about rats' appetites than humans'.

For a human perspective, it helps to listen to the experience of those who have benefited from regular exercise. Here's what one proud "loser," who also exercises faithfully, has to say.

"Exercise definitely does work as an appetite suppressant, but not immediately," says Marlin Groff, a 48-year-old resident of Lancaster, Pennsylvania, who lost 240 life-threatening extra pounds in three years. "I had to get into a consistent, regular exercise program before it became an effective appetite suppressant. For the first 100 pounds . . . when I would feel starved, like I just had to have something to eat, I would go for a long, brisk walk.

"I think the walk did two things: It relieved stress, which is what I think made me feel hungry, and it did something chemically in my brain. I would come back from my walk, and I just wouldn't have that tremendously empty feeling."

Plenty of people and scientific studies agree that during and for some time after exercise, overweight people do not feel hungry. The question is, Why? There are several theories about what the "something chemically" Marlin mentioned might be. Exercise, say the experts, may serve to normalize levels of insulin and other hormones that influence appetite. But the important thing is that for many overfat people, exercise can quell a prodding appetite both during the activity and for several hours thereafter.

No doubt about it, exercise makes you feel good. More self-confidence, pride in your appearance, a sense of control over different aspects of your life, reduced stress, and other feelings of increased self-esteem are some of the psychological rewards that you can expect.

What Kind, How Much?

Okay, you admit that dieting is a drag, and you're willing to work to see those pounds drop off. Now what do you do?

The first thing you need to find is an aerobic exercise that you can live with. Aerobic exercise is tantamount to weight loss, because that is what will really turn the burners up on your metabolism.

Sometime during the past decade the word "aerobic" became synonymous with "aerobic dance class," conjuring images of firm thighs carrying limber bodies through knee-jarring choreographed productions. That's fine for some, but what is aerobic exercise, really?

Aerobic exercise is any activity that

IN THE SWIM

If you're swimming to lose weight, experts say you may be all wet.

"Swimming is great exercise, but if weight loss is your objective, stay out of the water," says Grant Gwinup, M.D., chief of endocrinology and metabolism and professor of medicine at the University of California, Irvine, Medical Center. Dr. Gwinup studied the effects of 60 minutes a day of brisk walking, cycling, or swimming laps on three groups of moderately obese women. The women were told to eat whenever and whatever they desired. After six months, the walking women had lost 10 percent of their initial weight, the cyclists had lost 12 percent, and the swimmers had *gained* 3 percent. Why is this?

Dr. Gwinup speculates that because warm water (78° to 84°F in his study) takes heat away from the body much more rapidly than air of the same temperature, the body tries to preserve its heat-holding insulation (fat) by triggering its hunger or appetite mechanism. Result: Swimmers eat more than landlubbers who do the same amount of aerobic exercise. "People in swimming programs just don't lose weight . . . unless they make a concerted effort to restrict energy intake," Dr. Gwinup adds.

The good news is that Dr. Gwinup's swimmers gained the many other health benefits of aerobic exercise, as indicated by their reduced pulse rates and other simple measurements. "It's a fine exercise as far as cardiovascular fitness is concerned," says Dr. Gwinup, and it is frequently recommended as a form of exercise that bypasses the joint-jarring risks posed by, say, jogging. If weight loss is desired, though, swimmers are cautioned more than other exercisers to beware of overeating.

---

delivers a steady supply of oxygen to working muscles. This happens when activities are of low or moderate intensity, involve large muscle groups, and last long enough. Besides dancing, qualifiers for weight loss include jogging, bicycling, jumping rope, stair climbing, skating, rowing, cross-country skiing, and the exercise of choice for the 1990s and beyond: walking. Swimming is one aerobic exercise that, by itself, may not fill the bill for weight loss. (See "In the Swim" above.) When combined with restrained eating habits, however, swimming is a fine form of exercise for weight loss.

The universal prescription for effective aerobic exercise is at least 20 minutes of steady activity at least three times a week. The idea is to work out hard enough and long enough to get your heart pumping at 60 to 85 percent of your maximum heart rate. (See "How Good Is Your Workout?" on page 324.) Very overweight people should aim for 50 to 65 percent of their maximum heart rate, according to Herman Frankel, M.D., director of the Portland Health Institute in Portland, Oregon. Aiming for the higher rates might lead to injury, he says.

The second universal prescription regarding aerobics is to start slowly, and as with any exercise routine, always warm up with nonstrenuous exercises to avoid injury. "For very obese people, start by exercising at 50 percent maximum heart rate," cautions David J. Mersy, M.D., chairman of the Department of Family Medicine and director of the Family Medicine Residency Program at St. Paul–Ramsey Medical Center in Minnesota. The average, healthy adult should aim for the higher heart rates and gradually work up to them, Dr. Mersy recommends.

Turning Up the Juice

If you want to speed your losses and reach your ideal weight a little faster, it's okay to gradually increase your level of activity. "Start out easy, working up to 30 minutes every other day," advises Dr. Mirkin. "If you want to go beyond that, put *intensity* into your program by warming up slowly and increasing intensity gradually until you feel the least bit uncomfortable. Then back off and do a series of intervals where you accelerate and decelerate.

"When you use a program like this," Dr. Mirkin cautions, "do not do it more often than every other day, no matter who you are. If you want to do more than three workouts a week, you've got to alternate sports, because different sports stress different muscle groups.

"The best combination I know is to go rowing—which stresses your upper body—on Monday, Wednesday, and Friday, and cycling or walking—for your lower body—on Tuesday, Thursday, and Saturday. Choose two sports and do one *intense* workout in each sport only once a week."

Extremely obese people must use caution when increasing the intensity of an exercise routine. For instance, if your ex-

ercise of choice is walking and you have reached a point where trundling along on flat terrain is no longer a challenge, add interest and intensity to your program by tackling some hills or raising the incline level of your treadmill. That way, you can continue to move your limbs at a comfortable and nonjarring pace while using more energy, Dr. Frey-Hewitt explains.

Many people are dismayed by their inability to lose unwanted pounds without exercise, claiming that their day-to-day lifestyle is plenty active. Experts note that there is nothing that comes even close to aerobic exercise for losing weight.

"There is something about sustained aerobic activity that has a benefit that intermittent activity doesn't have," explains Grant Gwinup, M.D., chief of endocrinology and metabolism at the University of California, Irvine, Medical Center in Orange, California. "For example, I see people like nurses whose jobs keep them active off and on all day but who complain that they don't lose weight. But if they get on a sustained exercise program, like walking for an hour and a half every day, then they have a nice weight loss." (For information about starting and adopting a walking, bicycling, dancing, or running program, see the appropriate chapters in part 2.)

Have Fun

The activities you choose should not only use different parts of your body, they should also be fun to do both as part of your weight-loss campaign and later as part of your reactivated lifestyle.

"To be successful," says Dr. Mersy, "the

exercise must be something the person enjoys, or they won't keep doing it."

Perhaps a group of people working toward a common exercise and weight-loss goal can motivate you. "Get into a crowd of people who will do it with you. Looking forward to meeting other people is a definite advantage," says Dr. Mirkin.

Some suggestions: Join a hiking, canoeing, bicycling, or backpacking club. Too outdoorsy for you? There are people walking and jogging *en masse* during off-peak hours through shopping malls and airports throughout the country. The camaraderie of fellow fun-seekers and fat-combatants, plus the aesthetics of the outdoors (or shop windows), may be just the inspiration you need to maintain a lifelong active lifestyle. Don't forget to get your muscles moving on the other days if your group meets only once a week.

Some company fitness programs offer weight-loss teams. You may feel more comfortable using the buddy system for exercise, inspiring a friend or spouse to set and reach goals and likewise drawing inspiration from him or her.

If working out with exercise equipment keeps you motivated, consider circuit weight training—that is, a routine that alternates weight lifting with aerobic episodes. Gyms, health clubs, and fitness centers also employ staffs who can instruct you in using stationary bikes, rowing machines, stair-climbing simulators, and other equipment designed for aerobic workouts.

In many cities, there are exercise classes specifically for larger people. If this is not the case in your town, you may consider initiating one through your local Y, school, or community group. This type of program can be wonderful because the instructors are tuned in to the potential hazards and special needs that accompany extreme overweight—such as overheating, muscle and joint strain, arthritis, unsteady balance, poor circulation, coronary strain, and general discomfort (physical and psychological) about exercising. Such programs use particular caution with jogging or jumping activities that may injure knees, hips, and other joints. Also, since you'll be working out with other people who face the same physical challenges, you can help cheer each other on.

Maintaining Weight Loss

Let's jump ahead to the time when you have exercised yourself slim. How do you keep the fat at bay? Keep on exercising! Improvements in aerobic conditioning can be maintained by exercising aerobically just twice a week for 20 minutes. But laying off exercise for just two weeks can really reduce the fitness level you have worked so hard to attain; after five weeks of inactivity you will be back almost to your aerobic ground zero. Dr. Mersy sums it up this way: "If you give up the exercise, your weight may go right back up to where it was. When you use exercise to control weight, you must use it for the rest of your life. You can't expect to go back to your old habits and expect to keep the weight off."

And what about those last 10 stubborn pounds that are so difficult to drop? The underlying message is don't give up, and it applies to stubborn pounds as well as to the inevitable plateaus and reversals that successful losers experience.

A WORD ABOUT SPOT REDUCING: THERE'S NO SUCH THING

As you continue your exercise program and watch the fat begin to melt away, it's frustrating to note that it seems to cling more stubbornly to some areas than to others.

You may well wish for some magic little movement to deflate those spare tires, for example. Sorry.

There is no exercise that will remove fat from just one area. There is simply *no such thing* as spot reducing, says Wayne Sinning, Ph.D., exercise physiologist at Kent State University in Ohio.

"Weight training—an example of non-aerobic exercise—would have an effect if your flabbiness is due to poor muscle tone," he says. "It would improve the muscle tone and reduce body girth in that area—but it would not actually cause fat to be removed. It certainly would not spot-reduce the fat from any area."

Aerobic exercise, though, has demonstrated itself to be effective in reducing fat all over the body, including the dangerously unhealthy abdominal fat common in overweight men and some women, says David J. Mersy, M.D., chairman of the Department of Family Medicine and director of the Family Medicine Residency Program at St. Paul–Ramsey Medical Center in Minnesota. This type of fatty accumulation—known in both men and women as male-pattern obesity—can hardly be considered a "spot," however, as the fat is stored in the large area of the waist and abdomen.

A Spoonful of Inspiration

Still not inspired by the thought of how good you'll feel and how great you'll look when you exercise your way to weight loss? Take your cue from someone who has been there and back: At 6 feet 2 inches tall and more than 500 pounds, Howard Bennett of West Valley, Utah, had tried "every weight-loss diet in the book" without much success.

How did Howard finally lose more than 340 pounds? "The only thing I did differently with this regimen of losing weight was adding exercise to it . . . and I find that it's just so easy to keep it off with exercise." The only limitation he puts on his eating is steering clear of almost all fat. His personal motivator? "I just carry my old pictures with me." And his advice to other overweight people who wish to use exercise as a weight-loss aid? "Don't worry about how far you go or how fast you go when you start. Just do it. When I started out, I had to use a walker, and I could barely walk to the end of my driveway." Now, more than two years later, Howard never misses his hour-long walk every day.

People like Howard Bennett, who have renewed their life through exercise and gained so much through losing weight, seem to radiate joy. Imagine how great Howard felt about going to his recent class reunion: With his new, active lifestyle in full swing, he bicycled the entire 150-mile trip in one day.

No Pain, Everything to Gain

Beginning an exercise program can be difficult for almost anyone—but it's *particularly* difficult if you're overweight. Being very overweight puts added strain on you as you move, because of the way your body has to shift to balance those extra pounds. Your spine becomes swayed, adding stress to your lower back. Your hips, knees, and feet take an extra pounding, making joints painful and subjecting them to possible injury. Even moderate activity—such as walking or standing at the sink to do the dishes—may become synonymous with discomfort. Exercise is the best remedy, but how can you get started if every time you start to move your body, it screams *stop?*

The following set of exercises is designed to help you begin moving with a new sense of freedom and comfort. Herman Frankel, M.D., director of the Portland Health Institute in Portland, Oregon, and former chairman of the Obesity Foundation, has extensive experience in helping formerly inactive people develop appropriate exercise programs that enhance their health. The following exercises and suggestions for doing them comfortably and safely have been adapted from Dr. Frankel's videotape, "Warming Up: The Gentle Exercise Videotape for Formerly Inactive People." "In the course of mastering these exercises," says Dr. Frankel, "you will be taking an important step toward developing a sense of pleasure and ease in movement. You will begin to feel a new comfort in your body, a new confidence in your ability to do the things you want to

do without the kind of discomfort that may have caused you difficulty in the past."

Dr. Frankel recommends that you first get your physician's okay to do the exercises. If while exercising you develop breathlessness, pain, or persistent discomfort, be sure to report such symptoms to your physician.

Before you begin, change into loose, comfortable clothing and put on supportive aerobic shoes.

It's very important to warm up before you actually start the exercises, because warming up prepares the body to move more easily and safely. Start by taking small steps in place and swinging your arms smoothly for a few minutes.

Cooling down is also important. After you complete the full set of exercises, finish up with the series of gentle movements and stretches to help you cool down.

A few leg stretches require that you lie on the floor. To get down on the floor safely, place one foot far in front of the other. As you bend both knees, place both hands on the floor and gently lower your back knee to the floor. Now shift your weight onto one hip. Now you can roll onto your back. When you are ready to get up, first roll onto your side. Use your hands to push yourself into a sitting position. Get on all fours and place one foot in front of the other. Push down on that knee with your hand to help yourself up without straining.

When you're finished exercising, put on a long-sleeved shirt and long pants to

No Pain, Everything to Gain—Continued

prevent becoming chilled as you rest. Drink a tall glass of water to replace any fluids lost while exercising.

Here are some things to keep in mind while you're doing the exercises themselves. Do *all* the exercises slowly and deliberately, with no jerks or forcing. Your goal is to do each for a set of eight repetitions, says Dr. Frankel.

Don't worry if you can't do eight the first time out. You'll become stronger with practice.

It's important to be aware of your posture. While standing, pretend the top of your head is held up by a string suspended from the ceiling. Relax your shoulders, draw in your abdominal muscles, and tuck your bottom underneath you. Check your posture regularly while you're exercising to make sure you're standing tall.

Some people do all the exercises while standing, some find it more comfortable at first to do them sitting down, and others may prefer to do some standing and some

sitting. If you'll be sitting, you'll need a stable chair without arms.

When seated, be sure you sit tall, with your head erect, your abdominal muscles firm, your back straight, and your bottom tucked in.

Move your feet often during the exercise session, even if you are sitting. You can raise your heels off the floor one at a time or together, or for variety, lift the ball of your foot and keep your heel on the floor. This will help prevent your ankles from swelling.

Breathe regularly and deeply. If you become short of breath, slow down—or take a rest for a few moments. You may need a sip of water, so keep a glass handy.

These exercises are available on video-cassette from Dr. Frankel. If you wish to obtain a copy, write to The Portland Health Institute, 9045 S.W. Barbur Boulevard, Suite 4-B, Portland OR 97219-4028. Request a copy of "Warming Up: The Gentle Exercise Videotape for Formerly Inactive People."

Shoulder Shrug

Holding your head high, raise your shoulders as high as you can. Then lower your shoulders, keeping your head facing forward and your arms loose. Relax as you bring them down. Wait a moment before repeating.

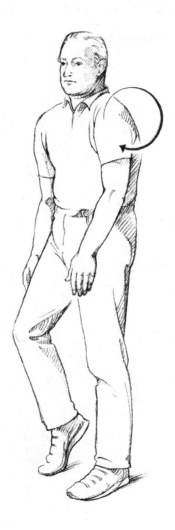

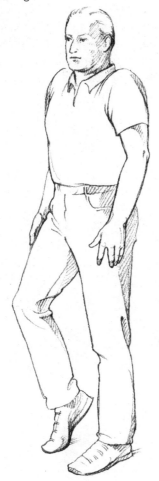

Shoulder Rolls

Bring both shoulders forward and up, then move them back and then down, making circular movements. Bend your elbows naturally as you move your shoulders. Then reverse the direction and repeat: Move your shoulders up, forward, and down, and then back, again letting your elbows bend naturally.

No Pain, Everything to Gain—Continued

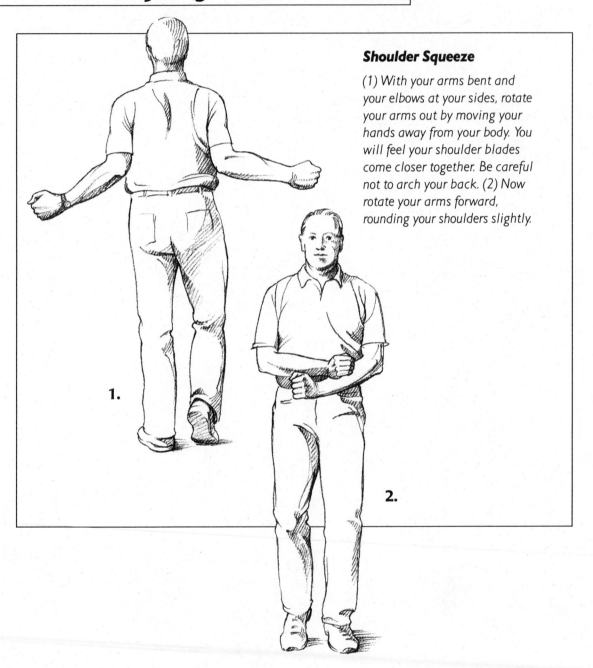

Shoulder Squeeze

(1) With your arms bent and your elbows at your sides, rotate your arms out by moving your hands away from your body. You will feel your shoulder blades come closer together. Be careful not to arch your back. (2) Now rotate your arms forward, rounding your shoulders slightly.

1.

2.

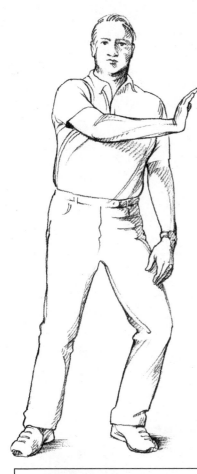

Side Reach

Keep your shoulders parallel to your hips. Sidestep to the left, at the same time reaching with your right hand across your chest as far as you can. Now bring your right arm and your left leg back to the starting position. Repeat on the other side, shifting your weight, stepping to the right, and reaching with your left hand. Do once on each side. When you feel comfortable with this exercise, add a little twist. As you reach to the side, rotate your shoulders slightly.

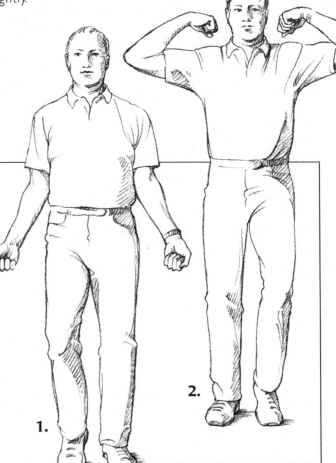

Biceps Curl

(1) Tighten your hands into fists and hold your arms at your sides. Then bend your elbows as if you were lifting something heavy. Lower your arms. Keep the movement slow and fluid. (2) From the starting position, raise your arms to shoulder height. Repeat, bending and straightening your arms like a he-man. Do two repetitions, one starting with your arms in the down position and one starting with your arms at shoulder height.

1.

2.

No Pain, Everything to Gain—Continued

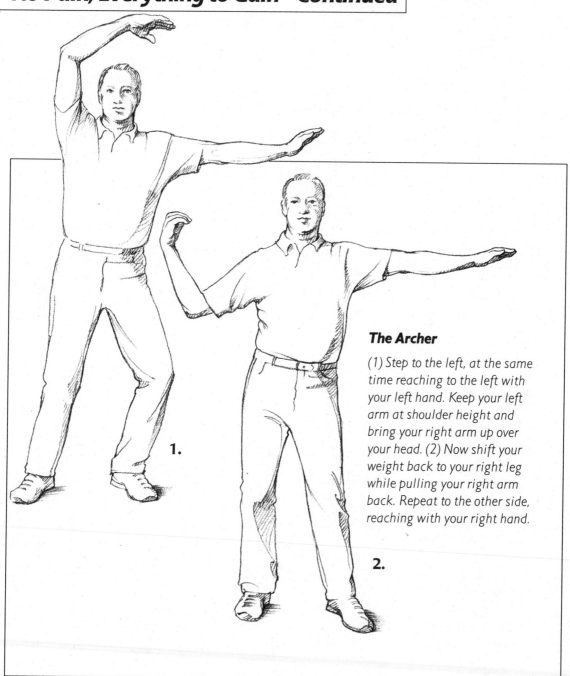

1.

2.

The Archer

(1) Step to the left, at the same time reaching to the left with your left hand. Keep your left arm at shoulder height and bring your right arm up over your head. (2) Now shift your weight back to your right leg while pulling your right arm back. Repeat to the other side, reaching with your right hand.

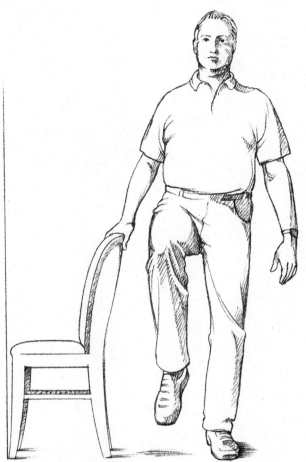

Leg Raise

Using a chair for support, lift your left leg as if you were going to take a step (below). Straighten your knee. Lower your foot gently to the floor. Repeat with the other leg.

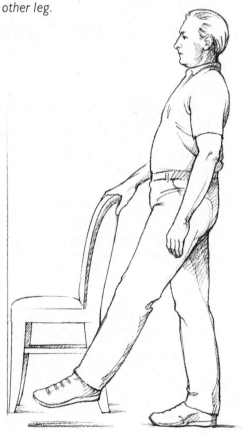

The March

Place the front of a chair against a wall (above). Holding the back of the chair with your right hand, lift your right knee as high as you comfortably can. Try to bring your thigh parallel to the floor. (Make that your goal, even if you don't succeed at first.) Lower your foot gently to the floor. You will need to shift your weight to your left leg as you lift your right knee. Then switch sides and repeat. To do a similar exercise sitting down, hold on to the seat of the chair. Lift one knee toward your chest as far as is comfortable for you. Don't strain, and don't lean forward. Lower your foot slowly to the floor, then repeat with the other leg.

No Pain, Everything to Gain—Continued

Cool-Down

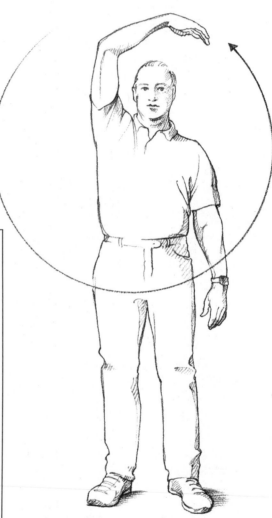

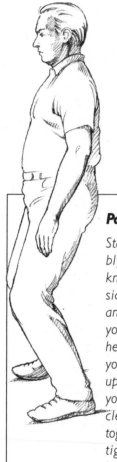

Partial Squat

Stand with your legs comfortably apart, with your feet and knees turned slightly out to the sides. Bend your knees partway and lower yourself slightly. Keep your back straight and your head erect. Then straighten your knees slowly. You can jazz up this exercise by pretending you're pumping up a flat bicycle tire. Bring your hands together in front of you and tighten them into fists. Now bend and straighten your elbows as you bend and straighten your knees.

Arm Sweep

Standing or sitting, sweep one arm forward, up over your head, then back and down. Pretend you're a ballerina. The movement is fluid and relaxed. Repeat with the other arm.

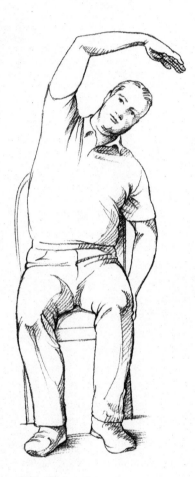

Shoulder Stretch

Sit erect and clasp your right elbow with your left hand. Gently pull your right arm across your chest, without twisting at the waist. Hold for a few seconds, then repeat to the other side.

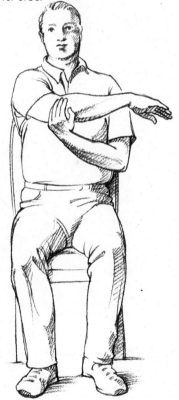

Side Stretch

Sit in a chair and hold the seat with your left hand. Lift your right arm over your head. At the same time, bend the elbow of your left arm and bend slowly to the left. Think of your back and neck curved like an ostrich plume. Hold for a few moments, sit up slowly, then repeat on the other side. Stretch each side once.

No Pain, Everything to Gain—Continued

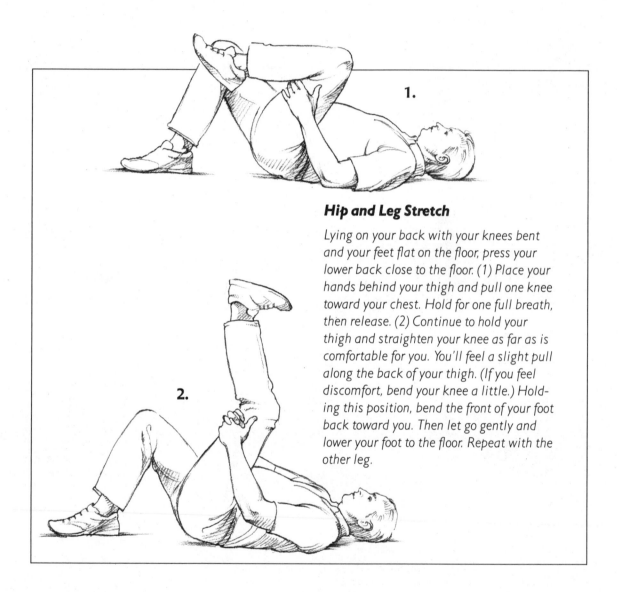

Hip and Leg Stretch

Lying on your back with your knees bent and your feet flat on the floor, press your lower back close to the floor. (1) Place your hands behind your thigh and pull one knee toward your chest. Hold for one full breath, then release. (2) Continue to hold your thigh and straighten your knee as far as is comfortable for you. You'll feel a slight pull along the back of your thigh. (If you feel discomfort, bend your knee a little.) Holding this position, bend the front of your foot back toward you. Then let go gently and lower your foot to the floor. Repeat with the other leg.

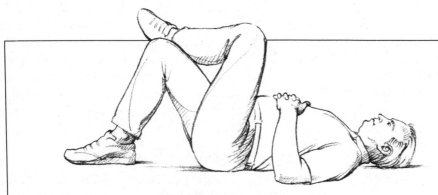

The Alphabet

Lying on your back with your knees bent and your lower back pressed close to the floor, rest your ankle on one knee. Draw the lowercase letters of the alphabet with your toes. (Pretend your big toe is a paintbrush.) Make the letters as big as possible. Repeat with the other foot. Before long, you can expect to get through the entire alphabet without becoming tired. Each time, remember where you stopped and see how far you get the next time.

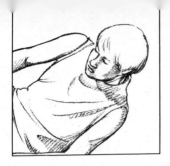

Pregnancy

One of the first purchases Beth Jackson made after becoming pregnant wasn't booties for the baby. Instead, she bought sneakers for herself. She also bought a swimsuit.

"I wanted a natural childbirth and knew I had to get in shape for it," she says. "Plus, I wanted to avoid gaining tons of weight." In consultation with her obstetrician, Beth planned an exercise regimen.

She swam three evenings a week and walked during each lunch hour—right up to the day her son was born. "I really approached exercise as if training for a race, except that I was training for childbirth," she says. "I firmly believe exercise helped me sail through pregnancy."

Although she had a long, arduous labor, Beth recalls feeling "energized even while pushing the baby out." As a bonus, she was able to fit back into her prepregnancy jeans just weeks after giving birth.

Beth thus joined a growing legion of women who have discovered that exercising during pregnancy means fewer aches and pains, more energy, extra push power during delivery, and a body that recovers quickly afterward.

Many obstetricians are cheering their efforts, thanks to mounting evidence showing that with moderation and monitoring, exercise can offer pregnant women a host of benefits with few risks.

"Delivering a baby is like performing in a marathon," says Douglas C. Hall, M.D., associate clinical professor of obstetrics and gynecology at the University of Florida in Gainesville. "Giving birth requires tremendous physical strength and mental stamina. Women who have exercised prior to childbirth seem to have an easier time of it."

Exercise Eases Delivery

During delivery, says Dr. Hall, it's apparent that women who stay fit during pregnancy have the cardiovascular strength to withstand labor and the muscle power to expel the baby.

In one study, Dr. Hall and his colleagues looked at 845 pregnant women engaged in low, medium, and high levels of exercise and compared them to pregnant women who did not exercise. Those who worked out on stationary bicycles and weight-lifting equipment three times a week, particularly those working at a high level, had shorter hospital stays and fewer incidences of Caesarean deliveries than the nonexercisers.

Other studies indicate that while exercise won't exactly make delivery a breeze, staying fit through pregnancy may help you cope better with the pain and hard work of childbirth.

James Clapp, M.D., professor of reproductive biology at Case Western Reserve University in Cleveland, found that physically fit women who continued to exercise during pregnancy used about half as much pain medication as nonexercisers in the study. And the women who stuck with exercise right up until delivery experienced a shorter labor than women who quit exercising.

What's most reassuring about this research is that exercise can help condition women for childbirth without harming mother or baby.

Many obstetricians have been concerned that overheating and other effects of exercise could harm the fetus, says Dr. Clapp. "Now there's good evidence that continuing moderate exercise during pregnancy does not have a detrimental effect. Although more information is needed to be sure, the benefits appear to outweigh the risks," he says.

Banish Those Aches and Pains

Aside from conditioning women for childbirth, another big plus for prenatal exercise is that it reduces the aches and pains in the months leading up to delivery, says Dr. Hall.

For many women, pregnancy can feel like nine *years* of hard work even before real labor begins. An ever-enlarging abdomen strains your back and compresses your internal organs. This may cause you shortness of breath and constipation and may give you heartburn and hemorrhoids. Lugging around some 20 or 30 extra pounds drains you of energy. Women report that engaging in regular activity reduces these common discomforts, says Dr. Hall.

"Moderate exercise doesn't interfere with the normal, necessary increase in a mother's body fat and weight," says Dr. Clapp. "But if continued, it appears to limit excess weight gain in late pregnancy."

Studies show that women who continued to exercise during pregnancy gained an average of 5 pounds less than women who stopped exercising for the duration.

Perhaps exercise's greatest gift to pregnant women is a positive boost in self-image. "Exercise helps women feel in control when their body seems to be growing out of control," says Dr. Hall.

As Beth Jackson puts it, "Exercising helped me feel graceful even though I looked like a clumsy blimp."

Selecting the Safest Exercise

Granted, prenatal exercise has a lot going for it. But it doesn't mean you should begin Rollerblading down the boardwalk if you're expecting.

"Some physical activities are more appropriate for pregnant women than others," says Dr. Hall. Ideally, he says, a prenatal exercise program should be aimed at correcting postural changes, minimizing discomforts, preparing muscles for delivery, and improving cardiovascular strength.

Of these, making postural changes is undoubtedly the most important prenatal exercise, according to Dr. Hall.

Improving your posture helps shore up the abdominal wall and eliminate constipation, heartburn, and hemorrhoids.

Half of all pregnant women are plagued with back pain. That's because the growing baby shifts the center of gravity forward, lengthening the abdominal muscles while shortening the back muscles. In other words, the muscles around your spine may bear the brunt of the load in front.

Pelvic tilt exercises can help prevent back pain and improve posture. This easy movement tightens and strengthens the abdominal muscles. At the same time the back muscles are lengthened, helping to align the body.

"Performing pelvic tilts helps you not only see the difference in posture but feel it," according to physical therapist Elizabeth Noble, founder of the Maternal and Child Health Center in Cambridge, Massachusetts, and author of *Essential Exercises for the Childbearing Year.* "Your back will feel better, and your posture will improve."

You can perform pelvic tilts while lying down, sitting, or standing. Simply tip your pelvis upward, flattening out the hollow at the small of your back. Your shoulders and knees should remain still as you perform this movement. Hold the tilt for 3 seconds and release. Repeat the movement eight to ten times, relaxing for a few moments between repetitions.

The Importance of Low-Impact Aerobics

Aerobic exercise—continuous activity that raises your heart rate—can help build the cardiovascular strength you'll need to handle the extra blood circulating in your system during pregnancy and the exertion of labor.

But when you're pregnant, you must exercise aerobically within reason. This means high-impact aerobics is out, says Noble. Hormones that are released during pregnancy help soften ligaments and loosen the joints to accommodate a growing baby. "Your joints are more prone to injury," says Noble.

Also, pregnancy is generally not the time to start new sports or set personal goals. "The goal of prenatal exercise is not to be faster or stronger but to feel more comfortable," reminds Dr. Hall.

Normal walking is fairly easy on the joints and helps tone the abdominal muscles, experts agree. Walking briskly for 20 to 45 minutes three times weekly provides a good cardiovascular workout and can help combat varicose veins and swollen ankles.

By about the fourth month, when your belly blots out the view of your feet and your center of gravity shifts forward, you may be more comfortable switching to stationary bicycling. Swimming in a warm pool is even better. "Swimming has the advantage of taking the load off and keeping you cool," says John Joseph Botti, M.D., director of the Division of Maternal and Fetal Medicine at Hershey Medical Center in Hershey, Pennsylvania. "Most women may be able to swim until late in pregnancy or even up until the day they deliver."

Do's and Don'ts

"There is no single exercise prescription that will meet the needs of all pregnant women," says Raul Artal, M.D., professor of obstetrics, gynecology, and exercise science at the University of Southern California School of Medicine in Los

Angeles. "You should consult your doctor to help you tailor an exercise program based on your own pregnancy and health status and activity level."

If you are very overweight or carrying twins, have a history of obstetric complications, or have a physical condition that affects your heart or lungs, all but the most mild stretching exercises may be off-limits.

Once you've consulted your doctor, you might consider joining a monitored prenatal exercise program sponsored by a hospital or the YWCA. Make sure it's supervised by a certified instructor knowledgeable in the postural changes that pregnancy causes, advises Dr. Hall.

While you have a wide range of beneficial exercises to choose from, there are a few that you'll want to avoid for safety reasons.

On the experts' list of exercises generally considered taboo are activities that may involve falling, such as horseback riding and downhill skiing. Activities involving bouncing and quick, jerky turns—such as racquet sports—are not recommended because of their potential to damage joints and ligaments, which are loosened by the hormonal changes of pregnancy. You should avoid lifting heavy weights for the same reason.

If you have been running on a regular basis, experts say you may continue running throughout your pregnancy, provided you get your doctor's approval and you moderate your pace. Some doctors recommend limiting running to no more than 2 miles daily during pregnancy.

"You should pace and distance yourself according to your own physical comfort and with the guidance of your doctor," says Dr. Botti.

Many runners find that the enlarging abdomen naturally slows them down around the fifth month of pregnancy and that walking regularly is easier during the remaining months, says Dr. Botti.

Whether you join a group or go solo, you should get approval from your obstetrician and follow these exercise guidelines set by the American College of Obstetrics and Gynecology (ACOG). They are aimed at minimizing overheating, dehydration, lowered oxygen, and injury to mother and baby.

- Don't exercise in hot, humid weather or when you have a fever. Avoid saunas and hot tubs.
- Don't exercise strenuously for prolonged periods. After 15 minutes stop and take your pulse. Your exercising heart rate should not exceed 140 beats per minute. The activity should not leave you gasping for breath; you should be able to talk and exercise at the same time.
- Don't exercise while lying on your back for prolonged periods. This position may be risky because the uterus cuts off blood flow to the heart.
- Do gentle warm-up stretches before aerobic exercise.
- Don't stretch to the point of pain.
- Do drink liquids before, during, and after exercise.
- Do listen to your body. What may be simple one day may be difficult the next.
- Do stop and consult your doctor if you have pain, bleeding, or unusual symptoms.

Postpregnancy Shape-Up Plan

A couple of decades ago, women who gave birth were instructed to stay in bed—for ten days. Now we know better. Once you have your baby, exercise helps to peel off those extra pounds you have been carrying around for the past several months, tones a saggy abdomen, improves posture, and helps you regain that lean look.

And the sooner you start moving, the better. Your postpartum program should be made up of toning exercises. Pelvic tilts will help you combat the back strain from carrying, then cradling, your baby.

Kegel exercises, named after the doctor who invented them, help keep the vagina elastic and prevent bladder problems. To perform them, imagine you are squeezing off your urine flow, then hold and release.

The following exercises, presented in *Essential Exercises for the Childbearing Year* by physical therapist Elizabeth Noble, will complete your postpartum exercise program. They help to restore sluggish leg circulation and shorten stretched abdominal muscles. Start out with five repetitions of each exercise. Increase the length of time you hold a position or increase the number of repetitions as your muscles regain their tone. Never hold your breath as you exercise, and remember to relax between repetitions. In a few weeks, you should be ready to add regular aerobics to your routine.

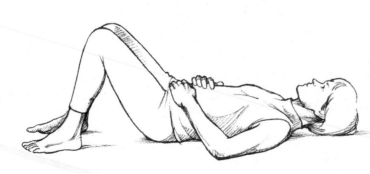

Lie on your back with your knees bent and place your hands on your abdomen. Feel your abdomen expand as you take in a deep breath through your nose. Exhale through pursed lips and force every last bit of air out as you tighten your abdominal muscles. Don't take too many breaths in succession—you may get dizzy. Once you get the hang of this exercise, tighten your muscles on a normal outward breath while you're standing or sitting.

Lie on your back with your knees bent.
Keep your lower back pressed against the
floor as you slide your feet out in front of
you. If you feel your lower spine begin to
arch, bring your feet back until your spine
is flat again. Try to move your feet a little
farther out each time you do the exercise,
progressing until you can keep your back
flat with your legs out straight.

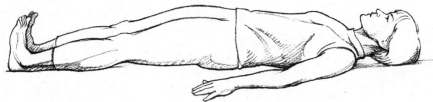

Lie on your back with your
knees bent and your lower back
pressed against the floor. Stretch
out your arms as you inhale.
Then exhale and tuck your
chin, rolling your head and
upper torso forward off the floor.
Slowly lower yourself down,
inhaling as you do. After this
becomes too easy, you can add
some difficulty, first by folding
your arms over your chest, then
by holding your hands at the
sides of your head.

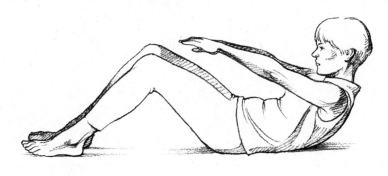

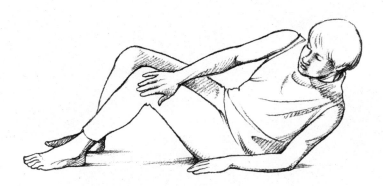

To strengthen the sides of your
abdomen (the obliques), do the
previous exercise, except curl
up toward your left knee, then
toward your right. Alternate
sides, doing one side for each
sit-up.

Postpregnancy Shape-Up Plan—Continued

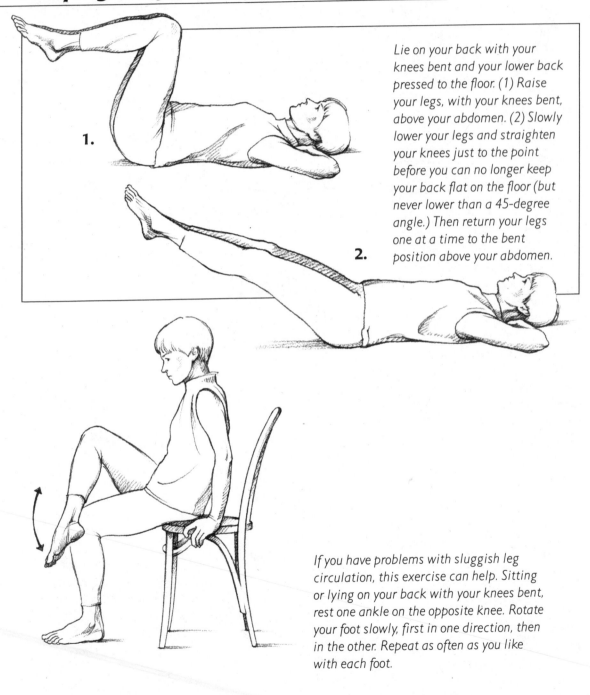

1.

2.

Lie on your back with your knees bent and your lower back pressed to the floor. (1) Raise your legs, with your knees bent, above your abdomen. (2) Slowly lower your legs and straighten your knees just to the point before you can no longer keep your back flat on the floor (but never lower than a 45-degree angle.) Then return your legs one at a time to the bent position above your abdomen.

If you have problems with sluggish leg circulation, this exercise can help. Sitting or lying on your back with your knees bent, rest one ankle on the opposite knee. Rotate your foot slowly, first in one direction, then in the other. Repeat as often as you like with each foot.

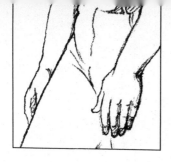

Raynaud's Disease

*I*f the hand life dealt you is a cold one, chances are you're a woman. That's because women are far more likely than men to experience Raynaud's disease—a numbing, sometimes painful coldness in the hands and fingers and, occasionally, the feet. Raynaud's is a common complaint that, fortunately, has an exercise prescription tailor-made to banish symptoms in most people.

Most of the people who complain about the condition are women between the ages of 15 and 45. Blood vessels in their extremities go into spasm and constrict excessively, according to John Abruzzo, M.D., professor of medicine at Thomas Jefferson University in Philadelphia. The skin of the fingers turns white, and in extended spasms, blue, he says.

Normally the condition is more of a painful nuisance than a real danger, but for some that nuisance can be a big one. Some people have such a low tolerance to low temperatures that their hands seem to freeze when they simply reach into the refrigerator for a snack, says Dr. Abruzzo.

Other than dressing warmly even when indoors and perhaps wearing gloves when you take those turkey breasts out of the freezer, little can be done to treat the problem, physicians say. Some people warm up with drug treatment, although others find drugs difficult to tolerate because of their side effects. There is, however, one verified way to snap the cold spell. That is, oddly enough, to imitate a windmill. "It sounds silly, but it works," says John P. Cooke, M.D., Ph.D., director of the Section of Vascular Medicine at Stanford University School of Medicine.

Whenever the blood seems to drain away from your fingers and your hand is about to go into the deep chill, extend your arm and very vigorously circle it around at about 80 revolutions per minute, as if winding up and throwing baseballs in rapid-fire succession.

Emphasize the downward swing of the exercise, and continue the exercise for about a minute or until the fingers warm up. "Centrifugal pressure increases, forcing more blood into the arm," Dr. Cooke says. "No one has studied finger blood flow with the movement, but I have patients who swear it works."

In some people, Raynaud's may be an early symptom of lupus or scleroderma, autoimmune diseases that attack the skin, or of rheumatoid arthritis, says Murray Hamlet, D.V.M., director of plans and operations at the U.S. Army Research Institute of Environmental Medicine and former director its cold research program. So it is important to see a doctor for a checkup and blood test if any limb coldness seems annoyingly frequent or persistent.

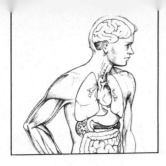

Rehabilitation

Some of us *don't* bounce back from an accident, operation, illness, or injury, at least not right away. Like Humpty-Dumpty, we land with a dull splat and need help putting the pieces together again. That's where rehabilitative medicine comes in.

Rehabilitation, or "rehab" for short, is designed to help someone return to his or her "maximum functional capacity"—to get as "better" as they're gonna get. And the right kind of movement and exercise is a vitally important part of every rehab program. Ideally, the program will restore someone to his or her level of activity before injury or illness intervened. If it can't, it shows the person the best ways to work around the new limitations. Someone who's had a stroke, for instance, may not regain the ability to walk without support. If that's the case, rehab will provide instruction in using a cane or walker.

Rehabilitation generally takes place over a period of weeks or months—sometimes even years. Rehab specialists—doctors, physical therapists, nurses, and others—have learned from experience that for many injuries, the earlier they intervene, the better.

"I'm with them the minute they roll through the doors," says physical therapist Tad Hardee about the people admitted to the regional burn center at the University of Virginia Medical Center in Charlottesville. With early intervention, both he and his patient can see, up front, exactly what the patient can or can't do. The next day, when pain, stiffness, and swelling have set in, Hardee is a familiar face that reminds his patients of what they could do the day before. "I try to make it our mutual goal to maintain the initial level of function," Hardee says.

Therapists say they also like to see an individual before a procedure such as a coronary bypass to show them how to breathe deeply and cough, and to explain why it's important to do so. "That way, when we see them after surgery, when they're in pain, on drugs, and scared, they don't think we're so crazy to suggest it," says Hardee.

If you're facing major surgery that will be followed by rehabilitation, ask your doctor whether it would be appropriate for you to meet your therapist ahead of time. It may make for a better working relationship, especially in those crucial first hours. (If you are going to be cared for by a nurse, ask the nurse to show you the exercises the night before your surgery.)

What about a presurgery exercise program? Physical therapists think it's a great idea but say that too often, they see people only after they've had their surgery. "I'd love to see someone who's going to have a knee or hip replacement before surgery," says Susan Bergholtz, a physical therapist in private practice in New York City. "It really helps a lot if we can get someone started on a strengthening program and teach them how to use a walker or crutches before their operation. It's a lot easier to get up with a walker post-op if you already know how to do it."

It might seem absolutely rude to be bullied out of bed the day after your surgery, and both therapists and nurses are used to a less-than-enthusiastic reception. "Someone might say to me, 'I can't get out of bed today. Come back tomorrow and I'll do it then,' " Hardee says. "Then I have to explain to them why it is going to be even harder to get out of bed tomorrow if they don't do it today."

As safe and warm as your bed may be, it's essential to leave it behind as soon as you can and take those first steps on the road back from injury or illness. Whether you're healing from something as devastating as a stroke or as painful as a broken bone, the right moves can speed your recovery. Let's look at some of the many ways that exercise can help in rehabilitation.

Mending Broken Bones

If you've ever broken an arm or leg, you know what your limb can look like the day the cast comes off—thin, pale, hairy, and flabby. Your bone may be healed, but your muscles have definitely taken a break.

Rehabilitation after a fracture is meant to reduce muscle wasting during the time an arm or leg is immobilized; it helps maintain range of motion in knees, elbows, shoulders, and hips; and it helps you safely regain full use and strength of an arm or leg after the cast has been removed.

Even while your cast is still on, a physical therapist may be able to teach you a number of isometric (nonmovement) exercises that will help preserve the strength of muscles inside the cast, says Mary Alexander, a senior physical therapist in the orthopedics division at the University of Virginia. For instance, if you break your tibia (the big bone in your lower leg), you may be able to do exercises to maintain strength in the muscles in the front and back of your thigh (the quadriceps and hamstrings).

Performing these exercises while the cast is on may help reduce scar-tissue formation, muscle wasting, swelling, and the risk of blood clots, Alexander says. They're especially important for someone who is stuck in bed for a while, as might be the case with a pelvic fracture or a break that requires traction. (In all rehabilitation cases, including these, you should be doing exercises only with your doctor's okay.)

You'll also learn to keep the joints above and below the cast moving by doing range-of-motion exercises while your limb is casted. These exercises keep adjacent joints from becoming stiff. "If you break your tibia, for instance, you may be able to keep your hip joint moving by gently moving your leg out to the side and back, or up and down," Alexander says.

And when your cast finally comes off for good, a physical therapist will help you loosen up tight joints, using range-of-motion exercises and perhaps some hands-on techniques that slowly stretch the tissues around the joint. This part of the process cannot be hurried.

If you've just had a cast removed from your leg, for example, it may take a while before you can straighten your knee and walk normally. The trick, therapists say, is to be patient but persistent, and to realize that you may have some additional pain during or after a therapy session. (Ice, aspirin, heat, ultrasound, and massage can all offer relief.)

"How long you take to recover fully depends on lots of things," Alexander says. "Different bones heal at different rates. Older people take longer to heal than younger people. Bad fractures take longer than clean ones. There's no simple formula for when someone is going to be better."

Recovering from Surgery

You've just experienced the physical trauma of surgery. You've lain helpless and unconscious while a team of doctors labored over you for hours. Now you've just awakened feeling nauseous and exhausted. And some enthusiastic therapist is hanging his face into yours, telling you he's going to help you breathe deeply, cough, and, horror of horrors, get out of bed. You'd rather die first! No, wait. You *wouldn't* rather die first! Okay, now, what's this guy saying?

Resting after surgery *is* important. But too much horizontal time has its hazards. It can lead to blood clots, pneumonia, muscle weakness, bone loss, and problems with low blood pressure when you finally try to stand. Oh, and there's also bedsores—a painful breakdown of tissue from constant pressure, usually on the buttocks. That's why getting out of bed, even if it's just to sit in a chair or shuffle to the bathroom, is so important. It helps counteract the negative effects of bed rest. And it's a start, however small, toward normal activities.

Therapists emphasize coughing and deep breathing right after surgery. Actually, this is a vitally important form of exercise because during any kind of surgery that requires general anesthesia, your lungs collect mucus. Mucus provides a rich growing medium for the bacteria that can cause pneumonia.

"Both coughing and deep breathing help bring mucus up and out," Bergholtz says. But after surgery, people tend to suppress coughing and to breathe shallowly, using only the upper portions of their lungs. That's because chest or abdominal surgery, or cracked ribs, makes it painful to cough or take a full breath. "People are not likely to do either on their own unless they're reminded that it's important for recovery," Bergholtz says. Some pain medications, especially narcotics, also depress breathing, so it may be important to find a happy balance between pain relief and sedation.

Anyone can do deep breathing after surgery, but learning and doing it *before* surgery is even better, Bergholtz says. That way, you get to practice before you really need it, and you can use the relaxation response brought on by deep breathing to get you through those tension-ridden presurgery hours.

To do deep breathing, it's easiest to lie flat. If you are sitting, make sure you sit up straight—not rigid, but not slumped over. You want your abdomen and chest to be able to expand easily. (If you have an incision that makes deep breathing painful, however, you may want to press a rolled-up towel or a pillow against the incision to relieve the pain.)

Put one hand on your abdomen just below your ribs. Take a slow breath in through your nose, hold it for a second, then let it out. If you are deep-breathing correctly, the hand on your belly will move out when inhaling, as the lower lungs fill with air. You might want to imagine you are blowing up a balloon in your belly. "We tell our patients to deep-breathe up to ten times an hour during the time they are awake, until they are fairly active again," says Cynthia Kane, R.N., clinical director of the Pulmonary Rehabilitation Program at Rehabilitation Institute of Chicago. "In actual practice, though, most are likely to deep-breathe three or four times every couple of hours." Usually, it's a nurse bringing in pain medications who reminds a patient to breathe deeply, and who may ask for a demonstration, she says. (See "Breathing Therapies" on page 333.)

To cough, try hugging a pillow—or better yet, a big teddy bear—against your incision to provide counterpressure and to feel more secure, Bergholtz suggests.

Most patients are encouraged to get moving within 24 hours of surgery. "We can show them ways to get in and out of bed that put very little strain on the chest and abdomen," Bergholtz says. For instance, a person can roll from his back to his side, drop his legs over the side of the bed, and then push up into a sitting position. "Once they see that they can get out of bed, into a chair, and walk without hurting much, people are willing to do it," she says.

Need more encouragement? "I tell people our bodies are designed to work in an upright position," Hardee says. That goes for the urinary and digestive tracts, as well. "Not having to use a bedpan is a great postoperative goal for most people," Hardee says. "And any patient with a urinary catheter wants it out. We say it will come out as soon as they start urinating on their own, and the best way to do that is to stand up, move around, and let gravity help." Lungs also begin to clear better once you're up and around, because physical activity forces you to breathe more deeply and gets air into more areas of your lungs than when you are lying down, Kane says.

Up and About

Sometimes people do have to stay in bed for weeks. As a result, they lose strength and endurance, and they can also develop a condition called orthostatic hypotension. That is, sitting up causes a sudden drop in blood pressure, and they get dizzy and nauseated. "That's because the heart loses some of its tone and strength because it's not doing much work when you are lying down," Hardee explains. "When you sit up, it doesn't respond as quickly as it normally would."

People can have a tough time with this one, Hardee says, but it just gets worse the longer they remain in bed. That's another reason why it's important to get up, with help, as soon as possible, even if it's initially just to sit or stand for a few minutes. Doing strengthening exercises in bed may also help, Hardee says.

After someone's up and moving, a gradual progressive walking program is often recommended to restore cardiovascular endurance and muscle strength. "It's something we push very strongly at our hospital because we think everyone can benefit from it," Hardee says. How fast someone progresses depends on that person's level of fitness before surgery and the length of time needed for his or her recovery.

Specific therapeutic exercises are recommended after some kinds of surgery. Women who have surgery for breast cancer, for example, are encouraged to do exercises that keep their shoulder flexible and reduce swelling in their arm. Those who've had heart bypass surgery may go through weeks of rehabilitation, during which they learn how to safely restore their cardiovascular strength.

Plan on taking three to six months to completely recover from major surgery that involves general anesthesia, Bergholtz says. Ask your doctor before your surgery what kind of recovery plan he or she has in mind and whether you'll be seeing a physical therapist. "Even a one-time consultation after surgery can be very helpful," Bergholtz says. People who have a solid recovery game plan are more likely to fully recover from surgery.

And that goes for strokes, too.

After a Stroke

A stroke is serious business, no doubt about that. A hemorrhage or blood clot that damages parts of the brain, a stroke can cause all sorts of problems. But one in every ten people who have a stroke returns to a normal life with no major impairment, and four out of ten have only mild disabilities. Even those with serious problems can improve with help from rehab specialists, says Julie Moreland, a physical therapist specializing in stroke rehabilita-

tion at Chedoke-McMaster Hospital in Hamilton, Ontario.

Unless a stroke is very mild, a certain amount of rehabilitation is standard practice. A stroke can damage parts of the brain that control muscle movements and body control, usually on one side only. That side of the body may feel heavy, useless, and unusually warm or cold, says Moreland.

After a stroke, an individual may have to relearn, step by step, many of the activities we all take for granted, such as grasping objects, getting out of bed, or walking up stairs. Sometimes parts of the brain that control a person's ability to learn or remember are also damaged by a stroke, which makes rehabilitation more difficult. "And sometimes a person begins to ignore, or neglect, his stroke-damaged side, almost as though it were no longer there," Moreland says. Then the therapist's job is to draw attention to the injured side so the person continues to try to use it.

"Some of these people are dealing with a great loss, so we feel it is very important to focus on what they *can* do," Moreland says.

Rehabilitation is started as soon as a stroke patient is stabilized and out of danger. That may take a few days to a number of weeks, Moreland says.

In the initial stages of rehabilitation, a person recovering from a stroke may be asked to or even helped to roll from side to side in bed or on a floor mat as a prelude to being able to rise to a sitting position without assistance. He may practice bending his knees and ankles before he begins walking. He may practice catching and throwing a ball to regain coordination.

STROLLING DOWN EASY STREET

Fran Roberts vividly recalls taking her father to a Chicago Cubs baseball game soon after he started using a walker to get around. Both her father and his walker got stuck in a turnstile, with an impatient crowd pressing in on him.

That was the last baseball game he attended, she says. "He won't even go near a turnstile."

It's those tight-squeeze situations that a rehabilitation program called Easy Street helps people to master. Now at 42 hospitals nationwide, the program is a veritable obstacle course of lifelike settings. A typical Easy Street may include curbs and bus steps; an automobile and a gas pump; a theater aisle and ramp; a bank; a grocery store complete with rolls of filmy plastic bags at the produce department; a restaurant with booths; and, for those who make it to the end, a bar stool.

Easy Streets are designed to be both challenging and fun. One at the Mid-Michigan Regional Medical Center in Midland has a greenhouse and a putting green where people work to improve their balance and eye-hand coordination. One in Boise, Idaho, has a simulated hiking trail, complete with rocks and a giant mural of the beautiful Sawtooth Mountains. And a Miami, Florida, course challenges people to get some sand between their toes.

"It makes therapy real," explains Pamela Gifford, director of rehabilitation services at the Mid-Michigan Medical Center. "It gives people a true-to-life experience in the same kind of environment they will be in when they leave the hospital.

"People really understand what therapy is all about within this environment. It's one thing to put a patient on a mat and tell her she needs to do exercises to strengthen her legs so that she can go food shopping when she gets home. It's completely different when you take someone into a store, have her load up the shopping cart with groceries, go through the checkout, then push the cart all the way down to the other end of the street and have her load the groceries into the car. All of a sudden those leg exercises take on true importance and new meaning."

"A variety of exercises help to keep arms and legs stronger and joints flexible and to minimize the severe muscle rigidity that sometimes occurs with a stroke," Moreland says.

Specific muscle-strengthening exercises may be done for a particular problem. People who "lock" their knees forcefully back when shifting their weight forward while walking, for instance, may benefit from exercises that strengthen the muscles in the front and back of the thighs (the quadriceps and hamstrings), he says.

Endurance training can benefit those who have enough muscle control to pedal a bicycle, Moreland says. They may find it helpful to use "arm bicycles" or exercise bikes modified to allow someone to pedal with his feet while sitting in a wheelchair.

People with serious head injuries often follow a rehab program similar to that for strokes. They may have to relearn simple actions like walking and may face problems with understanding, memory, and motivation. And people with spinal cord injuries that leave parts of their body

STAYING MOTIVATED ON THE ROAD TO RECOVERY

Professional athletes use all kinds of strategies to keep themselves going when injury cuts into their playing time—and their income. Those same methods can help you through a physical rehabilitation program, experts say. The top five can be adapted for your use.

Set realistic, fun goals. "I know I can't save money for a vacation unless I have the trip all planned," explains physical therapist Jennie Scipio, at the National Rehabilitation Hospital in Washington, D.C. "That's why I try to get my patients to plan something fun they can really work toward."

One stroke patient, for example, wasn't making much progress relearning to walk. Then his daughter became engaged and set a wedding date, and his walking program took off. His goal—to march his daughter down the aisle—made the difference.

Sometimes patients express goals that seem unrealistically high to those treating them, says Stanley F. Wainapel, M.D., associate director of the Department of Rehabilitation Medicine at St. Luke's–Roosevelt Hospital in New York City.

"When that happens, we defer their disappointment," he says. "Instead, we break down the goal into concrete tasks and then tackle them one at a time." It's hard to assess just how far a patient will get, he says, "and some surprise all of us by doing much better than anyone expected."

Other people undergoing rehab may not believe they can reach a goal a therapist has set for them, even though that goal is realistic, says Fred Cromes, Ph.D., associate professor in the Department of Physical Medicine and Rehabilitation at the University of Texas Southwestern Medical School in Dallas.

"None of us jump at something we think we are going to fail," he says. That's especially likely to happen if a person believes he can't do what the therapist is currently asking. To overcome this, patients need to express their concerns and fears to their therapist. The same strategy—breaking the goal down into smaller tasks, and tackling them one at a time—works here as well, Dr. Cromes says.

Some people aren't emotionally ready for rehab even though their bodies are. "Maybe they have to go home and decide for themselves that they don't want to sit

---

paralyzed often need extensive rehabilitation that focuses on adapting to their new limitations.

Getting the Best of Burns

Even people with burn injuries must do exercises. They must keep moving in order to counteract the tendency for burned skin to contract and shrink. Exercises that stretch the skin, especially over joints like knuckles or knees, and that keep joints

moving help to reduce swelling, minimize scar tissue, and encourage the maturation of a skin graft, explains occupational therapist Cheryl Leman, director of burn rehabilitation at the Washington Hospital Center's Burn Center in Washington, D.C.

People who have been severely burned may also be encouraged to participate in a general conditioning program during the time they are recovering, says Leman. "Exercising the entire body—using a sta-

around and do nothing," Dr. Wainapel says. "Then they come back for help." Part of getting ready for rehab may involve going through feelings of hurt, anger, and loss.

Don't let pain stop you. Rehab can hurt, no doubt about that. "Some people will go ahead and work even though it hurts. It's not a big deal to them," Dr. Cromes says. "Others are stopped by even a little pain. They are more motivated to avoid pain than to proceed toward something that they want." Finding ways to deal with the pain—relaxation training, deep breathing, pain medications, antidepressants, even making sure you get a good night's sleep—can help a person get fired up for a day's therapy. For most rehab patients, pain lessens with time, too, Dr. Cromes adds. "Patients have to believe that so they can move forward."

Know ahead of time what your rehabilitation should entail. Hang-ups in motivation often come from anxiety from not knowing what comes next, Dr. Wainapel says. So ask questions and get answers you can understand. He often sees patients who are going to have a leg amputated. "I tell them they may feel like their leg is still

there, and that that's common; they're not going crazy," he says. Before the surgery he also details their exercise rehabilitation program and discusses artificial legs at that time.

Beware of self-sabotage. People in hospitals often feel out of control. They're being awakened at night for blood pressure readings or pills and being told when to eat and when to go to the bathroom. "Some feel like the only control they have is their mouth—and they use it to say no," Dr. Wainapel says.

Make sure you're not refusing something that really is in your best interest and that will only help you regain control—like rehab.

Get support. Just as a professional athlete has people to turn to for help, so should you. "Being sick or injured can erode a person's sense of self-worth, and if you don't feel good about yourself, it's hard to be motivated," Dr. Wainapel says. The best help? Support groups of people in the same situation as you, experts say. These groups not only exchange valuable information about how to deal with a illness, they provide the empathy of someone who really has walked in your shoes.

tionary bicycle, for instance, and weight lifting—helps to preserve the body's muscle tissue." That's important because the body tends to rob itself of healthy muscle tissue in order to heal burned areas, she explains. Aerobic exercise also helps maintain strength and endurance. That's crucial for people who must return to a physically demanding job—shimmying up telephone poles and moving big spools of wire, for example.

Like all major injuries, recovery from burns continues long after someone leaves the hospital. "Most burn patients, for instance, follow a stretching and strengthening routine at home for about a year before they fully recover," Leman says.

People who know that exercises will help speed their recovery and live a normal life are more likely to make a commitment to a program and stick with it.

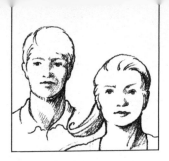

Sex Problems

It's as easy as climbing two flights of stairs, they say. Making love supposedly requires no more exertion than that needed to make a jaunt up to the third floor.

Sounds easy enough, but imagine making the climb if you're too depressed or stressed out to even try, or if you're uncertain of your ability to go all the way. Or if you're too tired. Or if you're ill or too overweight or out of shape to make the ascent easily. Those who can't climb the staircase may choose to remain on the ground floor and only occasionally, very self-consciously, perhaps unsuccessfully, and with much inept effort, make the trip up.

Sex is no stair climb, of course. It's a delicate dance of psychology and biology, athletics and artistry, a melding of two minds and two bodies. It's a warm, intimate, caressing mesh of flesh and fervor fraught with myth, fear, and even a few taboos.

Aerobic Aphrodisiac

But ultimately, making love is a physical act that requires a certain level of muscular and mental finesse and fitness. That's where exercise comes in.

Regular exercise helps prepare you for sexual intercourse both mentally and physically, according to Linda De Villers, Ph.D., a Santa Monica psychologist who specializes in sexuality and who leads workshops on increasing sexual confidence through exercise. Exercise, she maintains, helps counteract what she terms "the disease of the '90s"—inhibited sexual desire.

In people with inhibited sexual desire, an increasing number of whom are men, "the plumbing works. There's no dysfunction," Dr. De Villers says, but they are "actively inhibiting sexual impulses in a way that causes problems in their relationships." Even younger couples and couples in relatively new relationships "are going not just weeks but months without sex," she says. "It's a shocker to me."

The cure can be as shockingly simple: "I always manage to bring exercise up early on in therapy," says Dr. De Villers. While dark psychological problems may well lie behind a lazy libido, "it would be an exception to have somebody in therapy for low sexual desire who is a regular exerciser," she says.

The few studies conducted on the sex-exercise connection support that view. Almost half of more than 8,000 women polled by Dr. De Villers reported an increase in sexual activity and arousal after beginning regular exercise programs. Another study, done at the University of California, San Diego, looked at a group of sedentary, middle-aged men who were placed on a nine-month aerobic program of jogging, rebounding (jumping on a mini-trampoline), or stationary bicycling. During the study, the men "significantly" increased the frequency of their lovemaking encounters in comparison to a similar group that was not working out. Exercisers in the study who smoked less or completely quit increased both their desire to have sex and their number of satisfying sexual encounters more than all other men in the study. Not only that, researchers noted that "the degree of sexuality enhancement among exercisers correlated with the degree of their individual improvement in fitness." Talk about incentive to work out!

Similar findings came out of a study conducted at Harvard University. In that study, a group of competitive masters swimmers between the ages of 40 and 69 reported making love as frequently as people 20 to 30 years their junior, according to the study's principal author, Phillip Whitten, Ph.D., a behavioral scientist and research associate in Harvard's Department of Anthropology. The swimmers in their forties had sex more than seven times a month, he says, and those in their sixties were nearly as active.

Sexual Anorexia

The onus for a lax libido falls heavily on stress and depression, which "are devastating to sexual functioning," according to Helen Singer Kaplan, M.D., Ph.D, director of the Human Sexuality Program at the New York Hospital–Cornell Medical Center in New York City. Chronic stress turns lovemaking into an impossible act,

leading to what she calls "sexual anorexia." But even mild stress and low-grade chronic depression dull the libido, according to Shirley Zussman, Ed.D., a sex and marital therapist in New York City and a director of the Association for Male Sexual Dysfunction in New York. "You have very little appetite for anything—life in general and certainly sex," she says.

Stress and depression force the body to secrete more of the chemical cortisol, which suppresses the production of sex hormones, explains Barry J. Klyde, M.D., an endocrinologist with New York Hospital–Cornell Medical Center. The increased levels of this hormone upset the neurotransmitters in the brain responsible for stable emotions.

Stress also causes constriction of peripheral arteries, preventing blood from flowing to the genitals. Decreased blood flow also inhibits arousal.

"And what do we know about exercise and depression?" Dr. De Villers asks. "Exercise, particularly aerobic exercise, is an antidepressant. But it's not just an antidepressant. It's also great for relieving stress." Exercise promotes the release of endorphins, the body's own feel-good chemicals, and helps restore the neurochemical balance that affects emotions, she explains.

Weight and Your Mate

Body image also plays an enormous role in sexual feelings, Dr. Zussman says. The improved self-esteem that comes from a healthier, more attractive body carries over into sexual situations, she says. "The way you view yourself is just as important as—if not more important than—how your partner feels about you." An increasing number of women are becoming more self-conscious of how they appear in their mates' eyes while in bed as well, Dr. Zussman says. "It's not the sex itself, but the way they feel their partners respond to their desirability, which certainly influences their ability to free themselves and enjoy the sexual experience."

The men and women in Dr. Whitten's Harvard study of swimmers ranked themselves high in body image, but more important, he says, their partners gave them even greater marks.

Sexual confidence and satisfaction are highly correlated with weight, Dr. De Villers says. Many women, for example, are reluctant to assume the female-superior position, even though it offers many benefits for themselves and their mates, because their self-image is fragile and they feel too visible when on top. "They say, 'He can see my fat stomach. He can see my hanging breasts,' " she quotes them as complaining.

Losing fat and resculpting the body through diet and exercise, though, will shape self-perception and bring the mind more in tune with the body, Dr. De Villers says. "If you're not ashamed of your body, you'll be much less sexually inhibited and have a better time in bed," she says. (See "Overweight" on page 252 for information on how to use exercise to lose weight.)

Intense exercise elevates the amount of human growth hormone in the body, Dr. Whitten says. One study has indicated that men in their sixties injected with human growth hormone increased their muscle mass and reduced body fat, essentially reversing the aging process, he says.

While this study did not specifically examine sexuality, it may help explain what happened to the masters swimmers in Dr. Whitten's study. He says he suspects that his swimmers and others who work out regularly may be experiencing increased rates of release of human growth hormone, which results in higher levels of the hormone in the blood. "If they're physically active, they're exhibiting all the characteristics of someone who is younger," he says. "It seems to me reasonable that they would also behave that way."

While regular exercise apparently revs up the libido, too much exercise virtually shuts down the body's sex hormone factory in both men and women. "Fertility and sexuality can be impaired by exhaustive exercise," Dr. Kaplan says.

The personality traits of fanatic exercisers are, in fact, similar to those of anorexics, Dr. De Villers says. "If you're obsessive-compulsive about exercise, you'll have neither the interest in nor the energy for sex."

Rising to the Occasion

The right amount of exercise can also help prevent impotence.

Men who ignore cardiovascular health soon learn that the price may be a higher one than they are willing to pay. "A man can have a heart attack," says E. Douglas Whitehead, M.D., a New York City urologist who is co-founder and director (with Dr. Zussman) of the Association for Male Sexual Dysfunction in New York. "But he also can have a penis attack." He won't experience it as a sudden stab of pain, but rather as a gradual loss of function.

TAPPING THE KEGEL

Kegeling is not kegling—a game of ten-pins down at Lanes and Lounge—but it sure can bowl you over in bed.

To enhance sexual enjoyment for both men and women, some cultures emphasize exercising and learning to control the pelvic perineal and pubococcygeal (PC) muscles, according to Domeena Renshaw, M.D., a professor of psychiatry at Loyola University in Chicago. The PC muscles surround and support the genitals and anus. Oriental prostitutes are "legendary and much prized," says Dr. Renshaw, for their ability to seize the penis with their vagina.

But there's no real trick. All it takes is time and practice. Kegels, the same exercises that can cure urinary incontinence, can also heighten orgasmic pleasure and help prevent premature ejaculation.

When kegeling, you voluntarily tighten the same muscles that contract spasmodically during orgasm. Some men can train themselves to distinguish between orgasm and ejaculation, according to E. Douglas Whitehead, M.D., a New York City urologist who is co-founder and director of the Association for Male Sexual Dysfunction in New York.

Near the point at which ejaculation is inevitable, a man can tense the PC muscles in an internal variation of the old squeeze technique.

He prevents ejaculation but still feels the orgasm. "It's simple to do but takes a lot of willpower in sexual situations," Dr. Whitehead says. Although the man may briefly lose his erection, with an understanding partner he quickly regains it because he did not ejaculate.

Then, like the Energizer Bunny, he can keep going and going and going.

A woman can derive even greater benefits from kegeling than a man. While the squeeze of stronger PC muscles enhances the sensations of her partner, kegeling pulls more vaginal nerve endings around the penis, enhancing the sensation for the woman as well, according to Barbara DeBetz, M.D., a New York City psychiatrist and author of *Erotic Focus*.

Kegels also help a woman gain heightened vaginal awareness, says New York City sex and marital therapist Shirley Zussman, Ed.D. "Men, from birth on, have something visible and touchable. A vagina is hidden, not part of a woman's awareness for some time." And even then, women "are brought up almost to ignore vaginal feelings," she says. All of that tends to disassociate a woman from a part of her body, Dr. Zussman says, "and exercising the muscle and being aware of it has a real contribution in making a more complete body image and feeling." (Strengthening that muscle, according to Dr. Zussman, does not necessarily make a woman more orgasmic or contribute to more intense orgasms.)

Using Kegel exercises to enhance sexual pleasure involves experimenting with variations on the pace of contraction and relaxation. Once proficient at manipulating the muscle, you might try tightening and releasing in rapid-fire succession, mimicking the involuntary contraction of orgasm. Then when making love, you can opt to tighten the muscle when appropriate, either as a climax-builder or to prevent ejaculation. (To learn more about how to do these exercises, see "Kegel Exercises" on page 368.)

The risk factors that lead to coronary artery disease—smoking, a sedentary lifestyle, a diet high in fat and cholesterol—"are the same factors operative in patients who develop impotence due to impaired blood flow to the penis," Dr. Whitehead says. "Whatever is good for a healthy heart is good for a healthy penis."

Regular exercise is "extremely important," maintains Dr. Whitehead. In younger men, it may prevent impotence due to impaired blood flow and ensure sexual function well into the senior years, he says.

Being overweight also can lead to impotence, says Dr. Klyde. "I see that in many, many men," he says. Excess fat converts the male sex hormone testosterone into the female sex hormone estrogen. As a result, desire wanes, frequency and firmness of erections decrease, and the testicles may atrophy, explains Dr. Klyde. Men even can grow breasts—"not just fat tissue but actual glandular tissue." A weight-reducing exercise program, he says, will reverse the condition, shrinking the breasts, resuscitating the libido, and reviving the erections.

While too much body fat can damage a man's sexual response, too *little* endangers a woman's hormone balance and her ability to become sexually aroused, Dr. Klyde says. Overexercise can take the spin out of women's menstrual cycles, which eventually stop as estrogen diminishes. A lack of adequate estrogen supply can produce the symptoms of menopause in younger women. Sexual desire may diminish as the vagina shrinks. Vaginal linings thin and lubrication ceases. All of these effects contribute to one of the most common female sexual dysfunctions—painful or uncomfortable intercourse.

Again, the right kind of exercise—and not too much or too little—is the answer.

Aerobic exercises—the kind of activity recommended to improve sexual functioning—include walking, running, swimming, dancing, bicycling, cross-country skiing, and jumping. To start an appropriate exercise program, see chapters in part 2.

The only other exercise that's good for sex, Dr. Kaplan says, is sex itself. Postmenopausal women who remain sexually active don't lose as much vaginal lubrication, and sexually active men are much less likely to develop potency problems.

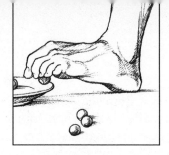

Shin Splints

You've taken up hiking around the block in the evenings in an attempt to decrease that stealthily increasing waistline. One day you notice a nagging pain in your shins that throbs with every step.

You've just encountered shin splints.

Although you may have thought that this persistent and annoying problem occurs only in hard-core athletes, shin splints can strike *anyone* doing unaccustomed or increased exercise.

"I see them in people who visit San Francisco," says Holly Wilson Greene, Ph.D., a certified athletic trainer and physical therapist who treats patients at Ortho-East Physical Therapy in Berkeley. "They get them from walking up and down the hills and doing more walking than usual."

So what exactly is this nagging pain in your shins? Although the term has been used to describe a sizable collection of conditions that cause shin pain—including stress fractures—your basic, aching shin splint results from a muscle strain. Your muscles have tugged at their attachments to the bone, resulting in tiny muscle tears and inflammation.

Shin splints may pop up any time you overstress the leg muscles, such as when you take up an unaccustomed activity,

increase your mileage, change your running surface, or even change your shoes. "A lot of it revolves around poor selection of shoes and poor flexibility and strength," says Jennifer Stone, head athletic trainer at the U.S. Olympic Training Center in Colorado Springs.

The good news is that simple shin splints respond well to at-home treatment—generally rest, ice, and an anti-inflammatory agent such as aspirin—and can usually be prevented through stretching, doing strengthening exercises, altering your exercise routine, and making sure your shoes fit properly and are in good shape.

Those Aching Shins

The bad news about shin splints is that if you have them, you'll have to cut back on the walking, jogging, or aerobics until the pain abates.

Forcing yourself to continue working out with shin splints is definitely not a good idea, says Thomas Hoerner, M.D., team physician at Merrimack College in North Andover, Massachusetts, and staff physician at Lawrence General Hospital. "If people run through shin splints, they're going to end up with periostitis [inflammation of the bone covering] and stress fractures," he says.

Complete rest is not necessary, but you should find activities that don't stress your legs. "Basically you rest the part that hurts," says Stone, "but try to keep everything else active."

The pain in your shins may reflect a more serious problem, and if it has not abated after two weeks of rest you should see a physician. You may have a stress fracture, periostitis, or compartment syndrome, a condition in which the muscles in the leg become so inflamed that blood flow is cut off or impeded. (If you have acute compartment syndrome, in addition to leg pain your foot will feel numb or cold, and you must seek emergency treatment.)

But in most cases the pain will greatly diminish after two weeks of decreased activity, and you can carefully begin exercising again as long as your activity doesn't cause your symptoms to return.

Once you've experienced shin splints, you should look into what caused them in the first place. Taking the proper preventive action can keep them from coming back. Here's what you need to know.

Why It Hurts

There are two common types of shin splints: posterior, with pain along the lower inside border of the shin, and anterior, with pain at the front of the leg down the outside border of the shin. The muscle involved in posterior shin splints— the tibialis posterior—holds up your arch and stabilizes the foot. It is easily overworked. Many people suffering from posterior shin splints, the more common type, are "overpronators." That means they roll their foot too far inward after it hits the ground.

Anterior shin splints occur because the anterior tibial muscles, which slow your

foot down and keep it from slapping on the ground, are usually weaker than your calf muscles. Because of this imbalance, the foot pulls downward, overworking your anterior muscles. This type of shin splint is common in uphill runners and people who work out on hard surfaces.

The simplest cause of shin splints is overuse. "People do a lot of running or walking too soon before they're in condition, particularly the first sunny day of the year," says Dr. Greene. Stone recommends you not vary your workout—in either intensity or distance—by more than 10 percent per week. "Increasing from 1 mile a week to 2 miles a week may not sound like much," she says, "but that's a 100 percent increase."

Fending Off the Pain

To avoid shin splints, stretching is important, as are muscle-strengthening exercises. Because you can damage cold muscles, it's important to warm up before you stretch. You can warm up by walking slowly, jogging gently, or riding a stationary bicycle. Dr. Greene recommends that you break into a sweat before you start stretching—about 5 minutes of warm-up is usually adequate. Stretching *after* your workout as well is highly recommended.

Remember to always stretch gently. "There shouldn't be so much force on the muscle tissue that you have to grit your teeth to tolerate it," says Dr. Greene. She recommends 15 minutes of stretching.

A good basic stretch to loosen calf muscles is to stand facing a wall, approximately an arm's length away, with one foot in front of the other. Keep your back leg straight and your front leg bent, with your toes pointed forward. Place your palms flat against the wall and lean forward by bending your elbows, keeping your back leg straight and both heels on the floor. Then switch leg positions and repeat. (See the illustrations on page 294 for additional stretches.)

If you are susceptible to shin splints, experts recommend that you strengthen the muscles on the front of your lower leg as well as the muscles in the arch and toes. You also need to stretch the muscles at the back of your legs. You can work the appropriate muscles in your foot and leg by repeatedly scrunching up a towel with your toes. To strengthen the muscles in the front of your leg, sit on a table with a handbag or other weight hung over your foot and slowly lift your foot repeatedly.

What's under Your Foot

All the strengthening exercises in the world, however, aren't going to help you if you're wearing the wrong shoes during your workouts. In general, you want a shoe with a wide, well-cushioned heel. Also, the back part of the shoe that supports the heel should be firm, not soft.

If you're doing uphill workouts, try a heel lift, which will reduce the strain on the anterior muscles. You can buy them, or make your own by cutting a piece of carpeting or cork to fit, says Maine podiatrist Roy Corbin, D.P.M., vice president of the American Academy of Podiatric Sports Medicine.

If you suffer from posterior shin splints, ask at a running shoe store for shoes that help prevent overpronation, he advises. Arch supports or custom-molded orthotic devices can also help.

Finally, you may have to bite the bullet and ditch your favorite shoes. If you've put in hundreds of miles, whether walking or running, it's time to head to the shoe store. Somewhere between 300 and 800 miles, the shoe is worn out, no matter what it looks like, says Stone. Likewise, aerobic shoes can lose their cushioning after four to six months of twice-a-week low-impact workouts.

It's important for you to wear well-constructed shoes. The upper isn't always set on the sole correctly, Stone points out. And it will take your leg whichever way the shoe goes. Before buying new shoes, set them on a table at eye level and look at the back of the shoe. Is the top part of the shoe—the upper—centered in relation to the heel? Also check to make sure the thickness of the sole is even on both sides of the heel. Stone says she has had to look at three or four pairs of shoes before she found ones constructed correctly.

Other factors that can prompt shin splints are running, walking, or dancing on a hard, unforgiving surface, and running or walking on a banked surface that pulls some muscles more than others.

If you're running around a track, says Dr. Greene, periodically reverse direction. Try to avoid walking or running on severely banked road shoulders. And look for the softest surface you can find: "The softer the surface, the less the foot will slap down, and the less shock your leg will experience," says Dr. Corbin. The best surfaces are wood chip, grass, dirt, and composite tracks; asphalt is better than concrete, but they're both hard on your legs.

With proper precautions and appropriate stretching and strengthening exercises, shin splints should definitely be a thing of the past.

Shooing Away Shin Splints

You've done all the right things to relieve that nagging ache from yet another bout of shin splints. You've rested; you've applied ice. Isn't there *something* you can do to keep them from returning? Yes.

After the pain has subsided, try out these exercises and stretches. These help keep shin splints at bay by balancing the strength and flexibility of the muscle groups of your leg and foot.

In general, hold each stretch for 30 seconds and then relax a moment before repeating it. It's helpful to do the stretches several times a day. Always stretch gently and slowly, and never stretch so much that it causes pain.

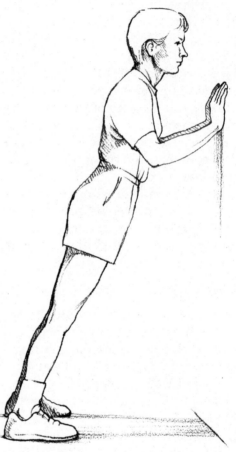

To stretch muscles in the ankles and calves, sit on the floor, a sofa, or a bed that supports your legs. Extend your legs straight in front of you and bend your feet back toward you. Then reverse the stretch by pointing your toes. Also practice these stretches while the soles of your feet are turned inward.

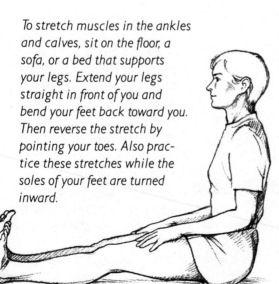

To loosen your calf muscles, stand facing a wall, about an arm's length away. Keep both feet flat on the floor. Place your palms on the wall and then lean forward by bending your elbows. Keep your legs straight and your toes pointed forward. You can stretch your calves more deeply by bending your knees slightly while keeping your heels on the floor.

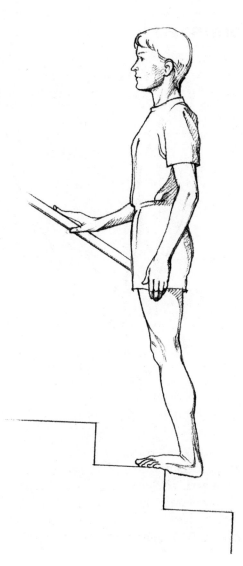

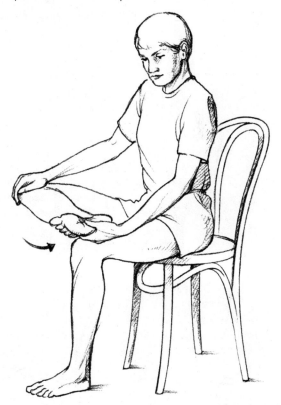

To stretch the muscles in your ankles and feet, sit on a chair and place one foot across the opposite knee. Grasp the foot from underneath and rotate it from the ankle so the sole faces up. Hold, then repeat with the other foot.

Another way to stretch the calf muscles is to stand on the edge of a step and slowly lower your heels below the edge.

Shooing Away Shin Splints—Continued

For another strengthening exercise, sit down and place a tennis ball between the soles of your feet. Practice rolling it from the ball of your foot to the heel and back again.

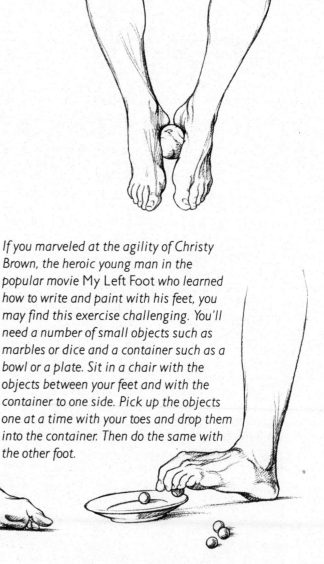

To further strengthen your ankles and feet, try to walk as far as you can on the sides of your feet, with the soles facing each other. Increase the distance as you feel able.

If you marveled at the agility of Christy Brown, the heroic young man in the popular movie My Left Foot who learned how to write and paint with his feet, you may find this exercise challenging. You'll need a number of small objects such as marbles or dice and a container such as a bowl or a plate. Sit in a chair with the objects between your feet and with the container to one side. Pick up the objects one at a time with your toes and drop them into the container. Then do the same with the other foot.

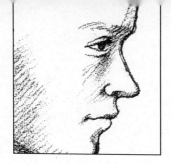

Sinusitis

When Stanley Farb, M.D., an avid tennis player, has sinus pressure and pain, his first inclination is to skip his game and take it easy for the day.

"But I know better," says Dr. Farb, chief of otolaryngology at Montgomery and Sacred Heart hospitals in Norristown, Pennsylvania. "I know that if I just start moving around the court, my sinus trouble will start to clear up."

If you wake up with sinus trouble, your first thought might be to take it easy, too.

Sinus pain and pressure feel like someone has pumped up a balloon inside your skull, one that presses against the back of your eyes, your cheeks, and your forehead. Sinus pain can get so bad, says one sinus sufferer, "you wish you could drill a hole in your skull to release the pressure."

Technically speaking, sinusitis is an inflammation in one of the more than eight small cavities within your head called the para-nasal sinuses. As is typically the case, nasal congestion from a cold or something in the environment that you're allergic to can swell the sinus linings and block the tiny openings that lead to the nose. When swelling occurs, air cannot move in, and mucus cannot move out. Over time, what was a simple case of clogged sinuses can turn into an ugly, raging infection that can be cleared up only with a course of antibiotics.

"Flowing mucus is part of your nose's built-in defense system," says Dr. Farb. A healthy flow of mucus helps filter incoming air and flush out bacteria and other debris. But when mucus stagnates, it becomes an ideal breeding ground for bacteria.

The good news is that when you get your body moving, you help get your nasal mucus moving again—and sinus pain and pressure are escorted out.

"People who exercise regularly seem to have fewer viral infections," says Robert S. Zeiger, M.D., chief of allergy at Kaiser Permanente Medical Center in San Diego.

A Natural Decongestant

"The notion that taking a walk clears your head takes on new meaning if you have sinusitis," says Charles Gross, M.D., professor of otolaryngology–head and neck surgery at the University of Virginia in Charlottesville.

Engaging in physical activity can open up your sinuses in two ways, says Dr. Gross. First, exercise increases the blood supply in your nostrils, flooding your nose with fresh, thin mucus. This fresh mucus helps flush out the stale mucus that's causing you all the trouble.

The second way exercise helps is that it works as a natural decongestant. "When you exercise, your body produces adrenaline, which shrinks swollen blood vessels all over your body, including those in and around your nose," explains Dr. Gross.

Certain types of exercise may be better for sinusitis than others. The slow, stretching movements of yoga, for example, may be ideal, especially if you have throbbing head pain. Brisk walking and bicycling are also good, says Dr. Gross.

While the best exercise prescription for sinus problems calls for staying active, there are a few activities you may want to avoid. You should stay away from any sport that might increase pressure in your sinus cavities—scuba diving or hang gliding, for example.

And don't even think of diving or swimming if you have a cold, says Dr. Farb. "The water going up your nose could push mucus farther back into the sinus cavities, where it can stagnate and trigger an infection," he says.

In general, you should pay close attention to your exercise environment if you're prone to sinusitis. "Most sinusitis is caused by airborne irritants that can make the mucous membranes swell, blocking the sinus cavity," says Dr. Gross.

For this reason, you should not exercise outdoors when the pollution or pollen count is high. Don't exercise in rooms that are overheated or excessively air-conditioned, either. "Low humidity can dry up nasal secretions and worsen sinusitis," says Dr. Gross.

Although regular exercise helps keep your sinus problems at bay, there is one quick relief technique that involves staying put—upside down. Here's what to do when the pressure in your face feels like you just went ten rounds with Sugar Ray.

"Try hanging your head and neck over the side of the bed facedown for a full 5 minutes," suggests Dr. Gross. "This posture will allow the maxillary sinuses, located in the cheekbones, to drain."

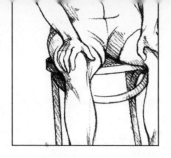

Sprains

So you've sprained your ankle . . . and your ego. And you've hobbled home in agony wondering what steps you should take *now*—and worrying if you'll ever take another step again!

Of course, like thousands of Americans who injure their ankles every year, you will recover. But how *well* you recover depends on what you do after the initial swelling has gone down. Experts agree that unless you strengthen the injured ankle, you're virtually destined to sprain it again.

"After people hurt their ankle, they tend to favor that leg," says physical therapist Cory Collins, of Fitcorp Physical Therapy Center in Boston. "And then the muscles get weak and resprains are likely to occur more frequently. This can spell disaster down the road if you're physically active."

"Exercising the ankle back into shape is *absolutely* the most important thing," says Gary M. Gordon, D.P.M., director of the running and walking clinic at the University of Pennsylvania Sports Medicine Center in Philadelphia. "Without rehabilitation, you're always going to have a weak ankle, one that won't function normally. And you may repeat the accident."

Sprained ankles typically occur when your foot lands on an uneven surface. Your ankle bone suddenly turns inward faster than your muscles are able to stop or slow down the motion. Because your muscles couldn't catch the motion, the ligaments that connect your bones stretch or tear.

Experts classify sprains into three levels—from moderate to severe—depending on whether the ligaments are partially or completely torn. "Think of your ligaments as a rubber band," says Dr. Gordon. "If you took a pair of scissors and cut partway through the rubber band, that's comparable to a moderate sprain. Cut halfway through, that's more severe. Cut all the way through the rubber band, and it's comparable to completely severing the ligament. Only your doctor will be able to determine how severe your injury is."

No matter what the degree of severity, however, the violent action against the ligaments will cause blood vessels to burst. That's why a sprained ankle swells—the area fills up with blood as well as other bodily fluids and waste products. The sprain can even rupture the tissue that covers the ankle bones.

If you injure your ankle to the point of swelling, your immediate medicine should be RICE, an acronym for *Rest, Ice, Compression,* and *Elevation.* Rest the joint, put ice on it (to help stop swelling), apply compression with an Ace-type bandage (but not so tight that you cut off circulation), and elevate the foot (above heart level) to help remove blood and other fluids from the area.

Depending on the severity of the sprain, it may be necessary to stay off that foot for up to four days until the swelling goes down, Dr. Gordon says. "If you walk too much you'll walk more stiff-legged, because the injury is putting more stress on your leg muscles," he says. "When your muscles aren't working right, more fluid accumulates in your ankle." Once you are able to walk with comfort, however, the pumping action of the muscles will help remove the accumulation of fluids and speed your recovery. It also helps during the initial stages of recovery to use a brace to support the ankle, says Dr. Gordon.

If your injury is extremely severe, you may need to wear a brace for up to a year, says Collins.

Once you're back on your feet, the fastest way to complete recovery is exercise, says Dr. Gordon. The longer you stay inactive, the longer your recovery time will be.

Be sure to start your exercise program with moderation. Ligaments take about six weeks to heal, and if you push too hard too soon, you're apt to land *off* your feet again.

First Step: Stretch It Out

"Before you work on strengthening your ankle, you need to get the movement back," says Dr. Gordon. Here are two stretching exercises that he has found most effective for treating his patients.

Stand about 1½ feet from a wall with your feet turned in, in pigeon-toed position. Now flatten both palms against the wall (at head level) and move your chest toward it, bending your elbows. Don't bend at the waist, keep your knees straight, and be sure to keep your heels on the ground. Hold this stretch for 10 to 30 seconds. Repeat five to ten times.

For the next exercise, stand with your feet approximately 6 inches apart. Keeping your back straight, bend at your knees until you feel tightness in the muscles of your lower leg. Hold this position for 10 to 30 seconds. Repeat five to ten times. Do this two or three times daily.

Second Step: Muscle Strengthening

You cannot strengthen damaged ligaments, Dr. Gordon says, but you can strengthen the muscles around them to help prevent future sprains. After you've worked on the stretches for two or three days, you can move on to resistance exercises including isometrics, exercises in the water, or working with a resistance band.

One particular isometric exercise serves as a good starting point, says Paul Sauer, a physical therapist at the Denver Sports Medicine Clinic. The idea is to push your foot against something that resists you— the floor, for example. Don't move your foot; just push back, forward, and from side to side for 5 to 10 seconds. Repeat several times and stop immediately if you experience any pain.

If you have access to a swimming pool, water therapy is an excellent way to strengthen the appropriate muscles, says Dr. Gordon.

"Get into a swimming pool with the water waist-deep and walk," he says.

Tame That Sprain

Ankle sprains are no fun any way you twist it. When you do take a turn for the worse, the right exercises can speed your recovery.

It's important to follow the progression of exercises from range of motion to stretching and strengthening. Balancing exercises should come last. Working too fast or too hard can cause further damage. Let pain be your guide as you perform each exercise. If it hurts, back off. Exercise four to six times a day, finishing each exercise session by applying ice to your ankle for 15 to 20 minutes to prevent any additional swelling. (You can wrap the ice in a towel or put it in a plastic bag.)

When you're ready to do the stretching and strengthening exercises, you'll need an elastic exercise band. You can purchase one at your local pharmacy or at a sporting goods store. An old bicycle inner tube will do as well. Hold the final position of each exercise for a count of three, doing 20 repetitions each unless otherwise indicated.

Once you can walk without a limp, you can add a few minutes of jogging in a straight line on a smooth surface; it will help you get yourself moving again. At the end of your rehabilitation program (when you can walk without a limp and feel no pain), you can add a few more maneuvers—jogging backward, in a figure eight and zig-zag fashion, and hopping.

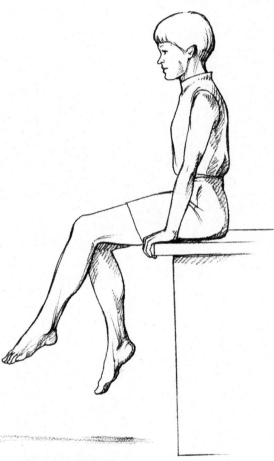

Range of Motion

Sit on a sturdy table or drape your leg over the arm of your sofa so that your leg hangs freely. First, slowly move your ankle up and down, pointing your toes up toward your chest, then down toward the floor. Hold each position for a count of three, then repeat. Do three sets of ten repetitions. Once you can easily move your ankle up and down, begin tracing the alphabet with your big toe, working through all the letters. Be sure to keep the movement slow, deliberate, and exaggerated.

Tame That Sprain—Continued

Stretching and Strengthening

After the pain and swelling subside, you can start to strengthen your ankle. Stand with the balls of your feet on the edge of a step and hold on to the handrail for balance. (1) With your toes pointing straight ahead, lower your heels past the step, then rise up on the balls of your feet. (2) Repeat the movement, but point your toes outward. (3) Finally, lower and raise your heels with your toes pointing inward. Repeat ten times in each position.

1.

2.

3.

Stretching and Strengthening

Hold the ends of the exercise band and loop it around the ball of your foot, keeping the band snug. Point your toes as far forward as you can. Hold, release, and repeat.

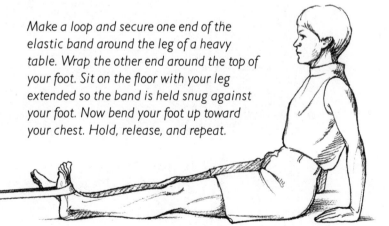

Make a loop and secure one end of the elastic band around the leg of a heavy table. Wrap the other end around the top of your foot. Sit on the floor with your leg extended so the band is held snug against your foot. Now bend your foot up toward your chest. Hold, release, and repeat.

Tame That Sprain—Continued

Stretching and Strengthening

With the looped band secured as in the previous exercise, sit in a sturdy chair and slip the end of the band around the outside of your foot. Sit far enough away from the table so that the band is snug. Keep your heel on the floor as you pivot your foot out to the side. Hold, release, and repeat.

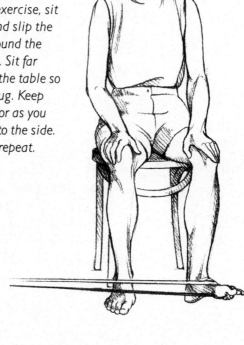

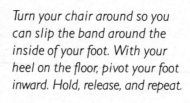

Turn your chair around so you can slip the band around the inside of your foot. With your heel on the floor, pivot your foot inward. Hold, release, and repeat.

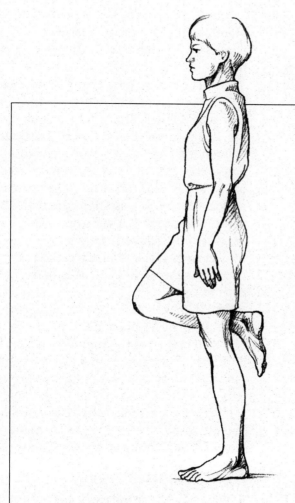

Balance

As you're building up the strength of your ankle, you also want to improve its coordination. Without holding on to anything, stand on the injured leg for 10 to 20 seconds. Do this first with your eyes open, then with your eyes closed. Keep practicing until you can maintain your balance for 2 minutes.

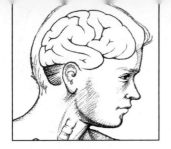

Stress

The cat's sick. Why did he have to start hacking up hairballs tonight of all nights? It's been difficult enough to concentrate on practicing for the recital and organizing the rest of the program, what with the mortgage problem and all. Now the headache's coming back, too, and your hands are starting to feel like cold chicken cutlets fresh from the fridge. Another night of restless sleep, probably. And will that nightmare return again? The one where you . . .

Don't even start to think about it. You'll be tired enough as it is when you go to work in the morning to tackle that new project. "Success" isn't doing you much good, either, when you're paying for it with high blood pressure, a high-idle pulse, and frayed nerves. At the slightest noise, you jolt from your seat as if it were The Chair at San Quentin. Wouldn't it be great to throw out the entire old wardrobe of woes and begin anew? Wouldn't it be great to free yourself from *stress?*

Good Stress, Bad Stress

Stress is any challenge to the body or mind. Things as minor as missing a meal or almost running a stop sign count as stress, as does the loss of a job or the death of a spouse. But oddly enough, how we cope with stress seems to depend on how often we endure a healthy form of physical challenge—the enjoyable, deep-breathing, noncompetitive workout.

"I've spent most of my career studying stress and ways of modifying it," says David S. Holmes, Ph.D., professor of psychology at the University of Kansas in Lawrence, "and I have never run across any stress-relief method as strong as aerobic fitness." Counteracting stress by improving the cardiovascular system and stimulating certain chemicals in the brain through exercise has "much more impact than psychotherapy, meditation, stress management, and biofeedback," he maintains.

Dr. Holmes likes to use himself as an example to prove his point.

"Say I've been at the computer all day," he offers. "I'm burned out, and the chapter I'm working on is looking old. So I go for a run.

"When I come back, my body's refreshed, and my mind is revved up. I'm going to have all kinds of mental energy to draw on."

Fight, Flight—or Fit

The body and mind experience a primitive response to stress called the "fight or flight response." This same powerful reflex allowed our prehistoric forbears to confront real physical dangers—marauding cavemen, growling gorillas, whatever.

When faced with such a challenge, the

body girds itself for action. Stress hormones are secreted. Blood sugar rises. Muscles tense up. Heart rate increases. Respiration becomes rapid and shallow. Circulation to the skin diminishes, as does blood flow to the digestive system.

Ideally, once the challenge is met, the body returns to its normally relaxed state to repair itself and rest, until the next threat—more gorillas, more cavemen.

Now that condos have replaced caves and beating the time clock has supplanted escaping the gorilla, many stressors are mental. The body's reaction remains the same—the fight or flight response—but because punching a time clock usually is more figurative than literal, you never actually flee or fight that immediate stress. That's where exercise comes in. It provides the perfect physical outlet for all that physical "readiness" that our modern society never puts to use.

Why Exercise Smooths Out Stress

Let's look at some of the physiological details of why exercise reverses stress. For one thing, when you exercise you deepen your breathing, and this deep breathing alters the shallow, quick breathing pattern that is characteristic of stress, according to Bonnie Berger, Ed.D., professor and director of the sports psychology laboratory at Brooklyn College of the City University of New York. The activity need not be conventional aerobic exercise (such as walking, bicycling, or swimming), she says, because other exercises such as yoga and circuit weight training also have proven helpful in deepening breathing and reducing stress.

Vigorous exercise also relaxes muscles by helping to eliminate any tension-causing stress hormones that may be surging through the bloodstream. In addition, it helps replenish brain levels of norepinephrine, an important emotion-stabilizing hormone. "If there's anything we know," says Dr. Holmes, "it's that stress lowers norepinephrine levels in the brain and that exercise increases norepinephrine in the brain."

Above All: Enjoy

The physical changes that exercise brings about are not the only factors in overcoming stress, however. There is also the sheer pleasure of exercise to consider.

"One overriding requirement for stress relief and exercise is that the activity has to be enjoyable," Dr. Berger says. Running on a miserably humid afternoon or swimming in water that is too cold may train your body, but it doesn't do much for your well-being. "It's not going to have a great psychological benefit that day," Dr. Berger says.

Other aspects of exercise also need to be considered. Competition, for example, can be counterproductive to stress reduction. Emphasis on winning and performance is a stressor, Dr. Berger says. While some people thrive on competition, others (especially if they are sore losers) find that the drive to win and fear of failure create more stress.

No matter what exercise you choose—competitive or noncompetitive—the idea is to stick with it. While a single exercise session can reduce tension temporarily, improving your overall fitness level is the best method of stress control.

Shifting Perspectives

Over time, as exercise produces noticeable physical changes, your entire perspective should improve, making you even more resilient to stress.

Women in particular seem to derive marked gains in emotional outlook. "And that may be related to achievement," Dr. Berger says. "We like to think there are no sex and gender roles, but they do exist.

"Women may experience even more stress reduction than men," she says, when they discover that developing a stronger body builds confidence and gives them a feeling of control over their lives.

For older people, "the psychological effects are as great, if not greater, than for younger age groups," Dr. Berger says. Those between the ages of 65 and 85 become encouraged when they see the benefits of exercise and what they still can accomplish, she explains. They can drive a car, walk to the store, carry a load of laundry up the basement steps—regular activities that grow increasingly difficult with age. Not having to worry about being able to accomplish such tasks automatically decreases stress in older people's lives, says Dr. Berger.

Exercise pays off in antistress benefits for both young and old, men and women. And it seems that almost *any* vigorous, enjoyable activity will do. You can run away from stress, walk away from stress, dance away . . . you get the picture.

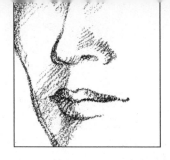

Stuttering

He worked in constant fear. But he wasn't a lion tamer or an undercover cop (and his boss wasn't *that* bad). He was an accountant, and he was afraid that one day he wouldn't be able to control his speech—that he would *stutter.*

It wasn't until the accountant retired that he got the courage to tackle his stuttering, says Hugo Gregory, Ph.D., professor and director of stuttering programs at Northwestern University in Evanston, Illinois, and a former stutterer. Many stutterers find ways to hide their problem, Dr. Gregory says, such as constantly thinking ahead to rephrase their speech or passing up job promotions that might force them to speak more.

But treatment for stuttering *is* available. Two ways to deal with the problem involve easily learned breathing techniques and tension-control exercises. There are many theories about the psychological causes of stuttering, but most professionals agree the *physical* cause is excess tension in the vocal cords or muscles involved in speech.

Smoothing Out Speech

"The simple definition of stuttering is excessive tension that interferes with the smooth movements in speech," explains Dr. Gregory.

One method of getting rid of this tension is the "airflow technique," taught by Martin F. Schwartz, Ph.D., executive director of The National Center for Stuttering, research professor in the Department of Surgery at New York University Medical Center, and author of *Stutter No More.* Most people tense their vocal cords as much as half a second before they speak; in a person who stutters the vocal cords can lock before speech occurs, explains Dr. Schwartz. By inhaling and then breathing out slightly before starting to talk, however, stutterers can keep the vocal cords from locking.

"Just before they speak they should let out from their mouths a very short, silent, passive flow of air," says Dr. Schwartz. (Don't force it; the idea is to stay relaxed.) It's also important to say that first word slowly, to avoid tension in the vocal cords. "You don't have to talk slowly, just start slowly," points out Dr. Schwartz.

Practice with the technique is required, however, and Dr. Schwartz recommends 45 minutes of daily practice for six months to a year. Speech, after all, is a lifelong habit, and it can be difficult to make changes. "Imagine if you've been playing the piano wrong for 16 hours a day all your life," he says. He also recommends joining support groups, since working on your stuttering alone can be frustrating and frightening.

Relaxation exercises can also be helpful

in reducing stuttering, according to Dr. Gregory. "We want the person to learn to sense the gradations of tension in the larger muscles of the body and to carry that over into modifying the tension in the smaller muscles involved in speech," he explains. The other function of relaxation exercises is to reduce body tension, which is thought to be a factor that contributes to stuttering.

"Relaxation is very helpful; it's tremendous," says Ted Price, director of the National Council on Stuttering, who has used relaxation to help control his own stuttering.

Here are some antistuttering relaxation exercises recommended by Dr. Gregory.

Extend your right foot. Gradually bend the foot up toward your shin, while increasing the tension in the leg all the way up to the hip. Then let the leg muscles relax and think about the tension flowing out of the leg. Repeat for the left leg.

Now hold your right arm extended in front of you. Make a fist while gradually increasing tension up your arm and into your shoulder. Then let the arm relax, and think about the tension flowing out of it. Repeat for the left arm.

Next, breathe in deeply and hold the breath for 1 second before exhaling. Breathe quietly for about 10 seconds, then repeat the whole procedure three times.

Now slowly and carefully roll your head from side to side. Start with your chin against your chest, then roll your head up so your right ear is over your right shoulder. Drop your chin down to the center again, then roll your head up so your left ear is over your left shoulder. Repeat several times. Finally, yawn two or three times, consciously relaxing as you yawn. (For more exercises, see "Relaxation Training" on page 399.)

Doing relaxation exercises in a tub of hot water may be helpful, says Dr. Schwartz. To reduce general muscle tension, he recommends any aerobic exercise, such as running, bicycling, or swimming. But stutterers should avoid weight-lifting exercises involving the upper neck and shoulder, he says, because the increased tension in the neck could hinder efforts to speak fluently.

Improving posture may also help control stuttering, according to Dr. Gregory. "The speech mechanism involves breathing," he says. "If you're slumped over, you're not in a good position for speech." (See "Posture Training" on page 387.)

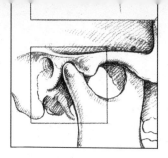

TMD and Bruxism

A few years ago Liza Frenette's life seemed an endless cycle of jaw pain, muscle inflammation, and headaches so severe that sometimes, in desperation, she headed to the emergency room for pain relief.

The Albany, New York, journalist was suffering from temporomandibular disorder (TMD), apparently triggered by stress-induced clenching of her teeth at night. Today she stays relatively symptom-free by avoiding getting overtired and by doing exercises prescribed by her physical therapist. "If I feel a little bit of a headache coming on, I get down on the floor and do my exercises," she says. She also finds that gentle swimming is a tremendous help.

While treatments for TMD vary greatly, many professionals are now steering sufferers toward exercises for both treatment and prevention.

"Exercise is a vital first step," declares Bernadette Jaeger, D.D.S., associate professor of orofacial pain and occlusion at UCLA's School of Dentistry and former director of the head and neck pain program in UCLA's Department of Anesthesiology.

Small Joint, Big Problems

You may be more familiar with the term TMJ, short for temporomandibular joint disorder. But because the problem so seldom involves only the joint itself, it is more correctly called TMD, for temporomandibular disorder, says Andrew S. Kaplan, D.M.D., director of Mount Sinai Hospital's TMD/Facial Pain Clinic in New York City. "It's a group of disorders," he explains, "that affect both the temporomandibular joint and the muscles that surround it."

The temporomandibular joint is a complex apparatus that connects your lower jaw with your skull. What's particularly distinctive is that it moves in two directions: up and down, like a hinge, and also from side to side. When the system is less than perfect—such as when your teeth and your temporomandibular joints don't fit together quite right—your jaw muscles may make minor corrections. In effect, your jaw "limps," and most people get through life just fine with their jaws limping a bit, says A. Richard Goldman, D.D.S., director of the Institute for the Treatment and Study of Headaches and Facial Pain, in Chicago.

For some people, however, the system goes haywire. Muscles go into cycle after cycle of painful spasm. These can spread to the neck, shoulders, back, or legs and, because of the intricate interlocking of the body's muscles and nerves, can even cause earaches or numbness in the feet and hands, according to Dr. Goldman.

TMD can be triggered by teeth clench-

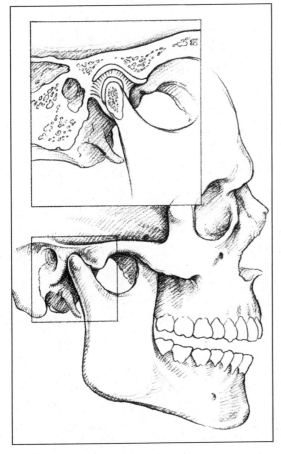

The temporomandibular joint (TMJ), like a hinge, allows you to move your mouth from side to side or back and forth. Any imbalance of the jaw or muscles surrounding the joint can trigger headache or joint or muscle pain.

tion of causes, explains Dr. Kaplan, author of *The TMJ Book.*

Exercises, say TMD experts, may help in a number of ways: They can improve posture, help build connective tissues, and in some cases retrain uncoordinated muscles of the jaw. They can also relieve the stress that causes clenching, grinding, and muscle tension, which in turn can lead to TMD problems.

Making the Right Moves

Because what triggers TMD can be so different from individual to individual, you need to have a health-care professional design an exercise treatment program tailored to meet your individual needs. Everything that moves in your body works together, so your whole musculoskeletal system must be considered in creating such a program, notes physical therapist Mariano Rocabado, director of the Head, Neck, and Maxillofacial Dysfunctions Program of the Dental School at the University of Chile, and coauthor of *Exercise and Total Well-Being for Vertebral and Craniomandibular Disorders.* Exercises based on Rocabado's system have become standard treatment for TMD throughout the United States.

Rocabado and physical therapist Terri Antoniotti are co-directors of the International Fundamental Orthopedics Rocabado Center in Tucson, Arizona, where they make extensive use of exercise in treating TMD. They've also designed a program to identify people with TMJ problems and treat them with exercise before the symptoms become apparent.

"We're seeing TMD, " says Antoniotti,

ing and an overstressed life, as in Liza Frenette's case. Other triggers can be a blow to the jaw, whiplash, misaligned teeth, teeth grinding (bruxism), poor posture, muscles that aren't coordinated, or ligaments and tendons that are too lax. In most cases, TMD results from a combina-

EASY DOES IT

Stressed out? Want to exercise your troubles away? Reconsider before you lace on a pair of running shoes or sign up for an aerobics class. Some exercises can actually *trigger* TMD outbreaks or worsen them.

A. Richard Goldman, D.D.S., author of *TMJ Syndrome: The Overlooked Diagnosis,* cautions against any types of exercises such as biking, jogging, aerobic dance, or roller skating that might cause you to clench your teeth. "When people tense their muscles, they tend to clench their teeth together, which has the potential of re-triggering some of the problems," he points out.

Other TMD experts don't rule out specific exercises, but they restrict the activities of some patients. They might tell swimmers, for example, to use a snorkel and mask so they don't rotate in the water to breathe. (Just make sure you don't clench down on the snorkel.)

Bernadette Jaeger, D.D.S., has a patient with an unstable temporomandibular joint. This woman opens her mouth so wide when she sings that she gets a sore jaw, so Dr. Jaeger limits her singing to a half hour.

Terri Antoniotti, co-director of the International Fundamental Orthopedics Rocabado Center in Tucson, Arizona, steers patients away from pounding, high-repetition exercises such as running and aerobic dance and toward gentler activities such as bicycling, swimming, and cross-country skiing. Many people who have TMD are overly flexible (hypermobile), with too-lax connective tissue and joints that already have increased movement and range of motion, she says. They should be screened by a knowledgeable physical therapist before beginning a stretching program. "Flexibility exercises may not be good in all people," she points out.

Some common sense is also involved, says Dr. Goldman. You should avoid activities that aggravate your condition. If you have neck-muscle spasms, aerobics will likely make those sore muscles hurt even more. It's better to try an alternate activity, or wait until the pain has subsided.

If any exercise or activity causes you pain, bring it to the attention of your doctor.

"in two types of people: in very loose-jointed people with a genetic problem that can be managed through exercises, and in people who aren't loose-jointed but who clench their teeth."

Adjusting the Jaw

If you visit a physical therapist who uses a Rocabado or Rocabado-based system, you'll learn a variety of exercises, including a simple series you can do on your own throughout the day. These "6 by 6" exercises are held for 6 seconds at a time and performed six times a day.

It's also possible that your dentist or therapist may prescribe jaw exercises to train muscles to manipulate the joint smoothly and without "limping." TMD is not so much a problem of muscle weakness as it is a lack of coordination, says A. Joseph Santiesteban, Ph.D., vice president for education for Healthmark Inc., and director of physical therapy at the Therapy Works Inc., in Indianapolis. "It's more training the muscles to open at the same

FINDING A COACH FOR YOUR JAW

What do you do if you want to put your jaw through its paces, but your dentist confines you to the bench? How do you find out whether exercise can help relieve *your* TMD symptoms?

Unless you've been properly diagnosed, you won't know for sure if you have the disorder, what triggers TMD in you, or what exercises might help you.

The trick, therefore, is to find the right professional to evaluate your symptoms.

Whether you go to a physical therapist, doctor, or dentist, you need to work with an individual experienced in treating TMD. This may require some leg work—or telephone work—on your part.

"You have to interview your doctor," says A. Richard Goldman, D.D.S., author of *TMJ Syndrome: The Overlooked Diagnosis.* "And if your doctor doesn't want to talk to you, maybe it's time to look for someone else." He recommends asking the doctor where the doctor learned about TMD, what his success rate is, how long he has treated TMD, and how many patients he currently has in treatment.

And you should always ask the doctor or dentist to explain how a TMD problem can give you headaches, neck aches, and shoulder aches. If the professional can't explain adequately, says Dr. Goldman, perhaps he or she doesn't fully understand the syndrome.

The same is true of physical therapists. Some have more experience than others in treating TMD; some may have received now-outdated TMD training. It's a good idea to seek a physical therapist specializing in "musculoskeletal dysfunction," recommends Terri Antoniotti, co-director of the International Fundamental Orthopedics Rocabado Center in Tucson, Arizona. Again, this means spending some time on the phone and asking a lot of questions.

time and to relax at the same time," he explains. Other exercises you might get from the dentist or therapist are designed to increase the mobility of the joint. And certain jaw-stretching exercises can help counteract the effects of bruxism.

Jaw exercises in particular are specific to each patient, and TMD sufferers shouldn't try them unless directed by a professional.

Tackling TMD at Home

While many TMD exercises must come from a medical professional, there are a number of exercises that are safe for you to do on your own. However, it's prudent to clear any exercise program with your doctor or therapist before starting. Posture correction is an important part of many therapies. "If you have poor posture, then you're setting yourself up for problems," says Dr. Jaeger. "I've had people come in with chronic headaches, and all I did was teach them correct posture and their headaches went away." (See "Posture Training" on page 387.)

Dr. Jaeger also suggests these exercises.

Squaring the shoulders. Stand with your feet 4 inches apart with your arms at your sides and your thumbs pointing forward. Tighten your buttocks, then turn your thumbs out and back. Now squeeze your shoulder blades together and down. Raise your chest and breathe in deeply. Hold for 6 seconds and repeat six times.

Neck and upper back stretch. Sit in a straight-backed chair. Inhale; then as you exhale, drop your head forward and try to touch your chin to your chest, keeping your mouth closed. Breathe regularly as you hold for 6 seconds, then slowly raise your head as you exhale. Repeat six times.

Positioning the tongue. Say the letter *N* with your teeth slightly apart. Now close your lips and breathe through your nose. Try to keep your tongue in this position any time you are not eating or talking.

Doing the exercises regularly throughout the day is more important than doing many repetitions at one time, explains Dr. Jaeger.

Deflating Stress

Because so many TMD patients suffer from stress that can trigger flare-ups, Dr. Jaeger also recommends general fitness activities. "Aerobic exercise is good," she says. "It gets your heart rate up and increases your sense of well-being."

It may be a good idea for some people with TMD to avoid certain exercises that involve jarring movements.

Antoniotti and Rocabado encourage their patients to do aerobic exercises for 15 to 45 minutes, four to five days a week. Good activities are bicycling, hiking, swimming, and gentle walking. You could also use exercise equipment: a rowing machine, stationary bicycle, stair-climber, or cross-country skiing machine.

For additional stress relief you might also try yoga or relaxation exercises. "Relaxation exercises are very beneficial," says Dr. Kaplan. Some people, he notes, don't have a good feel for their body and don't know when they're overstressed. If you fall into this category, working with a therapist may prove helpful.

Many people are surprised to learn how many things they can do on their own to help treat TMD, says Dr. Jaeger. "TMD problems don't lend themselves to passive therapy."

Just remember, she adds, whatever exercises you do, it's important to incorporate them into your lifestyle.

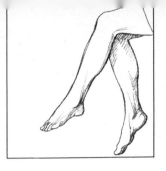

Varicose Veins

You've seen them in science textbooks: Those time lines that show an evolutionary parade of humanity with its ever-improving posture—from the knuckle-to-ground shuffle of our apelike ancestors to the proud, erect march of the Modern Person. There's just one small feature those charts always leave out.

The Modern Person's varicose veins.

Yes, we may have opposable thumbs, but we've paid the price. Scientists say that the change from all fours to all twos didn't do our legs much good—blood that used to move easily from heart to legs and back again now has to fight gravity harder. And in some of us, blood loses that fight—it pools in the vessels of the leg, resulting in ropey, bulging veins. Or tiny, overfilled blood vessels grow and expand, forming spidery, blue fireworks. In either case, you've got a "varicosity." What's a Modern Person to do?

Take the next step in evolution. Walk faster.

No New Veins, No Old Pain

"Think of exercise as preventive maintenance," says Luis Navarro, M.D., director of The Vein Treatment Center in New York City. "Though you can't get rid of the varicose veins you already have—only medical treatment can do that—exercising on a regular basis can keep you from aggravating the situation and might help you stave off getting new ones. At any rate, exercise can help you eliminate any discomfort you feel." (Not a small matter, since varicose veins can throb and ache.)

Dr. Navarro recommends brisk walking, jogging, bicycling, or swimming—anything that keeps your muscles in gear for 20 minutes or more. This extra dose of activity helps prevent varicosities for two reasons: It strengthens the muscles in your legs that push blood toward the heart, and it strengthens the heart itself, so that blood moves more quickly through your body, giving it less chance to pool in the legs.

"If you have large varicose veins, exercise without a graduated elastic stocking may make them worse," says Mitchel Goldman, M.D., assistant clinical professor of dermatology at the University of California, San Diego. Your physician can fit you with the appropriate type, he says. The stockings cost anywhere from $40 to $80. Once you're properly equipped, the right kind of movement can be helpful.

"Exercise pumps the blood out," he says. "If you're just standing, the blood doesn't get pumped out and continues to collect in the legs. I strongly believe that exercise is important." (To begin an exercise program, see the appropriate chapters in part 2.)

Besides brisk exercise, Dr. Navarro recommends specific movements to strengthen the legs. Here are four he finds particularly useful.

The curtsey. Stand with your feet shoulder-width apart and your hands on your hips. Now take a great big step forward with your right leg. Your right leg should now be bent and your right foot flat on the floor. Your left leg should be straight out behind you, and you should be up on the ball of your left foot. This is the starting position for the exercise. Lower yourself by bending the left knee, then return to an upright position. Move your left knee as close to the floor as possible before straightening up again.

In the advanced form of the exercise, the knee almost touches the floor. Don't be concerned if you can lower yourself only a couple of inches—you'll still benefit from the exercise. Remember, the knee behind you is the one that's going up and down. Your front knee will bend somewhat but should never push forward past your toes. Repeat the movement 10 to 15 times. (If you tire before 10 repetitions, just do what you can.) Then stand up, step out with your left leg, and repeat the exercise another 10 to 15 times, this time dropping your right knee toward the floor.

Sitting leg raise. Sit on the floor with your legs extended straight out. Bend your right knee, placing your right foot flat on the floor beside your left knee. Now, without pointing your toes, raise your left leg up as high as you can without bending the knee. (It's okay if you can lift it only a couple of inches.) Lower it slowly without touching the floor. Repeat 10 to 15 times. Now switch legs and repeat. You can either keep your hands flat on the floor or wrap your arms around the bent leg to brace yourself. Try to keep your back straight throughout the exercise.

Standing calf raise. Stand on a telephone book or on a two-by-four. Your toes and the balls of your feet should be planted firmly on the book or wood block, with your heels hanging over the edge. Your feet should be comfortably apart, and your toes pointed straight ahead. Hold on to the back of a sturdy chair to help you keep your balance. Now lower your heels until they're below your toes. The lower you can make your heels go, the better. Then, keeping your legs straight, raise yourself as high as you can by standing on your toes. Then lower your heels slowly to the starting position. Repeat 15 to 20 times.

Wide calf raise. This exercise is particularly good for the calf muscles. Stand facing the back of a sturdy chair. Hold on with both hands to help you keep your balance. Now spread your legs as far apart as you can and point your toes out. Lower your buttocks toward the floor by bending your legs until your buttocks are slightly higher than your knees. Raise your heels as high as you can, then lower them back to the floor. Repeat 15 to 20 times.

Part II
Exercise Therapies

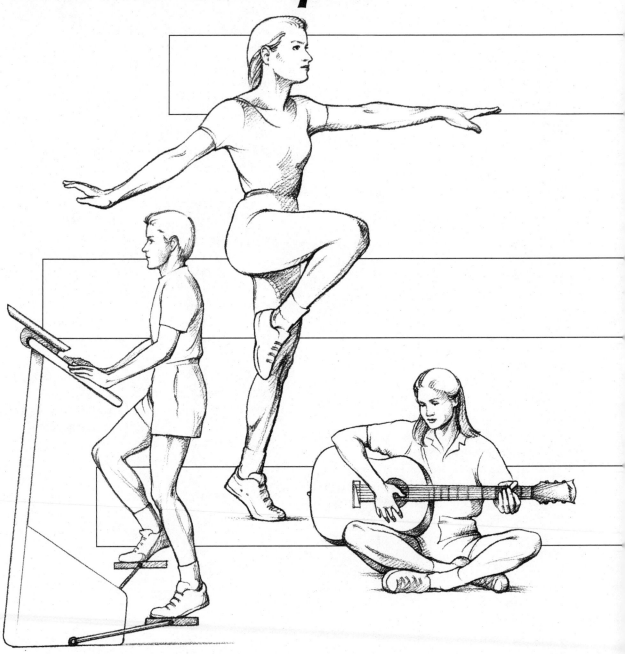

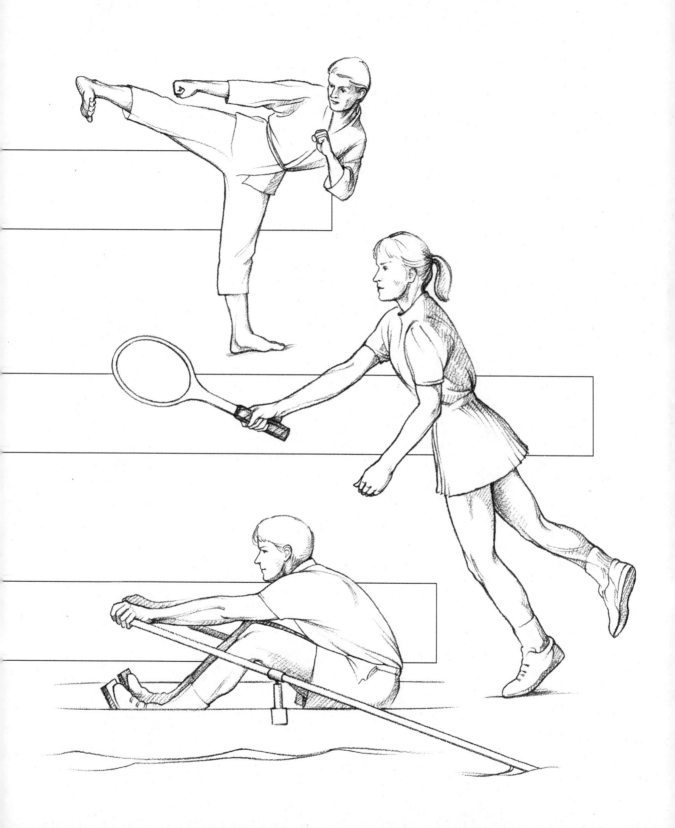

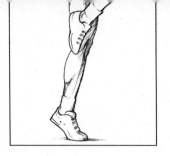

Aerobics

*B*ack in the old days, when Jane Fonda was better known for her acting than her exercising, both physical fitness and the English language were much more simple. *Impact* was something that occurred when a car hit a tree. *Intensity* usually referred to the behavior of car salesmen and those who drank too much coffee. And *cross-training?* Maybe that had something to do with Amtrak, but nobody was really sure.

Then in 1982 Fonda made her now-famous workout tape—the first of 14, we might add—sparking a revolution in physical fitness. Suddenly, "aerobics" became a household word. Normal, intelligent, even distinguished people were on all fours in front of the TV doing Donkey Kicks and The Hydrant. New "health clubs" (many of them teaching these same moves to people who preferred to get on all fours in public) sprouted up like weeds across the land.

The things that made this newfangled aerobic dance (simply called "aerobics" in those pioneering days) so darned appealing are the same things that *still* attract enthusiasts by the hundreds of thousands. Simply, aerobic dance does the same great stuff as running, swimming, or any good workout: It strengthens the heart and other muscles, helps weight control by burning calories and body fat, lowers blood pressure and cholesterol, helps control heart disease, boosts brainpower (regular exercisers have quicker reaction time, better memory, and better reasoning ability), improves one's sex life by bettering body image and increasing stamina (wink, wink), and even helps reduce pain by releasing endorphins—the body's natural painkillers.

And unlike the loneliness of long-distance running, aerobic dance is social. But it doesn't *have* to be. You can join a class, or you can go it solo in your living room—just you and Jane and your VCR. Unlike swimming or bicycling, it isn't dependent on weather conditions. It doesn't require expensive equipment like other sports—just a good pair of sneakers. It doesn't mandate that you be a certain age or height or weight. You don't have to be athletically inclined. Heck, you don't even have to like to exercise.

"Because aerobic dance is done to music, many people forget that they're actually exercising. They get caught up in the music and forget where the time went," says Elece Hempel, workshop coordinator of the National Dance-Exercise Instructors Training Association (NDEITA), which teaches the teachers what they need to know about aerobic dance.

And unlike some forms of exercise—such as running or bicycling—that give only one or two sets of muscles a good workout, aerobic dance works the entire body: arms, legs, torso, buttocks, you name it.

A problem did develop back when aerobic dance was taking those first well-publicized steps: Many people realized just how painful the steps could be. The funky, pounding music accompanying this new form of exercise prompted people to really shake their often out-of-shape body.

Unfortunately, about 40 percent of participants and three in four instructors wound up getting hurt—thanks to the high-energy steps, jumps, kicks, shuffles, and assorted gyrations that made up the typical aerobic dance class.

It seems that in their quest for stronger hearts and leaner frames, sharper minds and more exciting bedroom romps, America's newfound aerobics faddists "earned" untold numbers of shin splints, twisted ankles, stress fractures, burned-out knees, pulled ligaments, and other "overuse" injuries. Why? Because all those enthusiastic aerobics faddists told us (they've since changed both their philosophy and their exercises) that *no pain* would bring us *no gain* and *no burn* would give us *no earn.*

But what a difference a decade makes.

Intensity Beats Impact

Today, with a good ten years of study under their belts, sports medicine researchers and aerobic dance instructors now have a better idea of how to help keep everyone safe and injury-free while still reaping all those benefits that attracted so many people to aerobic dance in the first place.

What they've found is, unlike the message preached in those early days, you *don't* have to jump around like a frenzied cheerleader in order to have a body like one. In fact, the new direction is toward a kinder, gentler aerobic dance.

"It used to be that people thought they couldn't get a really good workout unless it was high impact," says Hempel, whose organization has taught more than 39,000 aerobic dance instructors how to instruct safely. "Although that's still a popular misconception, we now know that you can get a workout that's just as good, if not better, with a low-impact routine—as long as it's high intensity."

Huh? It seems your body isn't the only thing that gets a workout from aerobic dance. So does your vocabulary. Let us translate.

Impact refers to the force with which your feet hit the floor (usually to the beat of the music). You don't have to be Sir Isaac Newton to figure out that the higher the impact in your workout, the harder you're hitting the floor—and the greater your risk of overuse injury. With high-impact aerobics, there's a lot of jumping around, and sometimes both feet are off the floor simultaneously. With low impact, one foot *always* remains on the floor, which translates to a less jolting and safer workout.

Intensity refers to how hard you're working your cardiovascular system. (A cardiovascular workout is the whole point of *any* aerobic exercise.) So a *high*-intensity workout means that you're huffing and puffing your way to better cardiovascular health, whereas a *low*-intensity workout means you may not be working hard enough to reap the full benefits.

"More important than whether it's high or low *impact* is whether it's high or low *intensity*," says Hempel. For most healthy people looking to get maximum benefit from an aerobic dance class, high intensity is the way to go, say experts.

Lighten Up

Notice we said intensity, *not* impact. "Many people still have the misconception that high impact means working harder," says Hempel.

But the truth is, you may not be getting a better workout with a high-impact class because the momentum of your movements is moving your muscles more than you are. That momentum doesn't affect only arms and legs. Many women complain that the constant jumping of high-impact classes hurts their breasts; men might note it can have a similar affect on testicles.

A good sports bra or jockstrap can help those problems, but experts still recommend low-impact routines for most people—especially beginners and the sedentary. "The advantage of low impact is its reduced stress on the musculoskeletal system. There's less chance of getting hurt," says Charlene Prickètt, host of *It Figures*, a syndicated aerobics show broadcast on the Lifetime cable network.

Still, *less* chance doesn't mean *no* chance. "The best way to avoid injuries, whether it's high or low impact, is to land properly, wear proper athletic footwear, and exercise on a safe surface," says Peg Jordan, R.N., editor-in-chief of *American Fitness*, the official publication of the Aerobic and Fitness Association of America (AFAA),

one of the largest and most respected authorities on aerobic dance and other exercise. "You should land on your heel and then roll through to your toe," she says.

Another advantage of low-impact aerobics is that it provides the perfect "introduction" to aerobic exercise. That's one more reason that it's widely recommended for sedentary people just starting an exercise program.

Listen to Your Breathing

One way to determine that you're burning enough calories—and getting the high-intensity, low-impact workout you want—is through your breathing. "You should be breathing hard, but not so hard that you cannot speak," says Prickett.

Another way is by monitoring your heartbeats per minute. For a *good* aerobic workout, you should be within your target heart rate zone—a range that's between 60 and 85 percent of the *maximum* number of beats your heart can produce. (To determine your target heart rate zone, see "How Good is Your Workout?" on page 324.)

Just because your heart rate increases slightly doesn't mean you've reached your target zone or are getting a good workout. "Anytime you place your hands over your head or grip something tightly, your heart rate and blood pressure will increase somewhat—even if you're sitting down," says Prickett. "That's because of something called the Pressor Response. And in low-impact aerobic dance, there's a lot of above-the-chest arm work being done. While that may increase the heart rate, it

HOW GOOD IS YOUR WORKOUT?

You break a sweat. You're huffing and puffing. It *feels* like you're working your tail-feathers off, but is it enough? Or perhaps more important, is it too much?

The easiest and most accurate way to determine whether you're getting the most from your workout is to determine your target heart rate zone. To do that, here's the formula that experts recommend: Subtract your age from 220 and then multiply that number by 0.6 to get the low number for your range; then subtract your age from 220 and multiply by 0.85 to get the high number for your range: $(220 - age) \times 0.6 =$ low number for range; $(220 - age) \times 0.85 =$ high number for range.

Everything within those two numbers is your target heart rate zone—and ideally, your heartbeats per minute should be within those numbers. If it's too low, you're not exercising hard enough. If it's too high, slow down your workout.

To calculate your heartbeat, use your index and middle fingers to measure the pulse at your wrist. Count the number of beats for 10 seconds and multiply by 6. But be quick—your heart rate drops immediately when you *stop* exercising for as little as 10 seconds.

Warning: Don't use your thumb, since it has its own powerful pulse (which will differ from your wrist's). And don't take your pulse at your neck. If you have atherosclerosis (hardening of the arteries) or any other artery disease, the pressure on the neck can decrease blood flow to the brain. It could cause you to lose consciousness.

doesn't necessarily increase the rate of respiration."

The bottom line: You're getting a good workout if you're breathing hard *and* your heart's pumping—and experts generally say you should sustain it for at least 20 *continuous* minutes. "That's why a good aerobic dance class is usually at least 35 minutes long," says Jordan. "It includes 7 to 10 minutes each of warm-up and cool-down periods."

You don't have 35 minutes to spare at one shot? Fret not. Research reported in the *American Journal of Cardiology* shows that multiple, shorter bouts of aerobic activity may be just as beneficial—as long at you get in adequate workout time by doing *three* 10-minute bouts a day. The important thing is to get the time in, whether or not it's all in one chunk. And while the more you exercise, the better off you'll be, remember that you *can* get too much of a good thing.

Variety Prevents Injury

"The most prudent approach to aerobic dance *is* cross-training," says Prickett. "If you do any *single* activity related to aerobic dance without switching around, you'll likely find that somewhere along the line, you'll suffer an overuse injury or boredom."

While most people think of cross-training as "combining" different sports or activities—for instance, runners might run on Tuesday,

Thursday, and Saturday and swim or bicycle on Monday, Wednesday, and Friday—many aerobic dancers can practice cross-training while sticking completely with aerobic dance. In fact, it's strongly recommended.

Among the most popular choices:

Step-aerobics (sometimes affectionately called simply "step") consists of stepping up and down an elevated platform, usually 4 to 10 inches high. "Step is probably even easier for beginners or noncoordinated people because the choreography can be made extremely simple, yet the exertion level can be high or low—depending on the height of the step," says Prickett. "Ideally, step should be done so that the angle behind your knee is at least 90 degrees. When it's less than 90 degrees, you can hurt your knees."

Weights consists of using light (usually 1- to 5-pound) wrist or hand weights to strengthen both the arms and the cardio-vascular system. Weights are usually lifted in rhythm to music and can be used as part of a low-impact dance routine or floor exercises. *Note:* Stick to light weights. Even if they seem too light when you first begin, the fast-paced dance movements will soon make the weights seem heavier (and you'll burn out too quickly if you're hoisting a heavier load).

Toning consists of doing floor exercises such as abdominal curls, leg lifts, and push-ups. "Only it's more fun because they're done to music and with other people," quips one aerobics instructor.

Says Prickett: "The routine I recommend is the one we do on my show: Monday, aerobic dance; Tuesday, weight training; Wednesday, step; Thursday, weight training; and Friday, aerobics. The important thing is that you do something every day—but not the same activity two days in a row."

The Right Music, the Right Shoes

Speaking of music, there's a good reason why you never hear Pat Boone at the local health club. "The beats per minute for music used in aerobic dance is very important," says NDEITA's Hempel. "It should be between 128 and 135 beats per minute for low impact, and as high but no higher than 160 beats for high impact." Beats per minute refers to the drumbeat (which can be calculated by counting them while looking at your watch).

Moving to that Uzi-like beat is a lot easier, not to mention a whole lot safer, with the right shoes. Figure you'll pay at least $50 for a good pair. "You should be able to wiggle your toes slightly in an aerobics shoe, so it should have a squarish toe box," says Hempel. "Most people prefer high-tops because they provide better ankle support. You could wear cross-training shoes, but if you're going to participate in aerobic dance at least three times a week, you're better off buying a pair made specifically for aerobic dance."

Running shoes are not appropriate for aerobics class, she explains, because they inhibit sideways motion. You don't want to move sideways when you're running, but when you're doing aerobics, you have to.

FINDING A SAFE INSTRUCTOR

Although the obvious place to look for a good aerobic dance instructor is on the gym floor, experts suggest you first glance at the walls. You want to know if the instructor is certified by an appropriate professional organization. (See the list below.)

"A certification is especially important because it tells you that the instructor has been educated enough to pick and choose exercises that will be safe," says Elece Hempel, whose job is to educate and certify instructors for the National Dance-Exercise Instructors Training Association.

"Anything that causes the spine to get out of alignment with the neck and hips—like most of the exercises on earlier workout tapes—isn't [safe]," she says. Besides having a good handle on the correct way to exercise, certified instructors also undergo at least 15 hours of intense education in physiology, nutrition, anatomy, and related fields.

"But probably the biggest advantage is that a certified instructor knows he or she doesn't have all the answers—but they know the people to get in touch with who do," adds Hempel. "What you're also getting with a certified instructor is the inside track to answer all your questions that another instructor may not be able to answer."

Certification should come from one of the following organizations. Some of these groups can also tell you the names of certified instructors in your area.

- Aerobic and Fitness Association of America (AFFA): 1-800-445-5950
- National Dance-Exercise Instructors Training Association (NDEITA): 1-800-AEROBIC
- International Dance-Exercise Association: The Association for Fitness Professionals (IDEA): 1-800-999-IDEA
- American Council on Exercise: 1-800-234-9229
- Institute for Aerobics Research: 1-800-635-7050

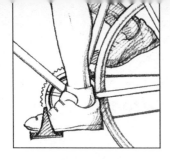

Bicycling

Remember learning to ride a bike when you were a kid? In that magical moment when your dad let go of the bike, your legs were pumping, the pedals were turning, and you were *riding* for the first time.

So now you're older and heavier and maybe a bit creakier—and it's been a long time since you first discovered the exhilaration of transporting yourself on two wheels. But the magic hasn't ever gone away. It's still there, just waiting for you to find it again.

Thomas C. Namey, M.D., rediscovered cycling when he was 32 and desperate to control an ongoing blood pressure problem. Not only did the cycling help his blood pressure, but Dr. Namey found a sport he still loves 13 years later.

"Suddenly this myriad of small roads and ways of getting out of the city opened up to me," says Dr. Namey, chief of the divisions of rheumatology and sports medicine at the University of Tennessee Graduate School of Medicine in Knoxville. "You see a side of the world you've never seen before."

Besides possibly helping to keep high blood pressure under control, cycling offers other enormous health benefits. It burns between 400 and 800 calories an hour (depending on how much effort you're putting out), benefits your heart and lungs, and tones up your muscles. Because the bicycle's saddle supports much of your weight, there's less stress on joints than in a sport such as running. For that reason, cycling is well suited even to people with arthritis or who are overweight, says Dr. Namey.

"I hear many people say, 'Oh, I can't ride a bike because of my knees,'" he says. "But *standing* places more weight on your knee joints than biking." He cautions, however, that people with high blood pressure or other health problems should consult their doctor before beginning cycling.

Back in the Saddle

Ready to try biking but don't want to spend any money for a bike just yet? The old bike stashed in the back of the garage may do just fine. Drag it out and pump up the tires (usually the correct pressure is embossed on the side of the tire). Check the brakes and try out the gears. If something doesn't work right or if the tires are cracked and worn, take the bike to a bike shop for a tune-up or a new set of tires.

The one item you shouldn't ride without, however, is a helmet. "I don't go out of the driveway without a helmet on," says Morris Mellion, M.D., medical director of the Sports Medicine Center and clinical associate professor at the University of

Nebraska Medical Center, both in Omaha. New models are lightweight, comfortable, and cool. (If you need convincing, consider that 75 percent of all biking deaths are from injuries to the head.)

Before you just leap onto your bike and take off, there are a couple of other points to consider. Three things in particular can cause you to conclude ruefully that biking's not for you: not adjusting the seat properly, riding in too high a gear, and overdoing it when you first start out.

Finding the right saddle height is easy, not to mention essential if you want to avoid knee pain. Hop on, pedal with the balls of your feet, and pause with one foot straight down. There should be only a slight bend in your knee, advises Dr. Mellion. If you find yourself rocking from side to side to reach the pedals, the saddle is definitely too high.

Check out the slant of the saddle as well. Most experts recommend a level saddle, or one with the nose pointing slightly up. You can eyeball this or use a carpenter's level.

Now you're up and rolling. Are you comfortable, or does it feel like you're working too hard? A big mistake many people make is using too high a gear and pedaling too slowly. People confuse pedaling slowly with easy cycling, says Dr. Namey. Pedaling too slowly not only is inefficient but can cause knee and muscle pain. Cranking it out in too high a gear ranks just behind improper bicycle fit as a major cause of knee overuse problems in cyclists. (More on this later.)

Another tip to increase your efficiency: Pedal with the *balls* of your feet, never your heels or insteps.

Planning a Program

When you're just starting, you may want to limit yourself to jaunts around your neighborhood. Lots of people simply overdo things that first time out. "The main mistake people make when they're starting an exercise program is getting too enthused on the first day and working too hard," says Don Cuerdon, East Coast editor of *Mountain Bike* magazine, who has been cycling for 20 years. Specifically, stay away from hills until you're a bit fitter.

If you want to get the best workout without overdoing it (and still enjoy yourself), you'll have to pay attention to how fast you pedal. Glance at your watch and count the number of times in 1 minute that either your right or left foot makes one complete circle. Optimal pedaling speed for most people is 60 to 80 revolutions per minute. This may feel ridiculously fast at first, and it may feel inefficient—but it's not. Studies confirm you're the most efficient at this cadence, and less prone to injury. Don't *push* yourself to cycle at this rate, however. You should feel a mild level of exertion, but you shouldn't be so out of breath that you can't carry on a conversation with a fellow cyclist.

The key to knowing how much to exert yourself is monitoring your heart rate. You can do this by checking your pulse against a watch, but because this can be dangerous while pedaling, you may want to stop to do it. Or you can spring for a heart rate monitor that straps to your chest, suggests Dr. Namey. (To calculate your maximum heart rate, see "How Good Is Your Workout?" on page 324.)

A basic minimum cycling program is

PAIN-FREE RIDING

For comfort during your ride and to avoid aches and pains afterward, follow these guidelines for bike fit and riding position:

Hands. Keep hands as relaxed as possible. If you have dropped handlebars, like those on a typical racing bike, move your hands frequently to different positions.

Arms. Your arms should be bent slightly, to aid in shock absorption.

Back. When you lean forward, your back should be straight or only slightly curved.

Knee. When your leg is fully extended, your knee should be bent slightly, about 10 to 15 degrees. Adjust your seat height accordingly.

Feet. You should pedal with the balls of your feet. Toe clips can help keep your feet in the right position and keep them from flying off—possibly into the front wheel.

Saddle. The saddle should be level, or with only a hint of a tilt up or down. You may prefer a slight nose-down tilt on mountain bikes and a slight nose-up tilt on road bikes.

Seatpost. Never raise your seatpost higher than its maximum—you'll find a small mark on the post indicating how high you can raise it.

Stem. The top of the handlebar stem should be level with or below the top of the saddle. A lower stem, however, will make your position more aerodynamic.

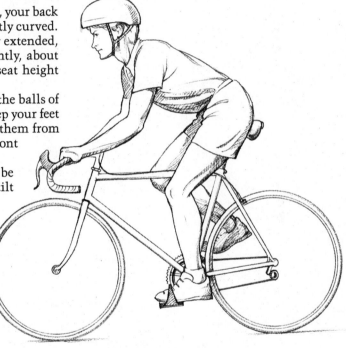

20 minutes, three times a week, reaching 60 to 85 percent of your maximum heart rate after you've warmed up. If 20 minutes feels like too much, you may want to start with 10 minutes at a time, three times a week, and increase that by 5 minutes each week. However much you ride, use the first 3 to 5 minutes as a warm-up, and end the ride with a 3- to 5-minute cool-down.

This means gliding along at an easy pace—and not huffing and puffing.

What Can Go Wrong

Most of the time bicycling is relatively trouble-free, but if you're troubled by lack of flexibility, for example, or find yourself tightening up from cycling, start stretching out after your workout—specifically your calves and your front and back thigh muscles (the quadriceps and hamstrings). Don't stretch before riding, when your muscles are cold, says Dr. Namey. (See "Stretching" on page 440.)

Much of what goes wrong in terms of bodily discomfort can be traced to improper bike fit or not using the right gear.

Not sure if your bike is the right size? Stand straddling the frame. On a road bike, you should have at least an inch of clearance between bike and crotch; on a mountain bike, 2 to 3 inches is appropriate.

Aching neck and back? You may be stretching too far to reach your handlebars. You should be able to reach them comfortably with your arms bent slightly (your bent elbows act as shock absorbers).

If your handlebars are too far away, you have two options—besides buying a new bike. You can buy a handlebar stem with a shorter extension, or if you have dropped handlebars, you can switch to standard, upright bars.

Back pain can also be caused by rocking back and forth because your saddle is too high. This motion can also cause chafing in your crotch area, or even bursitis in your hip.

Conversely, a saddle that's too low can cause tendinitis of the Achilles tendon or knee pain. Knee pain can also result from poor foot position or having the saddle too far forward, says Dr. Mellion.

Padded bike gloves can help relieve cyclist's palsy—a numbness in the hands—and also provide padding in case you take a tumble. Changing hand position frequently also helps relieve numbness, says Dr. Mellion.

If you experience numb toes or other foot problems, you may want to try shoes with a stiff sole that spreads the pressure around. "I tell people if they don't want to buy bike shoes to modify a regular pair of running or hiking shoes with a special plastic insole," says Dr. Namey. These insoles can be purchased at bike shops.

Realize that not all aches are avoidable: "People shouldn't be surprised if they have a little low-grade pain," says Dr. Namey. Muscles that haven't been used for a while will ache after suddenly being called into use. What's important to realize, he says, is that you shouldn't have a specific joint pain that doesn't go away. If you do, see your doctor.

If you're taking long excursions, dehydration can be a threat. Because the air blowing on you as you ride cools you and evaporates sweat, you may not realize how much liquid you're losing. By the time you feel thirsty, you may be a half gallon low on fluid. "Make sure you're well hydrated before you go out and drink at regular intervals along the way, before you get thirsty," says Dr. Namey.

Adding On Goodies

The great thing about biking is that you have a wonderful rationale for buying all kinds of extras. They'll not only make your ride more comfortable, they can often help motivate you.

Bike shorts, for example, have a padded, seamless crotch area, are worn without underwear, and won't hike up as you ride. They'll help prevent chafing, a sore bottom, and—*ouch*—saddle sores, uncomfortable bumps or boils caused by pressure and irritation in the crotch area.

CYCLING DO'S AND DON'TS

Here are some tips to remember—and follow—for maximum safety when riding.

- Do wear a helmet.
- Do ride with traffic, never against it.
- Do practice stopping as quickly as possible without skidding. Applying too much pressure to the front brakes can throw you over the handlebars.

- Don't wear headphones.
- Don't ride with a heavy backpack—it can upset your balance and strain your back.
- Do watch out for storm drains or railroad tracks that can catch your wheel.
- Do use hand signals to indicate turning and stopping.

Not all biking shorts are of the skin-clinging variety: Some are styled like hiking shorts.

While we're on the subject: If you find you just can't get comfortable on your bike saddle, you should consider a new saddle or a saddle cover with gel insert pads to relieve sore buttocks, according to John Schubert, author of *Richard's Cycling for Fitness*. There are also wider saddles designed especially for a woman's wider pelvis.

Cuerdon strongly recommends a good pair of sunglasses to help keep sun, wind, and flying matter out of your eyes.

And if you're ever going to take your bike farther than phone-home-for-help distance, you'll need a few other items. These include a frame pump, a patch kit, a spare inner tube, and basic tools. You can purchase all these items at your local bike shop.

Choosing a New Steed

After you've worked out for a while on your old bike and decided that, yes, this is the exercise of choice for you, you may want to buy yourself a brand-new bicycle.

It could be just the thing to keep you motivated. Okay, time to go shopping.

The number one rule is to go to a bicycle shop or a sports specialty store, says Dr. Namey. Cuerdon agrees: Sure, you can find a cheaper bike at a department store, but a cheap bike is just that—cheap. "It won't work as well, and you can't depend on it," Cuerson says. And bike store personnel know how to fit you with a bike that suits your needs *and* your body.

Expect to spend at least $300, says Cuerdon. You aren't likely to find a good, reliable bicycle for less. But mull things over before you start looking, or you may be dazzled by the choices. You can choose a standard multispeed bicycle, a mountain bike, or a cross bike. (Or a tandem, recumbent, tricycle, or recumbent tricycle!) All have particular advantages. (See "Which Bike Is Right for You?" on page 332.)

You can select a good bike shop through the recommendations of friends or by visiting a few stores. A good sales clerk will ask you lots of questions—such as what type of riding you'll be doing and how much you want to spend—and will

WHICH BIKE IS RIGHT FOR YOU?

Want to buy a bike? Boy, do you ever have a wide selection to choose from.

You can't just go out shopping for a 10-speed any more, because a lot of different bikes have 10 speeds—and more.

The basic sport bicycle with dropped handlebars—what we used to call a 10-speed—may have 12 speeds, 14, or more. A racing bike resembles a sport bike, but its components, frame, and price tag are more elite.

Mountain bikes, with fat tires, smaller wheels, straight handlebars, and low, low gears, are designed for rocketing down (and up) mountains. Some are specifically for off-road use, while others are intended mostly for road use. A hybrid bike, with standard-sized wheels, is a gentle combination of the two: You can ride it on dirt paths, but its narrower tires roll more smoothly on paved roads than does a mountain bike.

Mountain bikes and hybrid bikes are particularly well suited to older riders or those with physical limitations, says Thomas C. Namey, M.D., chief of the division of sports medicine at the University of Tennessee Graduate School of Medicine in Knoxville. Many people find the upright posture more comfortable, he says, and the fatter tires give a softer ride than other bikes.

If you like to ride with your spouse, a tandem bicycle might be the machine for you. These two-seaters naturally cost more, but they can be a lot of fun. They're also the perfect choice if one partner has limited vision, says Dr. Namey.

A recumbent or semirecumbent bicycle puts you in a stretched-out position, with your legs in front of you. Its seat provides back support, which many riders find much more comfortable than standard bike saddles, says Bob Goldman, D.O., Ph.D., president of the National Academy of Sports Medicine, director of sports medicine research at the Chicago College of Osteopathic Medicine, and director of the High Technology Fitness Research Institute in Chicago.

Tricycles—three-wheeled bikes—are heavier and slower than standard bikes but are a good option for people with balance problems, says Don Cuerdon, a cycling enthusiast for 20 years and East Coast editor of *Mountain Bike* magazine. Because of the weight and size of most trikes, you'll have to use them on flat roads with little traffic.

There are even recumbent tricycles, although they're a bit harder to find. And customized bicycles can be built for cyclists who are handicapped or have special needs.

Whatever your fancy, you'll find there's a bike somewhere out there that will suit you.

measure you for a correct fit.

Don't be put off by seemingly complicated gearing systems. The new index shifters are somewhat akin to using an automatic transmission: You push, it clicks, and *presto,* the gear changes. No finesse required.

Test-ride several bikes. If you don't like something in particular, ask whether it can be changed. When you find a bike that tickles your fancy, feels good, and suits your pocketbook, pull out the checkbook and take 'er home. You may have just found a life-long friend.

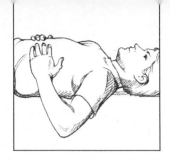

Breathing Therapies

To most people, learning how to breathe properly must seem about as useful and necessary as learning how to scratch an itch or blink.

Because we do it automatically from the moment we're born until the day we die, we may take for granted that we are breathing just fine, thank you. We use only about 10 percent of our lungs' available space, taking shallow breaths that fill only the upper portions of our lungs. When we play sports, we may hold our breath at crucial moments when our body most needs oxygen. These inadequacies can be remarkably easy to correct, but to do so you must at least be conscious that there is a problem that needs fixing.

Interestingly enough, what many of us think of as good posture—a sucked-in gut—can restrict your breath just as a tight belt does, according to Robert Fried, Ph.D., director and trainer at the Institute for Rational-Emotive Therapy in New York City and author of *The Breath Connection.* Even simply breathing through your nose—rather than your mouth—may be enough to normalize your breath, some experts say.

Doctors don't all agree on what it means to breathe improperly, but an increasing number of health-care and fitness professionals believe that improper breathing,

especially the rapid, shallow breathing associated with hyperventilation (over-breathing), heightens the body's response to stress. That in turn leads to a faster heart rate, higher blood pressure, more stress hormones circulating throughout the body, and possibly a vicious cycle of ever more rapid and shallow breathing.

These experts also believe that improper breathing may contribute to the development of many stress-related symptoms or ailments: fatigue, high blood pressure, migraine and tension headaches, seizure disorders, asthma, ulcers, gastritis, colitis, allergies, heart palpitations, angina-like chest pains, cold hands, panic attacks, even fear of flying! And that's just to name a few.

How could improper breathing cause such an array of symptoms? There are several possible ways, but perhaps most important is that it changes the pH (acid/base balance) in the body, making it slightly more alkaline than normal, says Dr. Fried. "The body is very intolerant of changes in pH," he says. "Ultimately, the result of this imbalance is that the kidneys have to work more and that the tissues of the body receive less oxygen."

Overbreathing (which blows off carbon dioxide) results in reduced levels of carbon dioxide in the blood, Dr. Fried explains. That means the blood is less likely to release its life-maintaining oxygen into the body. So you become slightly oxygen-deficient. That affects your heart, which uses 50 percent of the body's available oxygen, and your brain, which uses another 25 percent, Dr. Fried says.

These same health-care professionals also believe that learning how to breathe properly can often have a major impact on many illnesses and symptoms.

For Emphysema or Enlightenment

Who takes "breathing lessons"? Who teaches them? And what the heck is it they're learning and teaching, anyway?

The most likely students are people with asthma, chronic bronchitis, emphysema, and cystic fibrosis—all disorders that can make breathing more strenuous than hoisting the rear end of a pickup truck. These people are most likely to work with a respiratory therapist at a hospital, outpatient center, or doctor's office, says Ronald Adams, director of Therapeutic and Adapted Physical Education at the University of Virginia Medical Center in Charlottesville.

People with health problems—tension headaches, colitis, and the like—that are made worse by obnoxious in-laws, unreasonable deadlines, or exorbitant bills are most likely to visit a health-care professional who specializes in stress management, such as a psychologist or biofeedback therapist. People with stress-related health problems may have to learn tension-relieving breathing techniques along with other stress-management skills. Usually they're sent to a psychologist because the doctor treating their illness believes it would be helpful, says Dr. Fried.

Actually, he laughs, "they get sent to me because the doctor has had no luck treating their problem. I get all the failures." In more than one case, though, falling through the cracks of traditional medicine has led to breathing therapy and ultimately to a cure, says Dr. Fried.

Athletes, pro or amateur, who are having anxiety-related problems with performance may see a sports psychologist, and thus learn how to stay cool under pressure. And that "cool" inevitably involves correct breathing technique. "In sports, the word is 'choking,' and it means someone is actually holding his breath and so depriving his body of oxygen when he may need it most," says James E. Loehr, Ed.D., director of sports science for the U.S. Tennis Association and coauthor of *Take a Deep Breath.*

He likens proper breathing to an internal massage. "It relaxes muscles and improves blood flow, so it reduces cramping," he says. Breath control is considered important in just about every sport—from archery to scuba diving.

And any yoga student learns about breathing as a matter of course. Yoga, with its vast array of breathing exercises (called *pranayamas*) and poses that help expand the chest and stretch and strengthen the diaphragm, offers perhaps the most comprehensive study of the science of breath, says researcher John Clarke, M.D., chairman of the Himalayan Institute in Honesdale, Pennsylvania. Dr. Fried agrees. "Much of what we know about breathing comes from yoga," he says.

One study, for instance, showed that people who practiced yoga had an average 25 percent increase in vital capacity (the greatest volume of air that, following maximum inhalation, can be expelled during a complete, unforced exhalation), a 50 percent increase in the time they could hold their breath, and a 15 percent increase in chest expansion. All are important indicators of respiratory health.

Belly Breathing

Whether a person works with a respiratory therapist, psychologist, or yoga instructor, one of the first and most important breathing techniques taught is a process called diaphragmatic breathing. (It is also sometimes called belly breathing or abdominal or deep breathing.)

Diaphragmatic breathing exposes the areas of the lungs that have the richest supply of blood—the lower lobes—to a good blast of oxygen. (The blood then picks up a greater supply of energy-giving oxygen to feed the rest of the body.) And it pushes air out of the lungs, effectively helping to eliminate the feeling of shortness of breath. The result: almost instant relaxation, a signal to your brain that all's right with the world, Dr. Clarke says.

To check if you're doing diaphragmatic breathing correctly, put one hand on your abdomen just below your ribs. Put your other hand on your chest. When you inhale, the hand on your abdomen should rise; the hand on your chest should remain still. To help their patients do diaphragmatic breathing properly, some therapists tell them to imagine they are blowing up a balloon in their stomach. "Technically, however, no air is going into the stomach," Dr. Fried points out.

For maximum relaxation, therapists ask their patients to breathe in and out for equal amounts of time and then to work on slowly extending the amount of time they exhale. Initially, performing this exercise can make you feel faint. Perform these exercises only under the supervision and approval of your doctor. (People with certain conditions—diabetes or heart disease, for example—should not do these exercises.)

With proper instruction, anyone can do diaphragmatic breathing, but long-time chest breathers usually manage only a few deep breaths before they revert to their old ways, Dr. Fried says.

"The muscles of your chest and diaphragm have adapted to that way of breathing," he explains. "It has become automatic behavior that can be very hard to correct." A shortened or flattened diaphragm muscle does not have the capacity to work as hard, so you're working against it with each breath until you condition yourself to the new way of breathing.

Breathing therapy focuses on toning the diaphragm, strengthening or relaxing other muscles used for breathing, and practicing the technique until it's as natural as, well, breathing.

To teach correct breathing technique, Dr. Fried uses a biofeedback machine that monitors the amount of carbon dioxide in a person's breath (he considers that the best indicator of whether someone is breathing correctly). He also uses biofeedback to gauge tension in chest muscles, including the scalene muscles, which some people use to imperceptibly draw their shoulders up toward their ears and their chest toward their chin, Dr. Fried says.

BREATHING IN ACTION

Elite athletes know that coordinating breath and action improves their performance. The right breathing technique can do the same for you.

"We know that muscles become tighter and more rigid, that blood pressure is elevated, and that heart rate increases slightly as you inhale," says James E. Loehr, Ed.D., director of sports science for the U.S. Tennis Association and coauthor of *Take a Deep Breath.* "And we know that as you exhale, the opposite occurs. The body goes through a recovery process."

That's why accomplished athletes have learned to coordinate their "out" breath with the most critical moves of their sport, Dr. Loehr says. Doing that allows their body to stay relaxed during this critical time.

"So you'll see tennis players breathing out, or sometimes grunting, at the precise point of contact with the ball. (Some begin a split second before.) And skiers will breathe out as they go through a difficult turn," he says.

A poor athlete, on the other hand, tends to hold his breath at critical points, inhal-

ing without adequate exhalation. "He tires very quickly, gets tight, and loses balance," Dr. Loehr says.

It's possible for anyone to use his breath to increase his performance in, and enjoyment of, an activity, Dr. Loehr says. Whether you choose walking, biking, swimming, or running, start out just paying attention to your breath, and then try synchronizing your breath to the action.

Try to find a rhythm that is best for you, he suggests, such as a four-step exhale and a four-step inhale. Then experiment with relaxing with a longer exhale, or with deliberately speeding your body up with quick breaths.

"When you find a rhythm that fits your physiology and the work level at which you're going, it just makes everything flow," he says. "And that's what you are trying to do—to get an effortless sense of flow, where you are balancing stress and recovery."

Paying attention to your breath while you're exercising teaches you breath awareness in general, Dr. Loehr says. "And you begin to sense how breathing can help balance everything you do."

"Sometimes it looks like they are doing it correctly when it's all wrong on the inside," he says. "So one of the most important things in breath training is to make sure that the behavior you are teaching is the kind of behavior that is going to lead to the proper gas composition." The only guarantee he gives them is that if they're going to see results, they'll see them pretty quickly. "I say if we haven't made a dent in this in 5 to 10 sessions, we aren't going to do it in 50," he says.

Exercise Training for Weak Diaphragms

Someone who is working with a respiratory therapist may learn additional exercises in conjunction with diaphragmatic breathing, says Adams. They may learn elbow-assisted breathing or upper-chest breathing (see the illustrations on pages 339 and 340), exercises that help the chest expand fully. The therapist may help to stretch and strengthen the diaphragm by gently pushing the abdomen up and in with her hand as a person exhales, then putting light pressure on the abdomen during inhalation.

People learning stress management, however, are *not* encouraged to do upper-chest breathing exercises, Dr. Fried emphasizes. "It's exactly that sort of thing we're trying to get them to stop doing."

People finding it hard to breathe often automatically begin breathing through pursed lips to make breathing easier. And that's an exercise that's also taught by respiratory therapists and used in yoga. The theory is that pursed-lip breathing helps lungs by clearing out stale air better, by keeping airways open longer, and by

inducing the abdominal muscles to actively contract on exhalation.

To do pursed-lip breathing, inhale through your nose, pushing your belly out. Then exhale through tight, pursed lips as if you are trying to whistle. Extending your exhale will further deflate your lungs. Try breathing in for 2 seconds and out for 4 seconds. (Check with your doctor before doing pursed-lip breathing, since it can cause bronchial spasms.)

If you would like to study breathing therapies but do not have a lung condition that requires working with a therapist, your best bet would probably be classes in yoga. See "Breathing in Action" on the opposite page.

The Ins and Outs of Better Breathing

Breathing properly not only supplies your body with the oxygen you need to survive, it can be wonderfully relaxing as well. And paying attention to your breath while you're walking, swimming, or biking can help you get the most enjoyment, and benefit, from your favorite activity.

The first breathing exercise is designed to help you stretch and strengthen the diaphragm—the large, dome-shaped muscle that arcs from the bottom of your rib cage and along your back to your pelvis, and that helps draw air into your lungs and push it back out. The other exercises increase lung capacity and aid chest expansion. Stick with diaphragmatic breathing for stress relief. Check with your doctor before doing any pursed-lip exhalation exercises: They can trigger bronchial spasms.

Diaphragmatic (Belly) Breathing

Sit up straight in your chair. Place your right hand on your lower abdomen and your left hand on your chest. Slowly inhale through your nose to a count of ten, so that your right hand moves outward (your left hand stays still). Then exhale through your nose to a count of ten, pulling in your lower abdomen on the last few counts. Repeat three times and rest. Then do two more sets of three.

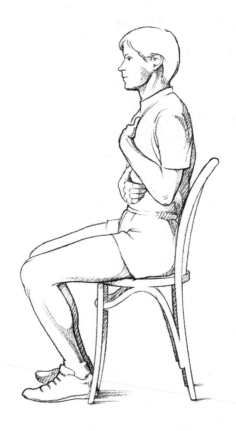

Elbow-Assisted Breathing

Lie on a flat surface with a folded towel placed between your shoulder blades. Bend your knees, keeping your feet flat on the floor. Bend your elbows and put your hands behind your head and your arms flat on the floor. Exhale, bringing your arms up toward your ears as though you are trying to touch your elbows together. Then, as you inhale, slowly bring your arms back down to the floor.

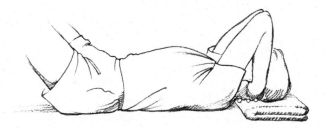

Rib Holding

Providing "resistance" to the muscles that help you breathe can make them stronger. Place a hand on either side of your chest, at the base of the rib cage. As you exhale fully, slowly press the ribs. Then, as you inhale, slowly reduce the pressure.

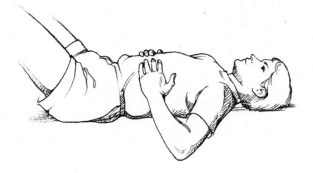

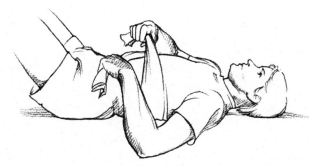

Towel Breathing

This exercise helps strengthen the diaphragm and the muscles around the rib cage. Wrap a towel around your abdomen. As you exhale slowly and fully, pull the ends of the towel to increase pressure. Then, as you inhale, slowly reduce pressure.

The Ins and Outs of Better Breathing—Continued

Upper-Chest Breathing

Most people don't need to practice upper-chest breathing. It's a bad habit they need to break! If you need all the lung capacity you can muster, though, try this exercise. Lie on the floor with your knees bent and your feet flat. Put one hand on your abdomen and one on your chest. Exhale fully. Then breathe in, but instead of filling your belly as with diaphragmatic breathing, concentrate on expanding and filling your upper chest. The hand on your chest should rise. The hand on your abdomen should remain still.

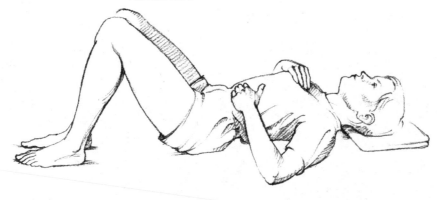

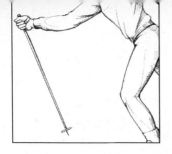

Cross-Country Skiing

*I*t's a clear, bright day, with the sun bouncing off new-fallen snow. You're gliding through the woods, in a world so still the only sound you hear is the whisper of your skis on snow and the faint thumping of your own heart.

Welcome to cross-country skiing.

"You can glide and think; you can be philosophical. You can enjoy it without getting very tired," says Per Renstrom, M.D., Ph.D., professor of orthopedics and sports medicine at the University of Vermont College of Medicine in Burlington.

But because you can tailor the intensity of your workout to your fitness level, you can also glide and sweat. "It's the best sport from a medical point of view," says Dr. Renstrom. While you're enjoying the great outdoors you'll be giving your body just about the best all-around workout you can get, experts agree. The rhythmic pumping of your arms and legs works most of your joints, tendons, and muscles, improving joint mobility and strengthening your entire musculoskeletal system.

More so than any other sport, cross-country skiing builds a strong heart and lungs. Because so many muscles are working, blood flow to the heart is increased, as is the heart's capacity to pump blood. Lungs must work hard to bring in oxygen and to get rid of the excess carbon dioxide created by that strenuous workout.

Because the gliding motion of cross-country skiing is easier on your body than the pounding of a sport such as running, doctors often recommend it as rehabilitation for people recovering from heart disease and knee and back problems.

Calorie counting? For most of us, cross-country skiing burns from 600 to 900 an hour. A world-class competitor can burn more than 1,000 calories an hour.

And this is a relatively inexpensive sport. You can outfit yourself for around $200.

Okay, what's the catch?

There are two. One is that snow is required, which means you're limited to winter months. The other is that unless you've caught on to the kick/glide/pole sequence that's the essence of cross-country skiing, you may not be having any fun. A lesson or two, however, can set you on the right track.

Before you spend any money on paraphernalia, it might be wise to give the sport a try. You may want to choose a cross-country ski resort, where you can rent properly fitted equipment, take those initial lessons, and ski on groomed trails. If you are a rank novice, just be sure you select beginner's trails, and before starting a loop find out how far it is—some trails are one way only.

Once you've caught the cross-country

skiing bug, you have a few decisions to make—decisions that will make a big difference in your future enjoyment of this delightfully challenging form of exercise.

Selecting Skis

First you need skis, boots, and poles, whether you choose to rent or buy. Go to a reputable ski touring center or ski shop, says Brian Delaney, ski instructor and owner of High Peak Cyclery, Ski, and Skate in Lake Placid, New York. Good, well-fitted equipment can make the difference between a pleasant outing and a terrible one, he says. Expect to spend $10 to $15 to rent and at least $175 to buy.

The skis, which snap on to the toes of special cross-country boots, come in two basic types: waxless, with serrations or patterns on the bottom, and waxable, to be used with waxes you apply as if you were rubbing with a big crayon. Both the grooves and the wax give you needed traction on the snow.

Waxable skis perform better than waxless because you can adjust the grip to fit conditions by applying different waxes. But while waxing itself is simple, picking the right wax may not be. "Waxes can be complicated—they can take away the interest in the sport," says Dr. Renstrom.

For that reason, waxless skis are easier for beginners. Even many accomplished skiers keep a pair on hand for rapidly changing snow conditions, says Delaney. "You'll always have a use for waxless skis," he says.

The length and flexibility of your skis is important so that they both grip and glide

properly. Proper selection depends on your height and weight. An indoor method of checking to see if you'll have enough grip, says Dr. Renstrom, is to stand in your skis with a sheet of paper directly under one foot. With all your weight on that foot, have someone try to pull the paper out. If the ski has enough grip, the paper should be held tight.

Confused? There's more: There are two distinct types of cross-country skiing. In the classic diagonal stride (shown on the opposite page), your skis move parallel to each other. In skate skiing, you use your skis as if they were huge skates. Skating uses shorter skis and longer poles, and it's faster and more efficient. But it may be a bit harder to learn, so it's better to start with the diagonal type, experts advise. (As you become more skilled, you can try skate skiing even on your diagonal skis.)

Getting a boot that fits right is also important. Boots should be snug in the heels, with some room in the toes. Many skiers like to wear a thin pair of liner socks with a medium-weight insulated outer pair. If you have perpetually cold toes, opt for overboots as well.

Once you've purchased or rented the equipment, you're almost ready to hit the trail. But first you need to put a little thought into what you're going to wear.

Dress for Success

Remember all the calories this sport burns? That means you generate a lot of heat, so leave those toasty downhill ski suits at home.

Layering is best, experts advise, and you

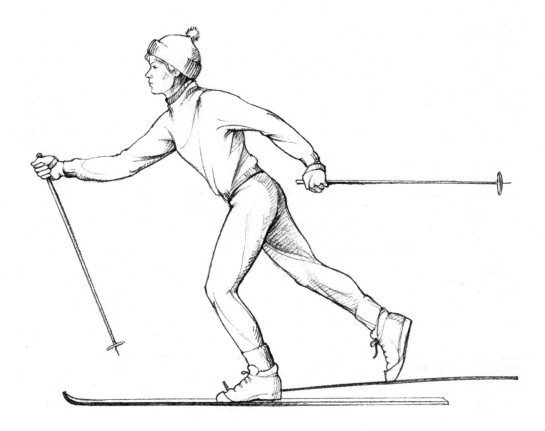

The diagonal stride is the basic technique for cross-country skiing. The skillful skier is able to give a strong kick that results in a long, smooth glide.

The secret to cross-country skiing is to learn to kick and glide—all the while using your poles as well. Sound complicated? It's not. First practice without your poles, transferring your weight from foot to foot while standing on your skis. Now kick back with one foot and glide forward on the other, leaning forward slightly and putting all your weight on that front ski. It's important to transfer your weight com-

pletely to the front ski, because otherwise you'll end up shuffling, not gliding.

Practice this a bit until the kick-and-glide seems natural, and then try it with your poles. Plant your right pole forward as you kick back with your right foot, then let that pole swing back and plant the left pole ahead of you as you kick back with your left foot. Don't lean on your poles—they're there to provide extra power, not to hold you upright. The whole routine should feel natural and smooth.

Congratulations! You've mastered the diagonal stride of cross-country skiing.

SKIING SANS SNOW

You like the idea of burning off lots of calories, strengthening your heart and lungs, and toning up muscles and tendons in a low-impact workout—but can't wait until winter?

A ski simulator may be just the thing for you.

Before you call in your order, however, think about what you're looking for in an exercise machine, advises exercise physiologist Dan Zeman, chief executive officer of the Institute for Health and Fitness in Minneapolis.

Some models require a certain amount of coordination, depending on whether the skis move independently or are linked together, notes Michael D. Wolf, Ph.D., president of Fitness Technologies in New York City. Until you've gotten the hang of it, there's a risk of falling when you use independent systems. That's because your feet might slide too far backward or forward, making it difficult for you to regain your balance.

And learning isn't instantaneous, says Michael Yessis, Ph.D., president of Sports Training Incorporated in Escondido, California. "You can't just jump on some of these machines and start using them," he says. He recommends working with an instructor until you're comfortable. You can get basic instruction at a gym or health club.

Once you've mastered the technique, however, you'll likely have no problem. The pioneer in ski simulators, NordicTrack, offers only independent systems, and a survey of owners five years after purchase reports a high degree of satisfaction.

Dependent systems, in contrast, are easily learned, notes Zeman. You jump on, and you're off and moving. The disadvantage is that they're less like actual cross-country skiing. Your best bet is to try both types—most likely at the local gym, or at exercise equipment stores.

Regardless, you should probably stay away from those handy-dandy $59.95 specials you see advertised on TV, cautions Patrick Netter, home exercise equipment

need far less clothing than you might think. Three layers of clothing are usually fine: long synthetic underwear, pants and a synthetic top or turtleneck, and a wind shell. For really frigid temperatures, add a wool or fleece sweater. The best choices for outer garments are ones that will shed moisture, such as nylon. Avoid jeans, which become soggy and heavy when wet. Wool is a good choice for socks, and gloves or mittens and a hat are a must.

A fanny pack, a small pouch that buckles around your waist, comes in handy for keys, waxes, a snack, and other odds and ends. You lose a lot of liquid while skiing, so drink plenty before leaving, and carry water if you're out for more than a very short jaunt.

Now you're ready to head for a local field or golf course that's fairly level. "It's difficult to go downhill at first," cautions Dr. Renstrom. "That's where you can get injured."

Getting Off on the Right Foot

While the kick/glide/pole sequence that moves you smoothly and easily across the snow isn't difficult to learn, it may not occur to you naturally. You'll get a better

expert and author of *Patrick Netter's High-Tech Fitness.*

You need to spend around $300 to get a sturdy machine, and you can shell out as much as $1,300 for a deluxe version. Solid construction is a must for safety reasons, advises Netter. Avoid models with exposed cables that could catch small, curious fingers.

The machine should have independent resistance settings for both arms and legs, with an adjustment for arm length. Finally, Netter says, the motion should feel smooth, particularly at higher settings. Having a feedback monitor that lets you know how you're doing is nice but by no means necessary.

When using a simulator, take it easy at first, advises Dr. Yessis. Start with no resistance, and learn the foot motion before you try to move your arms as well. As with real skiing, shift your weight from foot to foot as you stride. Be sure the hip-rest is flat against your abdomen.

Because a ski simulator uses so many muscles, give your body time to get used to it. Check your pulse to make sure you're not exceeding your target heart rate (see "How Good Is Your Workout?" on page 324), but don't force yourself to get your heart rate up to a certain level at first, says Dr. Yessis. "I've seen too many people who push too hard," he says. "They get sore, they get injured, and they decide this isn't for them."

Once you're confident and comfortable, you can increase your workouts to 20 to 30 minutes, including 5 to 10 minutes of warm-up and cool-down, advises Bob Goldman, D.O., Ph.D., president of the National Academy of Sports Medicine, director of sports medicine research at the Chicago College of Osteopathic Medicine, and director of the High Technology Fitness Research Institute in Chicago.

You won't have winter scenery to bolster your spirits, but you will find that a ski simulator provides the same physical benefits as cross-country skiing . . . even in July.

workout and enjoy the sport more if you learn to kick and glide and use your poles, experts agree. You *can* learn on your own, but getting some basic instruction can save time and frustration. You can pick up most of the basics in one lesson—at a cost of less than $10 for group instruction or $15 to $25 for an individual session. You might also plan to make that first outing with a buddy who is familiar with the basics.

Start out slowly to warm up, advises Michael Yessis, Ph.D., president of Sports Training Incorporated in Escondido, California, professor emeritus of California State University, Fullerton, and author of *Kinesiology of Exercise.* Some skiers like to stretch a bit before gliding away.

Get used to the feel of your skis and poles, and practice shifting your weight from one ski to the other. Remember how skis grip the snow? You need to have all your weight on one foot so the part of the ski directly under your foot will grab on to the snow and give you traction.

Lean forward a bit as you ski. Kick off on one foot as you glide forward on the other. Use your poles not as props to keep you from falling but to give additional power to your glide. When your right leg is behind you in a kick, your right pole should be planted ahead of you, ready to give impetus to your next glide. Top skiers get about 30 percent of their forward thrust from poling, according to Dr. Renstrom.

One way to achieve the right balance is to make sure your nose and the knee and toe of the gliding leg are all roughly aligned in the direction of the glide, advises Mike Gallagher, three-time Olympic ski competitor and Olympic ski coach.

Unfortunately, people tend to underestimate both the strenuousness of cross-country skiing and the speeds they can reach—and both can result in injury.

Injuries Do Occur

Tackling courses too difficult can cause painful falls, says Dr. Renstrom, so until you're skilled at turning and stopping, bypass any trails with hills. Other injuries—such as tendinitis of the shoulder, arm, and knee—can come from overuse. Overdoing it can be easy: "It feels so good you want to do more and more," says Dr. Yessis.

Overuse injuries can be avoided by limiting your early-season workouts and by strengthening your muscles *before* the season starts, says Dr. Yessis. He recom-

mends a strength-training program even during the season, specifically for shoulders and hips: Your cardiovascular and respiratory systems develop faster than your muscles, he says. You may *feel* like you can ski forever because you're not even out of breath, but the muscles of your arms and legs may not be ready for hours-long outings. This is where muscle injury comes in.

How to know when you've skied long enough? Easy, says Dr. Yessis. Stop *before* you get tired. You can check your heart rate regularly to ensure you aren't passing your target zone. (See "How Good Is Your Workout?" on page 324.) But pushing to reach that zone may be a mistake until your muscles are tuned up and you've become more skilled on skis.

Having poorly waxed or poorly fitted skis can also lead to muscle and tendon injuries, notes Dr. Renstrom. If your ski doesn't grip when you put your weight on it, you can find yourself doing the splits unexpectedly.

Finally, if you're completely out of shape, it may take a while to tune up your muscles enough to really enjoy the sport. Persevere for at least six weeks, says Dr. Yessis. "If you can hang in there, you'll find that you've fallen in love with it," he says.

Mastering the Ski Machine

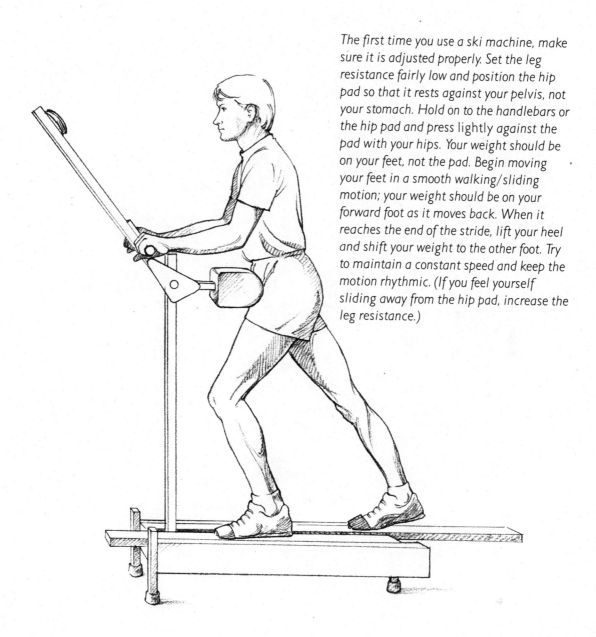

The first time you use a ski machine, make sure it is adjusted properly. Set the leg resistance fairly low and position the hip pad so that it rests against your pelvis, not your stomach. Hold on to the handlebars or the hip pad and press lightly against the pad with your hips. Your weight should be on your feet, not the pad. Begin moving your feet in a smooth walking/sliding motion; your weight should be on your forward foot as it moves back. When it reaches the end of the stride, lift your heel and shift your weight to the other foot. Try to maintain a constant speed and keep the motion rhythmic. (If you feel yourself sliding away from the hip pad, increase the leg resistance.)

Mastering the Ski Machine—Continued

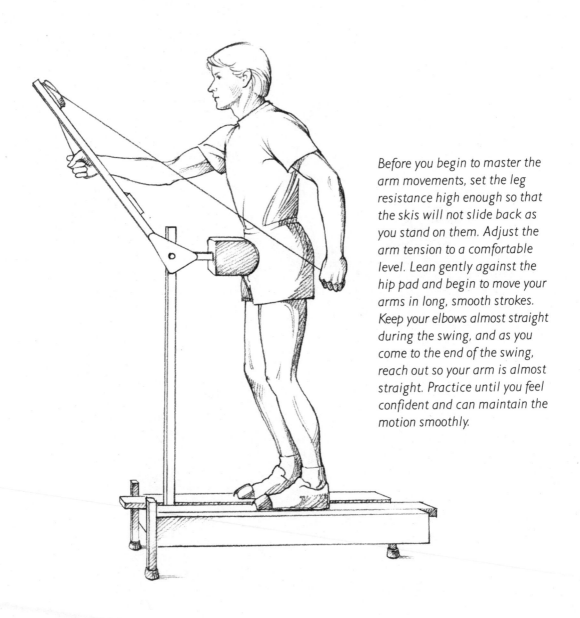

Before you begin to master the arm movements, set the leg resistance high enough so that the skis will not slide back as you stand on them. Adjust the arm tension to a comfortable level. Lean gently against the hip pad and begin to move your arms in long, smooth strokes. Keep your elbows almost straight during the swing, and as you come to the end of the swing, reach out so your arm is almost straight. Practice until you feel confident and can maintain the motion smoothly.

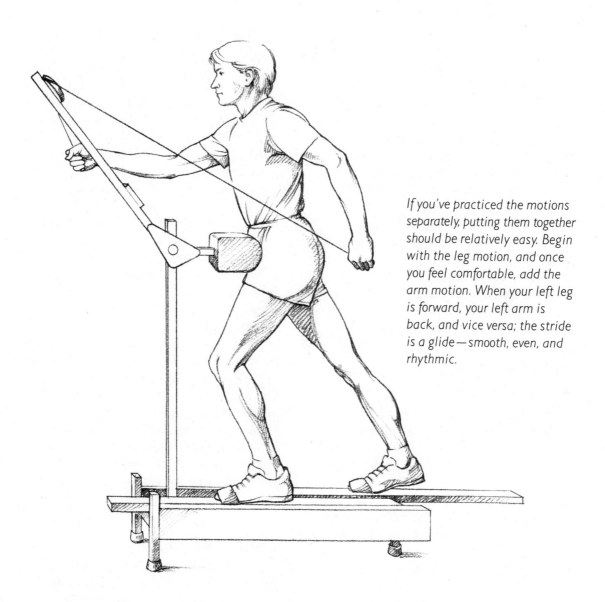

If you've practiced the motions separately, putting them together should be relatively easy. Begin with the leg motion, and once you feel comfortable, add the arm motion. When your left leg is forward, your left arm is back, and vice versa; the stride is a glide—smooth, even, and rhythmic.

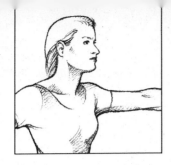

Dancing

*T*heir workouts used to take them miles apart. He'd jog left at the mailbox on a Saturday morning, she'd walk right. There was a lot of distance in their marriage in those days, too.

Then they tried something one weekend on a friend's advice. They skipped their Saturday morning workouts and went dancing Saturday night instead. And guess what? They've been burning calories cheek to cheek every Saturday night ever since. This is a modern-day romantic tale repeated just about every time a couple discovers that moving feet can draw people closer.

Why Sweat When You Can Swing?

"It's the ultimate togetherness workout," says Phil Martin, lecturer and dance instructor at California State University, Long Beach. "You move in a physical harmony that works toward an emotional harmony. You also tend to bring back a lot of fond memories. The dance floor can be a great place to give a tiring relationship second wind."

Not just the heartstrings get pulled by the likes of a good foxtrot, however. The heart itself gets a healthy push. "Studies show that steps such as the cha-cha, polka, samba, Viennese waltz, and East and West Coast swing easily can raise the average person's heart rate enough to achieve an aerobic conditioning effect," Martin says. "You tend not to realize it, though, because you are having so much fun."

Aha! Fun. That word seems to have gotten pushed aside in recent years by all the treadmills, gut busters, rowing machines, and stationary bikes. "No pain, no gain" was the cry heard throughout the land, but it seems that very little fitness has actually been gained.

"Surveys show that fewer than 15 percent of Americans have been successful at sticking to the kind of three-workout-a-week schedule currently recommended for good cardiovascular health," says Bryant A. Stamford, Ph.D., director of the Health Promotion and Wellness Center at the University of Louisville and coauthor of *Fitness without Exercise*. "We need more fitness activities that let people have a good time, that encourage them to be creative rather than compulsive, that encourage them to communicate and not just perspire."

5 Miles of Fun

Lee Walker, M.D., wholeheartedly agrees. The 75-year-old physician from LaFollette, Tennessee, traded his sweat suit for blue jeans years ago. Dr. Walker, you see, is a square dancer and has been for about 50

BEST STEPS TO STOMP CALORIES

Is it an exaggeration to call ballroom dancing "great exercise"?

Hardly. Tests by the Department of Human Movement and Recreation Studies at the University of West Australia have found that a robust rumba can be as aerobically demanding as running. That a torrid tango can raise the heart rate higher than a hot game of squash. That even just a well-done waltz can court the cardiovascular system as aggressively as a brisk walk. "Dancing several times per week can make a valuable training contribution . . . to persons seeking to . . . enhance their level of fitness," the researchers concluded.

And it can be a great way to step away from some unwanted body fat, too. Researchers from the Department of Physical Education at San Diego State University found that a 12-week program of low-impact aerobic dance resulted in body-fat losses averaging an impressive 7 pounds per participant. Plus, there were no injuries and no dropouts! Sessions lasted 45 minutes and were conducted three days a week.

Then, too, if you're out dancing on evenings when you might otherwise be home snacking, you're getting a double weight-loss benefit.

Which steps step up the heart best?

Based on a study of 45 dance-class students at California State University, Long Beach, the styles noted below raised the participants' heart rates to within their "target zones"—the level of exertion needed to produce an aerobic conditioning effect. "Any dance can be performed with different intensity, however," says Phil Martin, lecturer and dance instructor at the school. "The amount of exercise afforded ultimately depends as much on the dancer as the dance."

So go slowly or go wild, depending on what you're trying to achieve. And keep in mind that you tend to burn more calories, not fewer, the better you get at any given step. Some dances, more so than others, can help you achieve your target heart rate—60 percent or more of the estimated maximum heart rate. (To determine your target heart rate, see "How Good Is Your Workout?" on page 324.) Of those who did the East Coast swing (jitterbug, lindy, or bop), about 95 percent hit their target heart rate; 91 percent did so for the polka, 80 percent for the Viennese waltz, 75 percent for the samba, and 44 percent for the cha-cha. Other good aerobic workouts include the mambo and square dancing.

years. "It can be a heck of a good workout but also a heck of a good time," he says.

"Studies using pedometers have shown most square dancers cover about 5 miles in a single night," says Stan Burdick, coeditor of *American Square Dance* magazine.

Nice. And especially nice considering the social mileage that gets covered. "People bring their whole families," Dr. Walker says. "Children and grandparents alike take part. It's exercise, but it's also a form of celebration. Not a lot of other fitness activities can say that."

No, with most other fitness pursuits either you're alone or you're competing. But when you dance you're *cooperating*, Martin says. "The goal in dancing is to work *with* rather than against another person, and it can have very positive emotional spillovers."

Take Andy and Michelle Feldman, for example, who not only fell head over heels for each other at one of Martin's classes but decided to keep the ball rolling by spending their honeymoon at one of his week-long dance camps. "Dancing definitely revs up the romantic side," Martin says.

Not all dancers fire up as easily as the Feldmans, however. Some people need a little push. Consider 47-year-old George from California, who used to joke that, sure, he'd go dancing—if he could take his portable TV! But George's wife Diana finally broke him down, and bingo: Now George is the guy up there asking the band for "just one more" every Saturday night, brow sweating, shirttail on the loose. And he's *also* the guy now jogging or playing volleyball at least three times a week.

"The dancing makes me feel young—young enough to be a little bothered at how strenuous it seemed," George says. "It was a nice way to get kicked in the rear to get back in shape."

"I see it a lot," Martin says. "People get reawakened to the joy of physical movement, and it inspires them to want to do more. Many people even start making positive changes in their diet."

Boogying for the Brain

Maybe the most remarkable benefits to be gained through dance have to do with that area well above the feet—the mind. Researchers from the departments of psychology and dance at Reed College in Portland, Oregon, decided several years ago to study just that. They assigned a group of 133 college students to a sports class (which taught kayaking, fencing, and basketball), an academic class (with instruction in biology, religion, and American literature), or a dance class. Then the students were asked to respond to a 20-item self-evaluation both before and after their participation, as a way of measuring the influence of the class on their sense of well-being.

We'll let the authors themselves convey the study's results: "Relative to the academic students, dancers characterized themselves at the end of the class as more creative, happier, more secure, more confident, more relaxed, more coordinated, more exhilarated, healthier, and more competent."

And how did the dancers compare to the sports participants? "Dancers felt significantly more creative, confident, relaxed, excited, motivated, healthy, intelligent, and energetic."

Theories vary on exactly why dance has such mood-elevating powers, but central among them is that dance emphasizes expression and creativity more than competition. And that may have a very liberating effect.

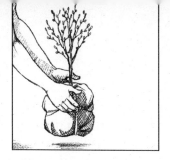

Gardening

Think of it as your own private health club, an invigorating open-air gym replete with bodybuilding equipment, aerobic sessions, resistance training—and an occasional squirrel.

Where else but a garden can you pump up your pecs amid the petunias, tone your triceps in a turnip patch? Forget the fancy treadmills, bikes, and barbells. You've got all the exercise "equipment" you need: a rake, a spade, a wheelbarrow—and that 10-pound sack of topsoil.

Seedy Alternatives

Time was when we didn't think of gardening as exercise. "People used to spend hours in their gardens, snipping, weeding, pruning the rose bushes, dusting for aphids, hustling in and out of the garage, and then later they'd be at some social gathering saying, 'I *hate* exercise!' " recalls ecologist and land management expert Charles Rhodehamel of Columbia, Maryland.

But clearly, they didn't hate exercise. They just didn't realize they were already doing what was good for them.

"Gardening is natural exercise," says Bryant A. Stamford, Ph.D., director of the Health Promotion and Wellness Center at the University of Louisville and coauthor of *Fitness without Exercise.* "Gardening takes you through a wide range of physical movements and works probably every single muscle in your body."

Not only are you toning your muscles when you garden, but you're pruning away excess pounds as well. Just the continuous action of raking, hoeing, and digging burns almost as many calories as a moderate aerobic dance workout. It's estimated that depending on your weight, you can burn anywhere from 300 to 470 calories an hour by gardening. (The dance routine burns 350 to 540.) In fact, if you want to lose 360 to 560 calories an hour, just cut your grass with a push mower.

Call a Spade a Spade

Put simply, gardening is good for your health. Studies show that moderate exercise such as hoeing, tilling, and raking helps lower your risk for a number of health problems, including high blood pressure, diabetes, and heart disease.

One large study conducted over a seven-year period and coordinated at the University of Minnesota found that activities such as gardening and yard work helped prevent heart attacks. Researchers studied more than 12,000 middle-aged men, comparing those who were sedentary with those who did light- to moderate-intensity activity, like gardening, for an average of

45 minutes a day. The results? Those who gardened lowered their risk of having a fatal heart attack by one-third.

Some experts suggest tilling the soil is an even *better* way to work out than other kinds of exercise. Why? Because your sense of accomplishment will encourage you to stick with it. "When you mulch the tomatoes and weed the flower bed, you're seeing immediate results you *don't* see when you're charging around a track or sitting on a stationary bike," says epidemiologist Ronald LaPorte, Ph.D., of the University of Pittsburgh's School of Public Health. "The biggest problem with traditional exercise is that people don't want to continue it. It's boring. But people *do* want to go back to their gardens."

Rhodehamel agrees. "All day long I shuffle papers or spew out reports," he says. "But after dragging home at the end of the day, I make a beeline to my garden, and suddenly I'm exhilarated. I'm working with nature, orchestrating a beautiful series of blooms here or creating massive swaths of color there. At the same time, I'm exercising, not sitting on my duff in front of the TV."

An extra benefit is that part of Rhodehamel's "workout" area is edible.

"What health club on earth," he asks, "is going to reward you with a basket of zucchini and a bouquet of fresh flowers at the end of a workout?"

SOWING THE SEEDS OF FITNESS . . . CAREFULLY

We're not suggesting that you tiptoe through the tulips, but you *should* be cautious about how you garden. The last thing you want to do is sprain your back lugging a 50-pound bag of fertilizer into the cabbage patch. Here are some tips to help you avoid injuries.

Stay straight. If you have back problems, or want to avoid them, always hold your back as straight as possible. If you must bend from the waist, never stand straight-legged, but rather bend your knees slightly. If you use a wheelbarrow, for example, bend your knees and lift as you straighten your legs.

Use a tube. If a bad back makes it particularly difficult to plant seeds, try using a long, thin tube and dropping seeds through it from a standing position.

Kneel in comfort. Always use foam-rubber knee pads. The ground can be rough on the knees and joints, but the soft cushion provides a protective buffer between you and the soil. You can pick up these pads at your local garden shop.

Think light. If your grip isn't great, use lightweight gardening tools. Children's tools or those made from aluminum are best.

Be easy on yourself. Remember, gardening *is* exercise. If you haven't been gardening regularly, treat it like any other exercise regimen. Use moderation, or you may pull a muscle. Try to space out your activities over the course of a week, seeding one day, weeding the next, and so forth.

Yard Work Made Easy

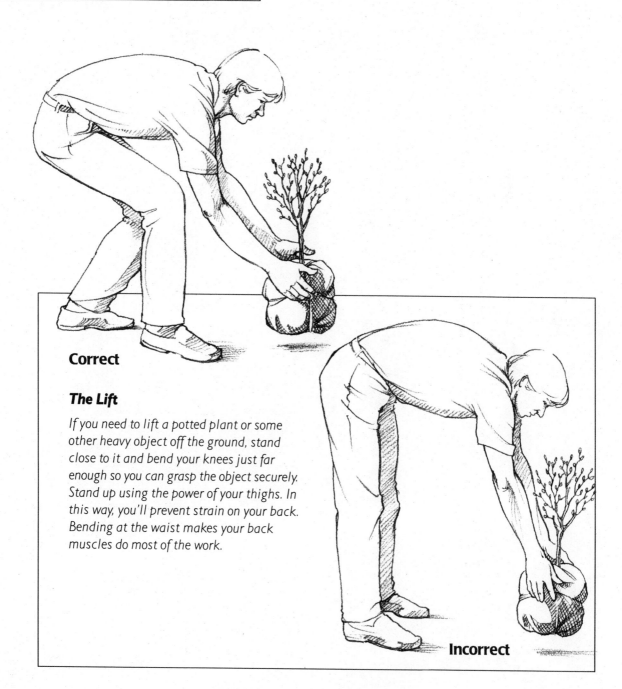

Correct

The Lift

If you need to lift a potted plant or some other heavy object off the ground, stand close to it and bend your knees just far enough so you can grasp the object securely. Stand up using the power of your thighs. In this way, you'll prevent strain on your back. Bending at the waist makes your back muscles do most of the work.

Incorrect

Yard Work Made Easy—Continued

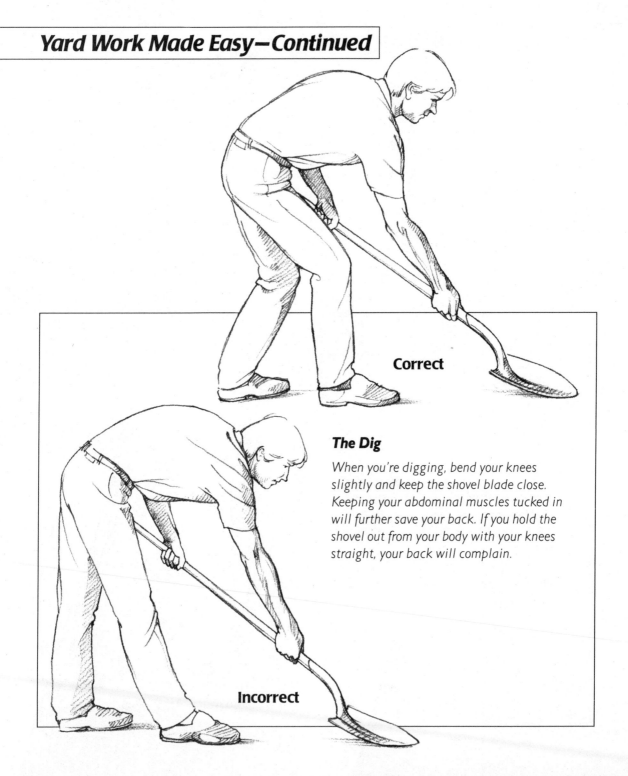

Correct

The Dig

When you're digging, bend your knees slightly and keep the shovel blade close. Keeping your abdominal muscles tucked in will further save your back. If you hold the shovel out from your body with your knees straight, your back will complain.

Incorrect

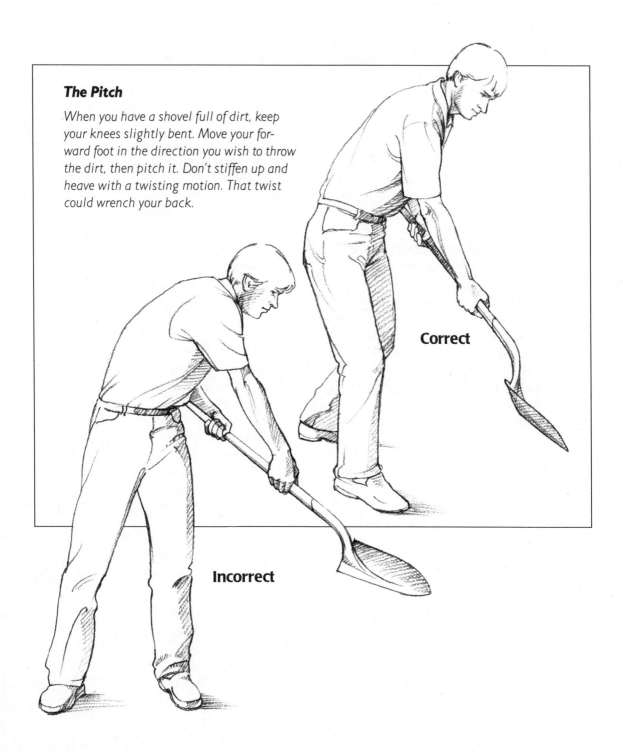

The Pitch

When you have a shovel full of dirt, keep your knees slightly bent. Move your forward foot in the direction you wish to throw the dirt, then pitch it. Don't stiffen up and heave with a twisting motion. That twist could wrench your back.

Correct

Incorrect

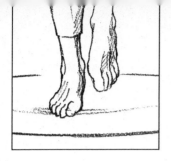

Jumping

Whether you skip rope or bounce on a mini-trampoline, jumping is a good aerobic workout for most people, experts say.

"Jumping, in the simplest sense, is like running without going anywhere. In terms of energy burned, there is very little difference between jumping and running. It provides an exercise alternative—other than walking or running—that people find satisfying," says Carl Foster, Ph.D., director of cardiac rehabilitation and exercise testing at Sinai-Samaritan Medical Center in Milwaukee.

Jumping rope for 30 minutes, for example, is the equivalent of 30 minutes of running an 8½-minute mile, says Kathleen Hargarten, M.D., medical director of AthleticForce at Columbia Hospital's Sports Medicine Center in Milwaukee.

"Jumping rope increases your endurance and your strength. It increases your aerobic conditioning. It also improves your coordination, agility, timing, and rhythm," she says.

Bouncing on a mini-trampoline, also called rebounding, offers many of the same physical benefits of jumping rope but with less impact on the joints, says James R. White, Ph.D., author of *Jump for Joy* and an exercise physiologist at the University of California, San Diego.

"Rebounding lowers resting heart rate, increases the number and size of blood vessels, decreases body fat, reduces total cholesterol, and increases the level of HDL cholesterol, the so-called good cholesterol," he says.

"It's not a miracle exercise, but it's a fun workout that has the capability of improving your cardiovascular system and your health in a nonimpactful way."

Give It a Twirl

Rope-jumping enthusiasts also stress the pleasurable aspects of their activity.

"You don't need a lot of equipment, and it's inexpensive. A good rope probably costs less than $10, and you can throw it in your suitcase when you travel," says Ken Solis, M.D., of Milwaukee, who along with Dr. Hargarten helped develop Ropics, an aerobic exercise program based on jumping rope.

"There are literally hundreds of techniques that are possible with a jump rope, and you can do them all indoors," he says. "That means you don't have to worry about falling in potholes to get a good aerobic workout."

Of course, jumping rope isn't the best exercise for everyone. Before you begin a jumping program you should see your doctor if you have a chronic ailment such as high blood pressure, heart disease, or diabetes or if you're older than 40 or haven't been exercising regularly.

Once you get the go-ahead, you need to learn how to jump rope properly, Dr. Hargarten says.

"Some people think they can just pick up a rope and start jumping," she says. "But they get frustrated very quickly because they keep missing, or they're so exhausted after jumping continuously for 4 minutes that they're ready to collapse."

A Little Hop Will Do It

"Most beginners jump too high. They also tend to use their shoulders and upper arms rather than their wrists and forearms to turn the rope," Dr. Hargarten says. "Jumping too high or landing wrong can cause injuries to the knees or other joint problems. Landing on the balls of the feet provides a certain amount of shock absorption.

"A lot of people think that jumping rope can cause a lot of wear and tear on the knees or other joints. In reality, if you jump correctly—less than an inch off the ground—it's actually a moderate-impact activity," Dr. Hargarten says.

She suggests renting an instructional video or enrolling in a rope-jumping course.

Choosing the right rope also is an important consideration, she says.

"You have to find a rope that isn't going to tangle easily and has the right amount of weight so you can swing it properly," Dr. Hargarten says. Segmented (beaded) or vinyl ropes are the most durable and are the best weight for jumping, she says.

"Personally, I like a segmented rope. To

adjust it, all you have to do to shorten the rope is untie an end and take out the number of beads necessary to make it the right length for you," Dr. Hargarten says.

To determine if the rope is the correct length, stand with one foot on the center of the rope. Then lift the rope. The ends of the handles should just reach your armpits.

Avoid weighted ropes, Dr. Hargarten warns. Some weigh up to 6 pounds and put excessive stress on muscles and joints.

"The risks of injury are too great to justify the minimal benefits (if any) from the additional weight," she says.

The proper shoes are vital, too, Dr. Hargarten says. Wear athletic shoes—such as good aerobic or cross-training shoes that have shock-absorbing cushioning in the forefoot and good lateral stability.

How to Skip and Jump

After you get the right equipment and have learned to jump correctly, how do you make rope jumping a regular part of your workout?

Start slowly, Dr. Hargarten recommends. You might begin by doing four 1-minute intervals of jumping rope, alternating with four 2-minute sessions of nonjumping activities such as marching in place while swinging the rope from side to side. This routine can be done three times a week. Gradually increase your jumping time over the next six weeks until you can jump rope 15 minutes per session, three to four times a week. You want to be jumping at a pace of 120 to 140 revolutions per minute.

"In Ropics, our beginner students might jump for 30 seconds to 1 minute, then they may do 2 to 3 minutes of nonjumping.

Then they do another minute of jumping and another interval of nonjumping," Dr. Hargarten says. "As they get in better shape, it's easier for them to jump, and it's not as stressful on their legs."

B Is for Bounce

Of course, if you really want to minimize the stress on your legs, you might consider jumping rope on a mini-trampoline, Dr. White says.

"You can skip rope on a rebounder. It's done for a longer time and at a slower pace, but rebounding and jumping rope are very compatible," he says.

"Actually, most of the exercises you see on television workout programs can be done on a rebounder with considerably less impact and much more fun."

Like jump ropes, mini-trampolines are fairly portable and can be used in your home, Dr. White says.

"Bouncing on a mini-tramp is like jumping rope without the disadvantages. You get an aerobic workout, but you don't have any trauma to your joints. It doesn't require as much coordination to do a mini-tramp as it does to do a rope," says James Peterson, Ph.D., author of *How to Jump Higher* and director of research and development at Randal Sports Medical Products in Kirkland, Washington.

In fact, people who can't do other aerobic exercises may be able to work out comfortably on a mini-trampoline.

"Originally, we thought rebounding wouldn't be good for people with back pain. But we found that most people with back problems can exercise on a rebounder with no pain," says Dr. White. "But if they try walking or running, they often experience significant discomfort. We also recommend it for people with arthritis. Swimming is the best exercise for them, but if they get a good rebounder, they can exercise very comfortably on it."

But jumping on a mini-trampoline does have its risks, Dr. Peterson says.

"You have to be careful," he says. "You can't ever lose track of where you are because if you do, there is a chance that you could hurt yourself.

"If you are bouncing and don't watch where you're going, you could hit the side of the trampoline and sprain your ankle or break your leg."

In addition, if you do have arthritis, joint problems, or another chronic illness such as heart disease, you should see your doctor before you start rebounding. You also shouldn't work out on a mini-trampoline if you experience balance problems or suffer from dizzy spells, Dr. White says.

Getting That Spring in Your Step

Mini-trampolines can be purchased for about $20, he says. But the best ones cost from $150 to $300.

"I personally like the rebounders that have springs in the legs in addition to springs on the mat," Dr. White says. "That way the whole rebounder gives when you bounce on it—you feel soft-yielding impact."

When you jump, keep your posture erect and your shoulders level. Try to keep your movements smooth and gentle, and remember that you can use your hands and arms for balance.

Up with Rebounding

Jumping on a mini-tramp is a fun and vigorous, yet gentle, exercise. Here's a moderately challenging beginners' routine to get you started.

A word about clothing: You really don't need a Lycra leotard to jump. Comfortable, loose cotton clothing is just fine. However, men should wear an athletic supporter, and women should wear a sports bra. Stockings or bare feet are okay, too. But if the mat feels slippery to you, you may be more secure wearing aerobic shoes.

As with any exercise program, it's important to warm up before and cool down after the routine. To do this, start with 3 to 12 minutes of stretching followed by 5 to 10 minutes of easy bouncing. After jumping, finish up with 5 to 10 minutes of easy bouncing followed by 3 to 5 minutes of stretching. (See "Stretching" on page 440.) The routine can be as long as you like. You might start with a goal of 10 minutes of vigorous exercise and adjust the length depending on how you feel.

There are only a few simple rules to jumping. Land on the heel and ball of your foot simultaneously as you jump. Landing on just the ball of your foot is reserved for advanced jumpers only and will help strengthen the front of your thighs. Jumping doesn't have to be done in a particular way, but you should become familiar with the two basic bounces shown in the first two illustrations. Start slowly and gain balancing experience before you jazz it up. Maintain good posture, and relax your arms so they can move freely to help keep your balance.

Good Warm-Up Jumps

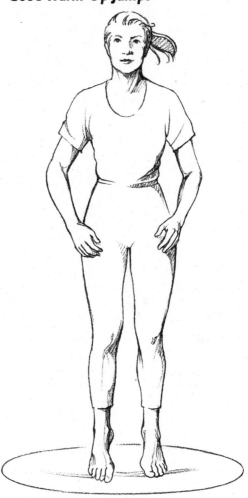

Stand on your mini-tramp with your feet shoulder-width apart. Start a gentle bounce, letting your arms swing freely. Bounce so that your heels lift off the tramp but your toes remain in contact. As you become more confident, increase the intensity of the bounce until your feet completely leave the tramp.

Up with Rebounding—Continued

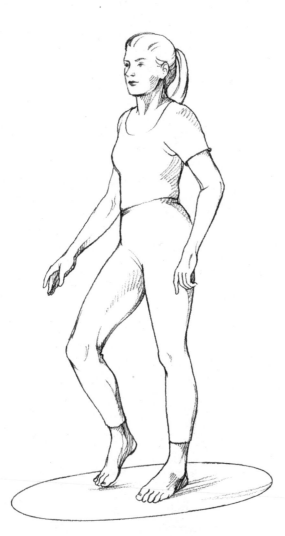

This jump is a more vigorous version of the previous jog bounce. Start with the easier movement and gradually increase your effort until you can alternately pick your feet up off the mini-tramp.

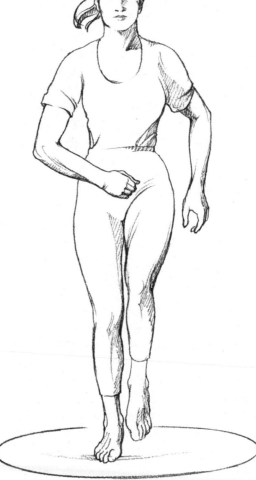

Bounce as in the previous exercise, but when you feel comfortable, alternately pick your heels up off the tramp. Keep your toes in contact. The movement is similar to an easy jog.

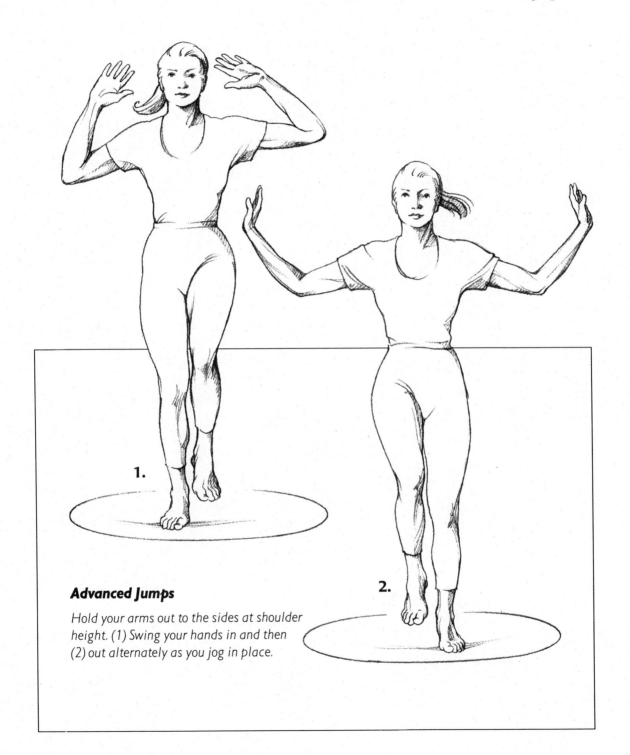

1.

2.

Advanced Jumps

Hold your arms out to the sides at shoulder height. (1) Swing your hands in and then (2) out alternately as you jog in place.

Up with Rebounding—Continued

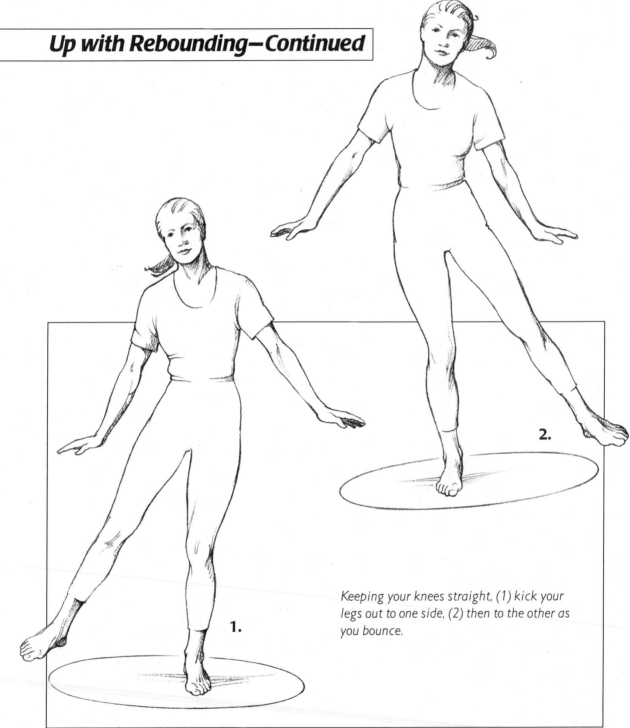

1.

2.

Keeping your knees straight, (1) kick your legs out to one side, (2) then to the other as you bounce.

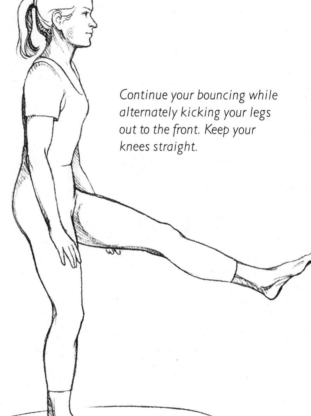

Continue your bouncing while alternately kicking your legs out to the front. Keep your knees straight.

Do jumping jacks. Keep your bounces low and your movements relaxed.

Up with Rebounding—Continued

Advanced Jumps

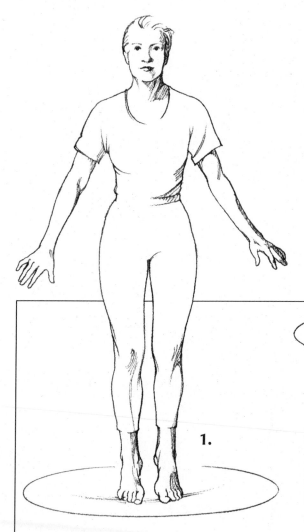

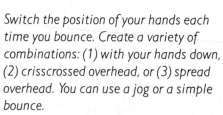

Switch the position of your hands each time you bounce. Create a variety of combinations: (1) with your hands down, (2) crisscrossed overhead, or (3) spread overhead. You can use a jog or a simple bounce.

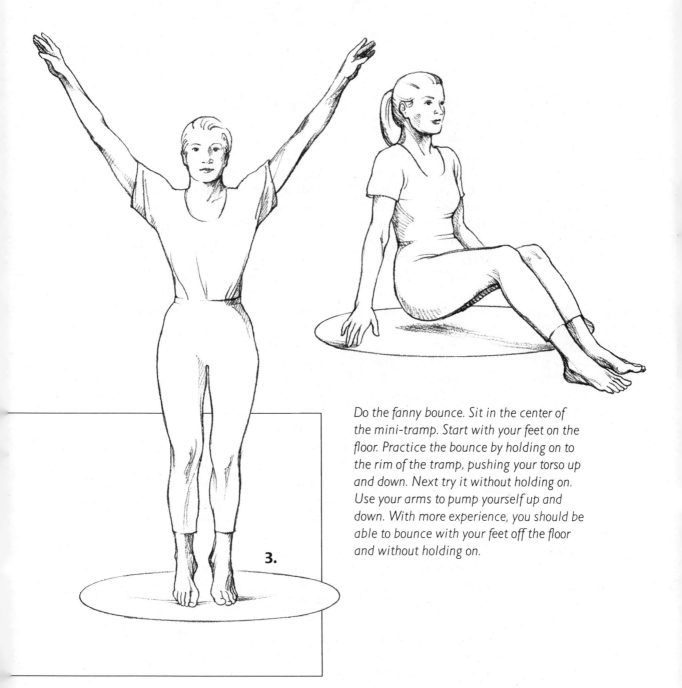

Do the fanny bounce. Sit in the center of the mini-tramp. Start with your feet on the floor. Practice the bounce by holding on to the rim of the tramp, pushing your torso up and down. Next try it without holding on. Use your arms to pump yourself up and down. With more experience, you should be able to bounce with your feet off the floor and without holding on.

3.

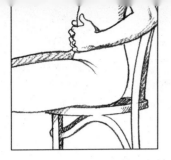

Kegel Exercises

They may bear his name, but Kegel exercises were around long before Arnold Kegel, M.D., was even born. There's evidence that women have been doing these pubic-muscle-tightening contractions for at least 100 years. But it was Dr. Kegel, a gynecologist from Los Angeles, who popularized the exercises when he found they had medical merit in the 1940s.

Kegel exercises are designed to strengthen a number of muscles, including the pubococcygeus (PC), or pelvic floor, muscles—a sling-shaped set of muscles that goes from the pubic bone to the tailbone, with openings for the urethra (bladder opening), vagina, and anus. These are the muscles that allow both men and women to stop the flow of urine and squeeze off gas. They also permit women to tighten the vagina.

Gaining Control

The exercises are often prescribed to help control urinary incontinence, which is related to weak urinary sphincter muscles. They are also used before and after delivery of a baby to help restore vaginal muscle tone, prevent urinary incontinence, and hold the uterus in its proper position.

Women can also use Kegels to enhance sexual pleasure for both themselves and their partner by creating a "tighter fit" that increases friction.

It is possible for many people to learn to do Kegels on their own, but doctors say that people whose muscles are so weak they can't stop the flow of urine can benefit greatly by working with a biofeedback specialist, physical therapist, or nurse who specializes in teaching Kegels. Such teachers are most likely to be associated with an incontinence clinic or a urology department at a major hospital.

Getting medical help means that if you have urinary incontinence, you'll first get a proper diagnosis. If you are a candidate for exercise therapy, you'll then be referred to a therapist, who will work with you for weeks or months.

"My sessions start off with an anatomy lesson," says Kathe Wallace, a Seattle physical therapist who specializes in Kegel training. "Lots of women don't even know that these muscles exist, much less what they look like or what they do."

Next, the therapist helps you identify and contract the PC muscles without using other muscles. She may insert a finger into the vagina or anus and lay her hand on your lower abdomen to feel if you are doing the exercise right. Or she may use a biofeedback machine to measure pressure or muscle activity within the vagina. (Biofeedback is a training technique that helps people gain conscious control of muscles or bodily functions.)

Once you've learned how to identify the correct muscles, the therapist will evaluate your muscle strength and design a daily strengthening program for you. Then you'll do a set of Kegel exercises as best you can with the therapist acting as coach. (You may need electrical stimulation to help you gain awareness of the muscles to be moved.) You may get a biofeedback machine to use at home, especially if your muscles are very weak. The machine can help tell you whether you are doing the exercises correctly.

If you want to try to do Kegel exercises at home, Wallace, an advisor with Help for Incontinent People (H.I.P.), suggests this procedure: First you need to locate the muscles to be exercised. Once you're about half finished urinating, try to stop or slow the urine without tensing the muscles of your legs, buttocks, or abdomen. (It's important *not* to use these other muscles, because only the pelvic floor muscles help with bladder control, and tightening the stomach muscles can increase pressure on the bladder, making an accident more likely.)

If you are able to slow or stop the stream of urine, you have located the correct muscles. Feel the sensation of the muscles pulling inward and upward.

When you have located the correct muscles, set aside several times a day for exercising: morning, midday, and evening.

There are two ways to exercise the muscles: a short contraction followed by a relaxation, and a holding contraction (work up to 10 to 15 seconds) followed by a relaxation. Both are important for pelvic muscle floor strength. Complete ten sets during each of your daily exercise sessions.

If you're not used to doing these exercises, perform them after you've finished urinating.

Practice Pays Off

In a few weeks, you should be able to increase the amount of time you are able to hold the contraction and the number of repetitions you are able to do. Your goal should be to work up to 10-second contractions, followed by 10 seconds of relaxation, and to complete as many repetitions as you can.

Like all other muscles, these muscles need to be challenged in order to gain strength. Each person responds differently. If this routine seems too easy for you, ask your therapist to help you develop a program that will provide a greater challenge.

In the beginning, check yourself frequently by looking in the mirror or by placing a hand on your abdomen and buttocks to ensure that you do not feel your belly, thigh, or buttock muscles move. There should be no visible movement. (In a man, though, the penis will lift slightly.)

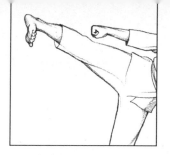

Martial Arts

Charles Richman was always slightly built. When he was younger, he turned to boxing to learn how to defend himself. Then when bullies started picking on his son, Adam, he naturally recommended boxing, but the boy wanted to learn martial arts. So Dr. Richman, who has a Ph.D. and is a professor of psychology at Wake Forest University in Winston-Salem, North Carolina, enrolled his son and himself in a tae kwon do (Korean karate) class. Eight weeks later, he saw a transformation in his son and other classmates so startling that his own study took a serious turn. And today he is a professional martial arts teacher.

"A lot of the kids," he remembers, "were having problems with school—discipline problems, learning problems, family problems. By the end of the course, there was, for the most part, an increase in their self-esteem. Their attitude in and toward school improved."

As a tae kwan do instructor, Dr. Richman says he *knows* martial arts trains the mind and body in ways few other exercise regimens can. For self-confidence, poise, flexibility, muscular and cardiovascular conditioning, and, yes, even the ability to bust a board with your bare hands, mar-

tial arts "offers incredible benefits for any age, either sex," he maintains.

Fight Doesn't Make Right

Forget about Bruce Lee, the Karate Kid, kickboxing tournaments, and those poorly dubbed fight movies from China shown Saturday afternoons on Kung Fu Theater. "That's not what it's about at all," says Peter Sherrill, D.O., an emergency and sports medicine physician at Door County Memorial Hospital in Oregon Bay, Wisconsin. "The better a martial artist you are, the less likely you are to need the art you've worked so hard to learn."

Physically and mentally, he says, "the word is empowerment. The discipline honed by martial arts training proves people do have some control over their lives, and they're not going to be victims." That empowerment applies whether you're rushing to your car in a dark parking lot or approaching the boss about a problem at work, he says.

For most people, martial arts "is not suiting up to spar and bang your head," Dr. Sherrill says. Learning one of the many forms of the ancient discipline, he says, translates into learning to control and coordinate body and brain for health—how to stand, how to breathe, how to move, how to concentrate, how to marshal the energy in your body and focus it for maximum effect.

Proponents of martial arts tend to tout their sport with what can only be called extravagant enthusiasm. "There's no comparison with the American system of sport and exercise, because Oriental arts develop the whole being and psyche," says Steven Schenkman, vice president of the New Center for Wholistic Health Education and Research in Manhasset, New York. When taught and learned properly, martial arts "towers over such things as tennis or weight lifting, which are useful but only deal with a fragment of being."

"Many ardent advocates of martial arts argue that it is all you need to develop the body," Dr. Sherrill says. "Depending on the school, it can be a total fitness program by itself."

The Art of Exercise

In martial arts, Dr. Sherrill says, "you use virtually every muscle in the body. . . . It's a wonderful way to condition the body with practically zero risk of injury." Uh, better make that zero risk of injury if you are taking instruction at a reputable school—we'll get to that shortly.

As an aerobic exercise, a martial arts workout increases heart rate, says Schenkman. Even with a slower, seemingly effortless t'ai chi routine that may take 16 or 17 minutes to complete, "you get an aerobic effect similar to jogging around the block," he says. Martial arts may also help lower high blood pressure, says Dr. Sherrill. He suggests, however, that anyone with high blood pressure talk with a

physician before signing up for martial arts classes.

No matter what the martial arts style, practitioners synchronize their movements with deep, slow abdominal breathing. The respiration is similar to that used in relaxation training, Dr. Sherrill says. Really advanced practitioners can inhale and exhale so slowly and so completely that they may take only two or three breaths a minute, maintains Schenkman.

Dr. Sherrill has found that the deep-breathing techniques he learned are useful in his everyday life. When he notices tension mounting within himself while working in the emergency room, he practices a tae kwon do deep-breathing exercise and wills serenity on his muscles and mind. "It makes me feel better," he says. "It makes an enormous difference. It's a clear health benefit in and of itself."

In addition to promoting healthy respiration, martial arts training "is a very good way of delaying aging," according to Alfredo Pauca, M.D., an associate professor at Bowman Gray Medical School at Wake Forest University and a 61-year-old tae kwon do instructor. The exercises expand and preserve flexibility, "something we lose as we get older," he says.

Poised for a Change

Although the physical benefits of martial arts require a greater amount of training to acquire, self-esteem and psychological outlook are buoyed within 8 to 12 weeks—about as long as it takes to earn the ranking of a novice in the field, Dr. Richman says. The increase in strength, the mastery of the body, the discipline of training, and the postural and emotional poise transform many people socially, academically, and professionally, he maintains.

Dr. Sherrill says that even though he stands 6 feet 2 inches tall and weighs 200 pounds, he always found himself "ill-equipped to deal with physically aggressive people" until he learned tae kwon do.

"But now I can," he adds. The self-control, discipline, and balance apply in nonphysical confrontations as well, he maintains.

"So much of what you learn is very subtle in body language, facial expression, gesture," says Dr. Sherrill. A meek posture, hunched-over shoulders, lack of eye contact, and other clues indicate to others passivity and submission. Once confidence becomes an innate part of your being, in a confrontation or an argument "you tend not to send out anxious messages, and people back off when they see they're not going to dominate you," he says.

Once you determine that you want to experience all these martial arts benefits for yourself, the next step is to select the kind of martial arts you want to study and find a school.

Now you have more than a few choices to make.

Hard Sell

Probably 150 martial arts styles exist. All teach defensive postures and fighting techniques. Differences between the styles often are subtle, having to do with such things as fighting stance and the height of kicks.

Broadly speaking, however, the martial arts can be divided into two categories—hard and soft. The hard styles are faster and more aggressive. The softer styles stress internal vital forces, fluid motions, and often defensive techniques.

Depending very much upon the skill of the instructor, age and health normally present no obstacle to learning martial arts in either style. Dr. Sherrill, who has taught people as young as 6 and as old as 80-plus, says he's sparred "with a number of grandmothers, and they're pretty good. They usually plop a couple of real good kicks on me before a round is over."

Nonetheless, people with heart problems or arthritis probably should avoid the hard styles and opt for a softer style, such as t'ai chi, Dr. Sherrill cautions. So should anyone who has rheumatoid arthritis, because "it will flare up if you work the joints hard," he advises. Those with osteoporosis can learn the fighting routines of hard styles but should not spar. (It goes without saying that they have no business breaking boards, either.)

The most popular hard style, tae kwon do, emphasizes spins, leaps, and kicks, often in dazzling combinations. This ancient Korean martial art has been accepted as a demonstration sport in the Olympics.

Karate, a Japanese form of self-defense, balances use of the upper and lower body in striking opponents. The student learns how to hit with hands and feet and even other parts of the body, such as elbows and knees.

Most hard-style schools avoid actual contact with the opponent, or else they stress the importance of *light* contact—barely touching the opponent. "The injury rate for light contact is about the same as for a softball game," Dr. Sherrill says. Wearing padding and protective gear helps further minimize the risk.

It's probably a good idea to avoid schools that advocate full contact—actual hitting. "All bets are off for the injury rate," says Dr. Sherrill.

Full-contact styles of martial arts, he says, "are for kids with more testosterone than brains. The body gets beat with injuries you'll carry to your grave. So much for the health benefits."

If you do elect to participate in martial arts classes that allow limited contact, make sure the instructor emphasizes safety and control during practice, advises Dr. Richman.

Easier Does It

Softer styles rely more on defensive techniques and use fewer kicks and punches. Some of these styles don't use kicks and punches at all. They're more likely to call for throwing, deflecting attacks, and unbalancing the opponent with leverage and evasion. Judo and jujitsu—the most aggressive nonhitting forms—rely on throws, holds, and nerve pinches to disable adversaries. Judo, the sports and Olympic form of jujitsu, prohibits punching and kicking altogether.

There are virtually hundreds of variants of kung fu—the soft martial arts from China. The one that's most popular and has the greatest claim to physical and emotional fitness is t'ai chi, often called "the grand dance for health."

In style, stance, and movement, t'ai chi "looks like a slow-motion ballet," Schenkman says.

"T'ai chi releases a tremendous amount of energy," he says. "As a result, vitality flows more freely."

And that energy, according to traditional Oriental healers, can be used to fight illness and heal the body. Some Western doctors trained in the martial arts actually agree that this may indeed be the case. And research in China is providing proof that qi gong, the grandfather of t'ai chi, has healing power, says Charles McGee, M.D., a qi gong student and physician in private practice in Coeur d'Alene, Idaho, who says he has seen dramatic proof of the art's curative power.

"Certainly this clashes with my training and background," he says. But he maintains that qi gong can help improve vision, clear the skin, and even slow the aging process. People who practice qi gong require less sleep, yet they have more energy and greater immunity to illness, he says.

Explanations for the reported restorative ability of qi gong and t'ai chi are speculative. Some physicians suspect the benefits may come from invigorated circulation and better oxygenation of the blood.

Class Acts

Learning a martial art thoroughly demands years of instruction and practice, as well as spiritual and financial commitment. Classes usually are held three times a week for about an hour each. Most schools require some practice away from the classroom.

Finding a good school, one that best meets your needs, can be difficult if you don't know what to look for—and look out for. You should visit several schools before you select one, says Dr. Richman. And don't disregard community colleges or the Y: Well-qualified teachers aren't associated solely with commercial operations. No matter what style of martial arts you choose, it is vitally important to study with a knowledgeable instructor who emphasizes safety during practice. Here are a few things to consider in a school.

No secret sessions. Ask to watch a class workout, says Dr. Richman, and don't be lured in or misled by claims of mysterious Asian techniques that cannot be divulged to outsiders. "There are no secret techniques," Dr. Sherrill says. If an instructor is reluctant to permit you to watch a class, "then there's a darn good reason to think he's hiding something."

Student behavior. Notice if class participants seem to enjoy themselves, Dr. Richman suggests. Do they pay attention and have a good rapport with the instructor? And does the instructor take part in the class, spending time with individual students? Do classes include a broad mix of people— young and old, male and female? Talk to them after a session for their views on the particular martial arts style and the school they've chosen.

A sense of order. Classes should be tightly structured, almost militaristic, Dr. Sherrill says, to instill a sense of discipline in students. The workout also should be ordered, starting with easy stretches and breathing exercises before proceeding to learning and practicing fighting techniques.

Established reputation. Select a school that has a track record and has been around for several years. "The failure rate for martial arts schools is high," Dr. Sherrill says. "It's something like 75 to 80 percent. They may not last a year."

Black-belt requirements. Some schools encourage students to sign a long-term contract to acquire a black belt. While it makes good business sense for the instructor, the agreement is not always in the best interest of the student, Dr. Sherrill says. Study the slant on the sales pitch for a black-belt contract. Is it offering you the chance to progress up to black-belt level, or is it guaranteeing you will possess the honor by the end of the contract? Realistically speaking, no one can provide an iron-clad promise of obtaining a black belt; if they do, it's worthless. (Note: Many Chinese styles do not offer black belts at all.)

Safety features. Inspect the school itself, says Dr. Sherrill. Is it clean and well lighted? Does it have dressing rooms and showers? Does it supply protective gear, such as pads for chest, knees, hands, and feet? Is the gear in good shape?

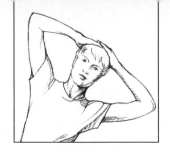

Physiatry

Go to a physiatrist for low back pain, and you'll likely be told to trade in your riding mower for a walking mower. Or you may find yourself with a "prescription" that forbids you to use the car for trips of ½ mile or less.

"That's our antitechnology treatment," says physiatrist Randall L. Braddom, M.D., medical director of Hook Rehabilitation Center in Indianapolis and chairman of the Department of Physical Medicine and Rehabilitation at Indiana University. Mechanization has "taken away all our exercise," he says. "Today we have many blue-collar workers doing only a little more manual work than their sedentary office counterparts." Sometimes all it takes to increase the level of physical activity in a person's life is to prohibit the use of machines, says Dr. Braddom. And sometimes, he adds, that's *all* that's needed to prevent or cure certain medical problems.

"When you're weak, there's more of a tendency to get injured," Dr. Braddom says. "Get a little stronger, and those aches, pains, and injuries all go away."

So what's a physiatrist? Who are these doctors with a propensity to prescribe push-ups instead of pills?

Don't worry about how to pronounce the descriptive word for the doctors who specialize in physical medicine and re-habilitation. Even the practitioners themselves can't agree. Some say "fiz-EYE-uh-trist," and some say "fiz-ee-AT-rist," but all say "exercise" for the prevention, rehabilitation, and cure of disease and disability.

Seeing the Big Picture

As physicians, physiatrists diagnose and treat muscle and skeletal ailments—everything from mild physical symptoms to severe medical problems. Conditions that might send a person to a physiatrist include sprains, tears, ligament and tendon problems, work-related injuries, spinal injuries, stroke, chronic pain, head injuries, even amputations. "We do a lot of what orthopedists do," Dr. Braddom says, "but we don't operate." If surgery is required, a referral will be made. A person with multiple debilitating injuries sustained in an automobile accident might see a physiatrist for long-term rehabilitation once the surgeons have finished their work. Even if a complete cure is not possible—in the case of a severe injury, for example—the physiatrist works to improve as many aspects of an individual's life as possible. After therapy, people "may be impaired, but they're not disabled," explains Dr. Braddom.

In a sense, a physiatrist is like a coach, directing the therapeutic work of a whole team of other medical specialists: social workers and physical, occupational, and speech therapists. "Some problems are too complicated to be solved by one physician," Dr. Braddom says.

Physiatry as a specialty got its start during World War II. The ugly, brutal disabilities and disfigurements inflicted during the war forced more and more physicians to realize they couldn't just fit people for wooden legs and let them hobble away to fend for themselves. Rehabilitation of war wounds also turned into a proving ground for the effectiveness of exercise and conditioning. Today, physiatry still emphasizes pain relief and physical function—whether the problem is as trivial as a sprain or as devastating as paralysis following a stroke.

An Office Visit to a Physiatrist

What do physiatrists actually do? If you strained your back lifting a suitcase, for example, the first thing a physiatrist would do during an office visit is conduct a thorough examination, says Albert O. Esquenazi, M.D., director of the Gait and Motion Analysis Laboratory and Regional Amputee Rehabilitation Center at Moss Rehabilitation Hospital in Philadelphia. He or she might use an electromyography machine—a device that measures how the nerves interact with the muscles. The physiatrist would also ask you about your work, your recreational habits, and your psychological health.

Besides trying to eliminate or ease the pain, the physiatrist would coordinate with physical and occupational therapists to create a treatment program. Your individualized program would probably include exercises for strengthening the back and some instruction in proper lifting techniques to prevent further injury. You might get a list of do's and don'ts to protect your back on the job, or even some back-saving techniques related to your particular profession. Depending on the extent of the pain, the physiatrist might consult with a neurologist, cardiologist, or orthopedic surgeon.

In more traumatic medical situations, such as an amputation, the physiatrist delves even deeper into the patient's life and family, Dr. Esquenazi says. "We assure them there will be life after the operation," he says. The physiatrist can provide detailed, accurate information assuring a person who has undergone an amputation that he or she will be able to make love, hold down a job, drive a car, and go to the bathroom without assistance. Following surgery, rehabilitation includes psychological and family counseling, job restructuring, and maintenance of a regular workout program. Exercise is *always* a part of the physiatrist's prescription, says Dr. Braddom.

Exercise: Empowering People

"For every specific medical condition, there's usually a specific exercise prescription," according to Dr. Braddom. And the more seemingly debilitating and disabling the problem, the greater the need for physical activity, he says.

"We're the champions of promoting early mobility," Dr. Esquenazi says. Without exercise to stimulate the production of

FINDING A PHYSIATRIST

A good physiatrist is hard to find. Actually, *any* physiatrist may be hard to find, because there are only a few thousand practitioners in the country.

Most rehabilitation hospitals and university hospitals with departments of rehabilitation have physiatrists on staff; other physiatrists are in private practice. Look in the Yellow Pages under "Physicians," then check these specialty listings: "Physiatrist," "Physical Medicine," "Rehabilitation." If the Yellow Pages don't provide you with a name or two—and depending on where you live, they may not—try contacting the American Academy of Physical Medicine and Rehabilitation, 122 South Michigan Avenue, Suite 1300, Chicago, IL 60603-6107. The Directory of Medical Specialists, available in many public libraries, also lists physiatrists by state.

While all physiatrists are trained in every aspect of the specialty, not all physiatrists practice in the full spectrum of the field. Some concentrate on the diagnosis and treatment of muscular and skeletal injuries; others focus on rehabilitation. Others specialize in electromyography, the electronic detection of nerve damage.

---

endorphins (the body's naturally occurring painkillers), to improve emotional health, and to take the edge off stress, people fall into a never-ending cycle of fatigue and depression, he says. Someone who has just had a leg amputated or has undergone heart surgery doesn't need to become any *more* tired or despondent, says Dr. Esquenazi.

As recently as 10 to 15 years ago, someone who had a heart attack or who broke a hip usually was kept in bed for weeks. "Now we have them exercising by day three," says Dr. Esquenazi. Heart disease, bone loss, and muscle atrophy all develop in the absence of physical activity. "Muscles need to push on veins to get blood back to the heart," Dr. Braddom says. "If there's no exercise, that muscle pump doesn't work." Blood that doesn't circulate clots and swells limbs. Bone and muscle "turn to Jell-O," he says. "And it happens quickly, even in a short period of time."

For people who are too injured or sick to lift even light weights, the physiatrist may use electrical stimulation to spark muscles to contract involuntarily, Dr. Esquenazi says. Others may be helped into a swimming pool to ease them into movement. People confined to a wheelchair because of hip surgery or amputation might be rigged up to a modified stationary bicycle and taught to pedal as soon as a week after the operation. Even people who are paralyzed can be strapped to a stationary bicycle that is wired to a computer that stimulates their muscles and allows them to pedal.

In less dramatic cases, the exercise prescription could be as simple as permanently parking the riding mower in the garage or walking 2 miles five times a week. Or it may require enrolling in a health club for an aerobics class.

Out of Shape, Out of Health

"Exercise is the single most important thing we can do," Dr. Braddom says. It's vital not only for relatively minor injuries or illnesses "but for people with severe medical problems." From a sore back to a heart attack, physical ailments are "treatable or preventable if you have adequate exercise," Dr. Braddom maintains.

Many problems a physiatrist treats stem from being out of shape, he says. Some people are weaker than they should be, which leaves them susceptible to muscle and skeletal injuries. Others lack endurance and "complain of being tired all the time," he says. Still others have low aerobic capacity because they don't tax their heart and lungs enough.

The potential for serious medical consequences multiplies the longer people remain out of shape and manifests itself in illness as they age. While growing older does have its own effect on the body, Dr. Braddom says, "a lot of what people believe is aging actually is a lack of activity." Whether they're young or not so young, though, many people's ailments ultimately can be traced to an absence of exercise. Strengthen the muscles and bones, become more aerobically fit, and "you'll function better in your life," Dr. Braddom says. A regular exercise program will help reduce aches and pains and help prevent heart problems, osteoporosis, arthritis, and many other health threats. In fact, if you exercise vigorously and regularly, you're far less likely to ever have to see a physiatrist in the first place, Dr. Braddom says.

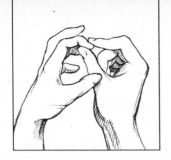

Physical Therapy

So you and your family *all* have your share of health woes. You've about had it with your aching back; your mother's arthritis has been acting up; your son can hardly move his shoulders after that tough weekend tennis match. And your out-of-shape spouse has just declared—for the zillionth time—that it's time to start a fitness program.

You may all end up in the same place for help: a physical therapist's office.

If you're not sure what physical therapy is, you're not alone. "Physical therapy is one of the best-kept secrets in the United States," says physical therapist Robert Burles, owner of Northwest Physical Therapy Clinic in Portland, Oregon.

Physical therapy is about motion—improving it, restoring it, encouraging it. People who can benefit from physical therapy include those with a sports injury or muscle pain, people who have had a stroke or been badly burned, children with birth defects, people who have had a heart attack—or anyone who wants to improve his or her physical conditioning.

How is this accomplished? Through exercises that improve strength, endurance, and coordination and through treatments that help relieve the pain that may be *preventing* movement.

An Evolving Profession

Part of the confusion surrounding physical therapy is because it's a rapidly evolving profession, says Burles.

Physical therapy began to develop around the turn of the century during epidemics of polio, an infectious disease that causes paralysis and muscle atrophy. It was in the 1940s, however, during World War II and yet another polio epidemic, that physical therapy began to boom. Many war victims as well as children stricken with polio needed help to regain mobility and to learn to function with crippled limbs.

Originally assistants to physicians, physical therapists are now licensed health-care professionals who are well trained in understanding the nervous and musculo-skeletal systems. Although they work closely with doctors and other health-care professionals, they function on their own.

"We've gone from being in a very subservient role to physicians to being decision makers," says Burles.

But people still tend to confuse physical therapists with chiropractors or even masseuses. "Some people think all we do is massage," says Dwight Kelsey of Atlantis Physical Therapy Associates in Torrance, California. Physical therapists do use therapeutic massage, as well as some treatment methods that are the same as or similar to those used by chiropractors, but their training is based on a traditional medical background, and their focus is treating the musculoskeletal system.

A physical therapist isn't a doctor and can't prescribe medicine. Physical therapy, according to the American Physical Therapy Association, involves "treating through physical therapeutic measures as opposed to medicines, surgery, or radiation."

What a physical therapist can do, however, is improve movement, relieve pain, and improve physical mobility. You can find physical therapists at work in a variety of places—including schools, nursing homes, hospitals, private practices, industrial rehabilitation centers, and spinal cord injury centers. Some work with outpatients at home, and others visit workplaces to suggest modifications in workers' movements to help reduce the chance of injuries.

Physical therapy can be broken down into three basic types of treatment: prevention, rehabilitation, and long-term care.

Prevention through Exercise

You say you've tried time after time to start a fitness program—but every time you get sore and discouraged and drop out? Physical therapists specialize in developing gradual and varied "preventive" fitness programs aimed at keeping you healthy.

"First we request that a person see a physician, in case there are any medical problems," says Neva Greenwald, chairman of the Department of Physical Therapy at the University of Mississippi in Jackson and president of the geriatric section of the American Physical Therapy Association. The physical therapist then conducts an extensive interview. The ther-

apist will also determine the types of activities you like to do.

Next comes testing to determine your capabilities. This varies but might include a treadmill test, a step test, or muscle testing on exercise equipment. Your balance and coordination may also be checked, as well as postural alignment and joint mobility. "This gives the therapist an overall idea of a person's strength, flexibility, and endurance," Greenwald says.

Next the physical therapist sits down with you and sets up a specific exercise program—which may include a variety of activities and exercises. You'll be taught how to warm up and cool down, and how to check your pulse and breathing rate.

Goals are established, along with a schedule to help meet them. For example, your exercise program might include walking 30 minutes three times a week, and you could progress by adding 5 minutes to each workout every week until a goal of 60 minutes daily is reached.

"We ask that you always keep a log of the kinds of things you're doing and how you're feeling," says Greenwald, "also if you noticed pain or fatigue or excess perspiration." Based on the information in the log and periodic examinations, your physical therapist might decide to modify your program.

Exercise As Treatment

Injuries also can land you in a physical therapist's office, or a doctor might send you there for muscle pain, tendinitis, or postural problems. In these cases, your initial interview will include questions about your injury or problem—how and when it occurred, and how long it's been bothering you.

WHERE TO LOOK

So you think you want to visit a physical therapist, but have no idea where to start? In 26 states, you can proceed directly to a physical therapist. These states are: Alaska, Arizona, California, Colorado, Idaho, Iowa, Illinois, Kentucky, Maine, Maryland, Massachusetts, Minnesota, Montana, Nebraska, Nevada, New Hampshire, New Mexico, North Carolina, North Dakota, South Dakota, Texas, Utah, Vermont, Washington, West Virginia, and Wisconsin.

If your state isn't on this list, you'll need a referral from your doctor or dentist to be treated by a physical therapist.

In most states, however, you can visit a physical therapist for an evaluation without a referral. (Only eight states—Alabama, Arkansas, Delaware, Indiana, Missouri, Ohio, Oregon, and South Carolina—require a referral for an evaluation.) The advantage to this is that the physical therapist can refer you to another health-care professional if physical therapy isn't warranted. But if physical therapy is recommended, you'll still need a physician's referral before treatment can begin if you're not in one of the 26 states listed above.

After evaluation, the physical therapist either will design a treatment program for you or, if your problem requires different treatment than he or she can provide, will refer you to another health-care professional.

Your physical therapy program will include specific exercises for you to do. Some may require exercise equipment or assistance from the physical therapist, while others you can do on your own at home.

The purpose of these exercises is to improve or maintain the range of motion of your joints and to strengthen specific muscles or tendons to avoid further problems. As much as possible, exercises are done on your own and made a part of your lifestyle.

"The aim is to have the patient working independently," says Sandra Curwin, Ph.D., assistant professor in the School of Physiotherapy at Dalhousie University in Nova Scotia. To treat tendinitis, Dr. Curwin creates individual exercise programs designed to strengthen the tendons.

The physical therapist will discuss the treatment program with you and write out the entire program, including diagrams of how to do the home exercises. He or she will discuss how long recovery is expected to take and will set both long- and short-term goals.

How long does physical therapy continue? It depends on the type of injury, the condition of the injured person, and sometimes how motivated the patient is to follow his or her program.

Providing Long-Term Therapy

Finally, physical therapy is used in rehabilitation of people with severe or debilitating problems such as spinal cord injury or severe head injury. People who have progressive diseases such as Alzheimer's and Parkinson's receive long-term physical therapy, as do those recovering from strokes. "Some of these chronic problems are progressive," notes Greenwald.

"You work with the patient, family members, and caregivers to help the patient function at an optimal level for as long as possible."

In some cases, treatment is designed to help people adapt to permanent changes in their physical abilities, such as helping them learn to use artificial limbs. Therapists can also prescribe items such as braces or wheelchairs and help families make the home better suited for the patient. The therapist may suggest grab bars in the bathroom, an elevated toilet seat that is easier to reach, and rearranged furniture that will make using devices such as a walker or wheelchair easier.

So What Exactly Do They Do?

Okay, down to the nitty-gritty of treatment. When you walk into a physical therapy facility, you'll likely find three major treatment areas: a therapeutic gym, an electrotherapy area, and a hydrotherapy area. Electrotherapy areas have treatment cubicles or room for treatment tables and various machines or equipment: ultrasound, traction, hot pack, or cold pack. Hydrotherapy areas may include whirlpools or swimming pools.

All rehabilitation programs emphasize exercise. Some exercises are passive—the therapist moves your limb for you—and in others, you provide some of the motion, and the therapist provides the rest. There are also exercises you do entirely on your own and others that are performed against a weight.

Massage and mobilization are common physical therapy techniques. In mobilization the therapist gently stretches and manipulates stiff or immobile joints to increase the range of motion. Massage is particularly helpful with muscle strains or tendinitis.

Physical therapists also use many other treatment methods to help decrease pain and increase mobility. These include applications of heat and cold, such as hot packs, ice packs to reduce swelling, or vapocoolant sprays that cool the skin. Vapocoolant is used in the "spray and stretch" procedure: The muscle is sprayed to decrease pain, then gently stretched.

Soothing Water, Soothing Sound

Hydrotherapy—treatment in water—is usually in a heated pool or whirlpool. Because water helps support your weight, movements are easier in water than on land. Gentle exercises in warm water can increase your range of motion and improve your circulation and coordination. Or your physical therapist may use contrast baths—alternating immersion in cold and hot water—to decrease swelling of painful hands or feet.

Other treatment methods you may encounter include ultrasound, traction, biofeedback, electrical stimulation, and TENS (transcutaneous electrical nerve stimulation). Confused? Don't worry—your physical therapist will explain everything.

In brief, ultrasound—high-frequency sound waves that penetrate tissue and raise temperature—can relieve pain and soften scar tissue and is used primarily for tight muscles and tendons. Biofeedback involves electrodes that are attached to your skin and a device that records electri-

CHOOSING YOUR THERAPIST

As you stare at the bewildering and lengthy display under the "Physical Therapists" listing in the Yellow Pages, you realize you have no idea how to pick a therapist.

The phone book is a fine place to start, says the American Physical Therapy Association, but don't just make an appointment with the first therapist listed. Instead, pick up the phone, call a few, and ask some pointed questions.

Is the therapist licensed? Your initial evaluation and treatment should be done by a licensed physical therapist.

What are their credentials, and have they treated this type of problem before? Physical therapists have different areas of specialty.

Is the facility owned by the physical therapist or by an outside company or provider such as medical doctors or a hospital? You want independent, unbiased treatment; you should ask if the referring physician gains financially by referring you.

What are their financial policies? You need to know what your insurance company pays and what it doesn't, and if payment is required to the physical therapist up front.

What's the facility like? Ask about office hours, parking facilities, whether there are individual treatment rooms, and so forth.

What type of equipment is used? This can be important if your injury or problem requires a specific piece of equipment.

Will your progress and evaluation be communicated to your other health-care providers? Your progress should be reported to other doctors or professionals involved in your health care.

Can you meet with the therapist or the staff regarding the facility? Your physical therapist should be willing to meet with you and answer any questions.

Will you get an evaluation and the opportunity to discuss treatment goals with a therapist, and will that same person be responsible for your treatment? Your evaluation should include a personal history, a list of findings, a list of problems to be treated, a plan of treatment, and a timetable.

cal signals as your muscle fibers contract. You can use these signals to learn to relax or contract the muscle. And if you have jaw or dental problems, your physical therapist may use TENS, which uses electrical stimulation to decrease pain.

Meet Your Physical Therapist

Wondering what type of training that white-coated person leading you through your physical therapy program has had?

Aspiring physical therapists study psychology, anatomy, physiology, chemistry, and medical sciences and acquire clinical experience. To qualify as physical therapists they must receive a baccalaureate or post-baccalaureate degree and pass a state licensing exam. (Physical therapist assistants, however, have associate degrees and are not always required to be licensed.)

A physical therapist can choose to specialize in a specific area such as pediatrics, sports physical therapy, orthopedics, neurology, cardiopulmonary, geriatrics, obstetrics and gynecology, hand rehabilitation, or oncology (working with cancer patients). Specialization generally requires further study, more clinical experience, and possibly passing a board exam.

Practicing physical therapists regularly participate in educational courses and programs. "They know the knowledge in the field is changing rapidly and wish to offer their patients the most effective treatment programs," says Greenwald.

But a physical therapist's job involves more than understanding your musculoskeletal system and being able to prescribe exercises. Sometimes the therapist may serve as coach or cheerleader as well. Restoring motion to painful limbs or sticking to an exercise program can be tough, and the physical therapist has to help the patient through.

"You need to know how to motivate people," says Greenwald. "You may have to help the patient work through pain or emotional crisis as a part of the rehabilitation process."

A good physical therapist, she says, is a good listener and a good communicator. And in many cases, a good therapist becomes a good friend.

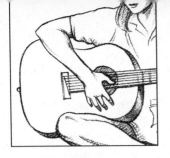

Playing a Musical Instrument

When Ken Finch practices his "sport," his heart rate goes up, adrenaline flows, and beads of sweat form on his brow. And by the time he makes the final sweeping movement of the bow on his cello, he knows he's had a terrific workout.

Ken, a 32-year-old cellist with the Oregon Symphony Orchestra in Portland, practices twice a day. It's a routine that not only keeps his musical talents in tune but also, he says, contributes to his mental and physical well-being.

"It seems that musicians tend to live longer. I don't know why that is, but if you talk to any of my colleagues in the orchestra, they'd tell you that their job is beneficial to their health," he says.

Doctors agree. In fact, some doctors say musical performance may contribute to mental health and, in some cases, actually help relieve a few chronic illnesses.

"I think there are many positive aspects of playing a musical instrument," says Alice G. Brandfonbrener, M.D., director of the Medical Program for Performing Artists at the Rehabilitation Institute of Chicago.

"If you have something like asthma, blowing on a wind instrument that doesn't require tremendously high air pressure or high air volume (such as a clarinet) may be helpful for your pulmonary function," Dr. Brandfonbrener says.

Playing music also may improve finger dexterity, says Robert Markison, M.D., an associate clinical professor of surgery at the University of California, San Francisco, School of Medicine.

"I find that my surgery goes much better and more efficiently because I've practiced my music early in the morning," says Dr. Markison, a professional clarinet and saxophone player. "My hands are toned, limber, and ready to work."

The act of playing a musical instrument also may decrease the disability of arthritis, Dr. Brandfonbrener says. "I have quite a few patients who have moderately severe degenerative arthritis. I think if they keep playing their instruments and keep their soft tissue moving, they'll be more comfortable."

"The stresses involved in playing a musical instrument aren't tremendous," she says, "and doing it promotes blood flow, muscle tone, and movement."

Singing in the Brain

There's more. Playing a musical instrument may help boost your brainpower and even improve your mood, says John Kella, Ph.D., coordinator of the Music Rehabilitation program at Miller Health Care Institute for Performing Artists in New York City, a center that has treated more than 6,000 musicians, dancers, and other performing artists.

"Practicing an instrument makes problem solving a natural part of who you are," Dr. Kella says. "If you're confronted with a demanding artistic problem and are able to work through it, that may help you in everyday life."

"The opportunity to play, to make music, offers a tremendous emotional lift that I think is important," says Ephraim Engleman, M.D., director of the Rosalind Russell Arthritis Center at the University of California, San Francisco, School of Medicine.

That type of emotional boost can influence your physical health, Dr. Brandfonbrener says.

When selecting an instrument, you should keep in mind that some put more strain on the hands than others, says Dr. Markison, who specializes in hand surgery.

For example, instruments that have keys positioned vertically, such as a clarinet, saxophone, accordion, or French horn, are less stressful on the hands than horizontal instruments such as the piano, Dr. Markison says. That's because when you're playing a vertical instrument, you're holding your hands in the same natural position that you do when your hands are at your sides. When you play a horizontal instrument such as a violin, you move your hands into more stressful positions, he says.

"The ideal instrument to take up is the recorder," Dr. Markison says. That's because this lightweight wind instrument, which has been popular for centuries, requires little finger pressure over the holes and can be purchased for less than $100.

And unless you have a chronic ailment,

getting started is less difficult than you may think, says Dr. Kella, a violist with the Metropolitan Opera in New York City.

"Don't be afraid of doing it. It's never too late to start," he says. "The rewards are more than being able to sit down at a party and play the piano. Playing music is a wonderful way to relieve stress after a long day of work. It's liberating for the soul."

A Few Precautions

If you do have a chronic ailment such as arthritis, however, doctors urge you to see your physician before you take up playing an instrument that may stress the joints. The instrument you play, even the music that you choose to perform, may have an impact on your condition.

"In selected instances, playing a musical instrument can be good physical therapy," says Dr. Engleman.

"If your arthritis is in your legs, then playing the piano not only offers an emotional lift, it can provide a certain type of exercise for your hands and upper extremities that you might not otherwise get.

"But if you have arthritis in your fingers, playing a piano may be helpful, or it may be harmful, depending on how much time you spend doing it."

In some cases, you may need to make a few changes in your repertoire, says Richard Hoppmann, M.D., a rheumatologist at the University of South Carolina School of Medicine in Columbia.

"The repertoire is very important because there are some pieces that are more technically difficult than others. You don't want to push yourself too hard because it may just aggravate your condition."

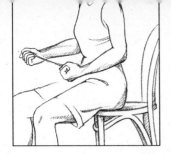

Posture Training

J ane Meryll clearly remembers her first lesson in posture training: "I went to that session in pain and walked out 45 minutes later feeling like I was floating," she says. "I knew there was a possibility that my back pain could be controlled."

She was in her early thirties then, a professional pianist diagnosed with two degenerated disks in her lower back. "I couldn't work. I was flat on my back, in the hospital, on painkillers," she says. Her doctor recommended surgery. But she was looking for anything else that might help her.

What she found was a posture training program. Using its concepts, Jane learned a better way to breathe, stand, walk, sit at a piano, sing, and do everything else she needs to do. The training taught her a way of thinking about her body during daily activities that helps keep her back correctly aligned, with muscles working efficiently to create less tension.

Poor posture is the source of many aches and pains, says physical therapist Deborah Caplan, author of *Back Trouble: A New Approach to Prevention and Recovery* and a teacher of the Alexander Technique, the posture training program that Jane Meryll used to alleviate her back pain. And for many people, getting rid of chronic pain is simply a matter of learning how to breathe, sit, stand, and walk correctly.

Learn from the Leaning Tower of Pisa

Think poor posture doesn't have anything to do with your aches, pain, or fatigue? Try this easy, at-home experiment.

Take a mop or broom. Hold it upright by the end of the handle, with the business end up in the air. Notice how little effort this takes, as long as it remains perfectly upright.

Now allow the mop or broom to lean slightly to one side and try to hold it in that position. Feel how much tighter your grip becomes? Feel how your arm muscles tense up? Feel how your whole arm starts trembling? That's how much harder your back muscles must work when you slouch or overarch your back, says physical therapist Tom Lorren, director of rehabilitation services at the Texas Back Institute in Plano, a suburb of Dallas. "Your body really wants to be efficient. Poor posture makes the muscles work *so* much harder." No wonder they get tired; no wonder they rebel or just plain quit.

Unlike an injury, back damage from poor posture can take years to develop, Caplan says. Over time, ligaments supporting the back stretch like an old girdle; muscle tone fades. "The whole support system of the back is undermined," she says. Then one day, when you lift something heavy, turn over in bed, sneeze, or get up after a long train or plane ride, you suddenly have severe pain in your back muscles.

Poor posture contributes to backaches two other ways, says Charles Steiner, D.O., chairman of the Department of Osteopathic Sciences at the University of Medicine and Dentistry of New Jersey in Stratford. It reduces the space between the vertebrae, the bones of the spine, putting the squeeze on the cushioning disks between them. As anyone who has had a herniated disk—literally, one that has been partly squeezed out of place—can tell you, it hurts.

And poor posture can lead to the painful compression of spine-stabilizing bony projections called facets. Good posture, on the other hand, helps maintain adequate space between facets.

The facets help to keep the spine stacked in place by resting one on top of another, but they also need to glide across each other when you twist and turn, Dr. Steiner explains. Facets are covered with cartilage, just like other joints, and they are lubricated with your spine's specially produced lubricant—the synovial fluid. When facets get jammed together because of poor posture, your vertebrae lock, which can throw back muscles into painful spasms.

Not Just Backaches

Many doctors think poor posture can also contribute to certain kinds of headaches. Muscle tension headaches, which can creep up the base of your head, can start from overwrought neck muscles. Disk

problems in the neck can also cause nerve pain that radiates into the head, says Dr. Steiner. Learning to maintain your head upright without taxing your neck muscles is a major part of posture training, Caplan says. Balancing your head properly while consciously letting go of the tension in your neck muscles can do wonders for this kind of headache, she says.

Jaw joint pain—temporomandibular disorder (TMD)—sometimes finds its source in poor posture, Dr. Steiner says. "The position of your head on your spine affects how your jaw hangs," he explains. If you drop your head forward from your shoulders, the slight change in the position of your jaw can be enough to cause muscle tension and jaw and neck pain.

"Improved head/neck/spine alignment is beneficial to TMD whether the cause is structural or related mainly to muscle tension," Caplan contends.

And some doctors believe fatigue is related to posture. Poor posture directly interferes with our ability to breathe efficiently, which means it inhibits our ability to provide oxygen to all parts of our body, including our oxygen-demanding brain.

"Efficient breathing is not characterized by being able to blow the chest up and take in a lot of air," Caplan explains. "It's characterized by the degree of difference between breathing in and breathing out—by lung expansion and contraction, just like a bellows. The more the bellows move to open and close, the more movement of air occurs."

If you are sitting or standing slumped over, your rib cage cannot move as freely on the sides and the front, your diaphragm

Standing

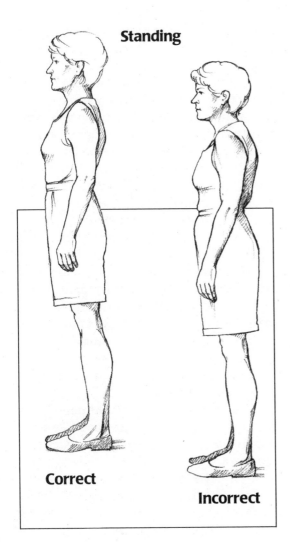

Correct

Incorrect

Sitting

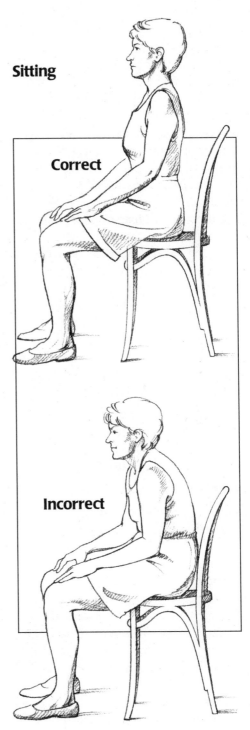

Correct

Incorrect

The elements of good posture are the same whether you're standing or sitting. Imagine your head is suspended from the ceiling by a thread. Picture a plumb line that runs down your spine from that point. By using it as a guide to align yourself, your head will be erect, your shoulders will be back and relaxed, and your buttocks will be tucked in to flatten your lower spine.

cannot freely move up and down, and thus your lungs cannot fully expand and contract. "And if you're sitting up too straight, with your back overarched, your rib cage in back cannot move as freely, either, so that stance also interferes with breathing," Caplan says. Correct posture allows maximum lung movement, at rest or when you're walking, biking, or running. And deep, slow, effortless breaths lead to instant relaxation.

Muscle tension can lead to poor posture, and when muscles go into spasm they consume energy and take away vitality, maintains Dr. Steiner. The vicious cycle of muscle spasm, pain, and loss of motion is reflected in the slumped look of a person in pain, he says.

No wonder the simple act of straightening up like the graceful dancer whose head and body seem to be held by an unseen force makes us feel so much better, says Dr. Steiner.

The Perfect Complement to Sit-Ups

Exercises that stretch or strengthen your back-supporting muscles may help relieve your back pain. But don't think doing these exercises automatically leads to better posture, Caplan says. You can have the shoulder muscles of Johnny Weismuller or an abdomen like Bo Derek's and still look like Quasimodo if you haven't straightened up your act. "If you want better posture, you have to learn and practice better posture. You don't get it doing sit-ups," Caplan insists.

In fact, posture training can be the perfect complement to an exercise program, because it helps you learn to move in a way that doesn't injure, or reinjure, your back. (Once injured, a back is much more prone to reinjury, experts say.)

Posture training can help you walk in a way that eases back and neck pain and tension, for instance. And good posture is imperative for people who lift weights. Overarching during a heavy lift can lead to painful injuries. "Too often, people begin an exercise program with little instruction and end up getting hurt," Caplan says.

Good posture minimizes strain on back ligaments and muscles and enhances an exercise program. Poor posture, on the other hand, can undo even the most ambitious back-building program, tiring out some muscles while allowing others to weaken, says Caplan. If you do stretches to relieve tense neck and shoulder muscles but then spend many hours hunched over reading a book or with the phone squeezed between your head and shoulder, your tension will be right back.

Strong, flexible muscles can help you maintain good posture. Most people have weaker front muscles than back muscles, so strengthening abdominal muscles becomes a major component of most back exercise programs. (See also "Resistance Training" on page 404, "Stretching" on page 440, and "Yoga" on page 480.)

Basic Training

If all of this sounds like a lot to tackle on your own, take heart. There are a number of health-care professionals who can give you special training and coaching in the basics of good posture.

Jane Meryll improved her posture and achieved pain relief with a program that has been popular for a number of years with singers, actors, and other stage performers.

Jane's "good posture" resembles more the stance of a dancer than that of a soldier. With the Alexander Technique, a popular form of posture training, you learn how to "release" your head upward and hold it as though it's floating or being drawn upward by a string, Caplan explains. You learn to allow your torso to elongate and to let your shoulders "widen" outward in a way that allows the whole body to be comfortably erect without excess muscle tension. The result, says Caplan, is a graceful, fluid way of moving, perhaps even a slimmer, taller, more composed look.

Now in her mid-forties and a composer and music teacher, Jane still practices daily what she learned. Whenever her back pain returns, she does her prescribed posture exercises and finds quick relief, she says.

For a referral to a certified teacher of the Alexander Technique, contact The North American Society of Teachers of the Alexander Technique (NASTAT), P.O. Box 3992, Champaign, IL 61826-3992.

Posture training is also taught by osteopaths, chiropractors, physical therapists, and physiatrists. Back schools—intensive back rehabilitation programs, for instance—usually include training in posture, movement, and correct ways to lift and bend.

Posture Perfect

Poor posture does more than just make you look sluggish—it makes you feel sluggish, too. When your posture isn't up to par, it can contribute to backache, headache, and jaw pain.

To start you on the road to better posture, practice balancing a folded towel on the top of your head.

This balancing act will teach you the basics of good posture. You will be forced to relax your shoulders, hold your head high, and bend without straining. Try the towel trick for a few minutes each day as you go about your normal routine.

The following set of exercises is designed to help improve your posture by strengthening your upper back and shoulders. Each exercise should be done using the "6 by 6" rule: Hold each for 6 seconds at a time and do them six times a day. You will need an elastic exercise band or bicycle inner tube to perform these exercises.

To help bring your lower back into proper alignment, you should practice the pelvic tilt and abdominal exercises described on page 79.

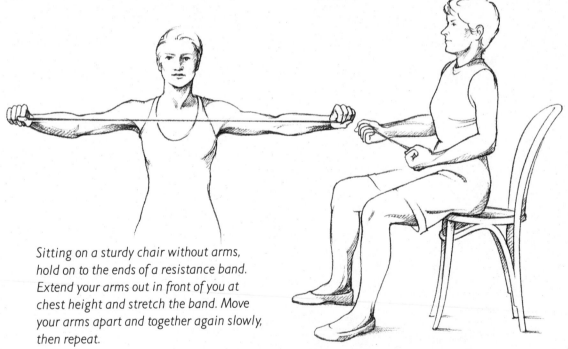

Sitting on a sturdy chair without arms, hold on to the ends of a resistance band. Extend your arms out in front of you at chest height and stretch the band. Move your arms apart and together again slowly, then repeat.

Bend your elbows 90 degrees and hold them in to your sides. Hold the ends of the elastic band with palms up and stretch the band, then return to the starting position and repeat.

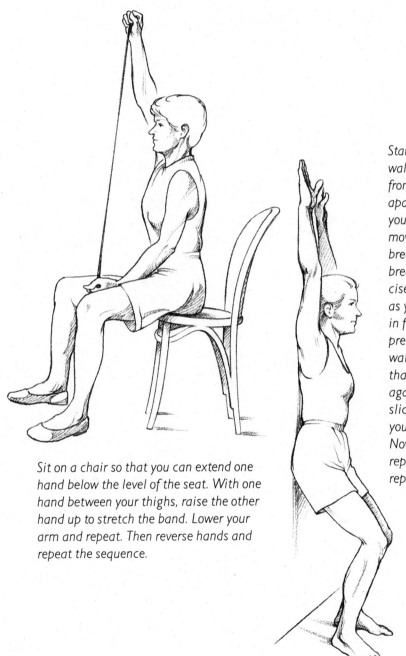

Sit on a chair so that you can extend one hand below the level of the seat. With one hand between your thighs, raise the other hand up to stretch the band. Lower your arm and repeat. Then reverse hands and repeat the sequence.

Stand with your back against a wall. Move your feet 12 inches from the wall and 12 inches apart. Breathe deeply through your nose so that your stomach moves in and out with each breath. Maintain this deep breathing throughout the exercise. Keep your arms straight as you gradually lift them out in front, then overhead, finally pressing your arms into the wall. Tilt your pelvis forward so that your lower back is flat against the wall, then slowly slide down the wall as you bend your knees. Hold for 6 seconds. Now straighten your knees and repeat. Do three sets of six repetitions.

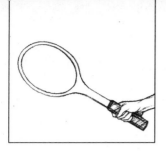

Racquet Sports

Jogging bores you, the chlorine in the pool annoys you, and working out on exercise machines makes you feel you're trapped on a medieval torture apparatus.

Fortunately, these are not your only options. A racquet sport may be the answer to your exercise woes.

Racquet sports can not only supply a great workout but also allow you to enjoy some friendly competition—and maybe unleash some pent-up frustration as well.

Hammering at a ball or shuttlecock can be a great anxiety reducer, says Jim Hiser, Ph.D., assistant director of the American Amateur Racquetball Association. "A lot of people come in and play on their lunch hour—then they go back to work in the afternoon with their problem solved," he says.

But not all racquet sports are created equal: There are significant differences among racquetball, badminton, squash, and tennis. For instance, racquetball and badminton are easier to learn, but squash or tennis may be more challenging. Squash gives the most demanding workout, while tennis, particularly doubles, can be downright lackadaisical.

Let's take a closer look at these sports.

The wonderful appeal of racquetball is that you can pick up a racquet and a ball,
step onto a court, and boom, you're playing the game. No lessons required. "You can get in there and do it right off the bat and have a good time," says Linda Mojer, spokeswoman for the American Amateur Racquetball Association, in Colorado Springs.

Ripping into Racquetball

But because it's so easy, you may be tempted to overexert yourself—particularly if you have a competitive personality or a sports background. "We get some ex-jocks who come in and try to run hard and hit every shot," says Dr. Hiser. "This is a very strenuous sport if you go in and try to go all out at it." The result? Pulled muscles, or worse.

He recommends that beginners work with a club pro, who can help them get started slowly.

The workout potential of racquetball is enormous. While racquetball does require frequent short bursts of energy, you're moving constantly enough to keep your heart rate high. "If you play for 40 minutes, you're playing 40 minutes with your heart rate at 70 percent of its maximum," says Dr. Hiser.

If you're playing intensively, you're burning lots of calories: from 600 to 850 per hour.

If you have ready access to a court, start-up costs can be relatively low: A

ARE YOU UP TO IT?

Racquet sports, as delightful as they are, may not be the best possible tonic for the individual who's main form of recreation tends to be late-night TV. Although these sports vary in intensity—according to which game you're playing as well as how you're playing it—none provides a gentle workout.

You may need to get in shape in order to be able to play a racquet sport—or at the very least get an okay from your physician or physical therapist, particularly if you are over 50.

"Older persons usually have medical and musculoskeletal deficiencies they bring to the sport," points out Robert P. Nirschl, M.D., medical director of Virginia Sports-medicine and Rehabilitation Institute in Arlington. The demands of a racquet sport can cause injury to tissues that may already be vulnerable from prior injury or stress or simple aging, he says.

Squash in particular is an intensive game. It developed a grim reputation after reports were released detailing fatal on-court cardiac arrests. Most players who had heart attacks during squash, however, had had previous coronary problems and prior cardiac symptoms. This makes a fine case for having a physical before taking up squash—or any vigorous activity, for that matter.

In some cases, a physical may not be enough. The American College of Sports Medicine recommends that adults over 44 have an exercise tolerance test before starting a vigorous exercise program. This may alert you to symptom-free coronary disease you aren't aware of. It will also assess your fitness level and tell you how much exercise will be safe.

But if you're healthy and sensible enough to ease into a program slowly—and with proper instruction—you may be able to forgo a tolerance test, according to E. Randy Eichner, M.D., professor of medicine in the Hematology-Oncology Section at the University of Oklahoma Health Sciences Center in Oklahoma City. He suggests that a healthy person can begin a gradual racquet sport program without testing, *provided* he or she has none of the following: history of heart trouble, hypertension, arthritis, or diabetes; any family history of premature coronary artery disease; or breathlessness, dizziness, or exercise-related pain or pressure in the chest, neck, shoulder, or arm.

But when in doubt, consult your doctor.

---

racquet will run $25 to $250, and balls $3 a can. Protective eyewear is essential. (See "The Eyes Have It" on page 396.)

Swinging at Squash

Squash, an older, elitist cousin of racquetball, is played with a smaller, less bouncy ball and a longer-necked racquet with a smaller head. So—no surprise—it's more difficult to learn.

But squash offers a particular mental challenge, says Douglas Smyth, technical director of Squash Canada in Toronto. "It's like chess on a physical level," he says.

You can't just whale away at the ball, explains Darwin Kingsley III, managing director of the U.S. Squash Racquets Association. "You plan your shots two or three ahead; you plan a series of shots so you can get a winner," he says.

You also don't want to walk onto a squash court in poor shape. "To play

THE EYES HAVE IT

You've got your shiny new racquet, spiffy sport togs, and deluxe cushioned shoes, and you're ready to step onto the court. Hold on! You've forgotten the most important piece of gear—goggles.

A racquetball or tennis ball can zoom through the air at 110 miles per hour, and a squash ball can accelerate to 140 mph. And our innocent-looking feathered friend, the badminton shuttlecock, can hit speeds of *200 mph.*

Don't assume that recreational or beginning players aren't at risk. "Someone who has never hit a squash ball before can still hit at 80 mph," says Michael Easterbrook, M.D., associate professor of ophthalmology at the University of Toronto and consultant to Canadian and American squash, badminton, and racquetball clubs and associations.

Likewise, don't assume that your normal eyeglasses will protect you—that's a common misconception, says Dr. Easterbrook. "People wearing safety glass or plastic lenses think they're impact-resistant," he says. Such lenses may not break in a simple fall, but they *won't* stand up to the force of a speeding ball. Such an impact can result in serious injury: Of 685 eye injuries at Canadian squash and racquetball clubs in eight years, 31 resulted in blinded eyes.

What you need is polycarbonate plastic—which will stop a .22-caliber bullet, not to mention a speeding ball, says Dr. Easterbrook. You can choose standard goggles, goggles that fit over your eyeglasses, or prescription protective eyewear. Open eyeguards, which do not have lenses, may help protect you from racquet injury but not from speeding balls: A racquetball or squash ball can squeeze through the opening.

Who needs protective eyewear? Anyone who plays squash or racquetball, and in some cases, badminton and tennis players.

"We're recommending that people who play a high level of competitive badminton, particularly doubles, wear eye protection," says Dr. Easterbrook. Protective eyewear for tennis players who play aggressive competitive doubles at the net may also be a good idea.

Protective eyewear may not be particularly glamorous, but it's effective. If you're hesitant to don yours, consider that no player in North America wearing a polycarbonate eye protector has ever lost an eye or had any serious loss of vision, says Dr. Easterbrook.

squash, you should be fit," cautions Smyth. Studies have shown that no matter what your fitness level, during a game your heart rate will reach at least 150 beats per minute—a workout comparable to moderate or intense running. It burns slightly more calories than competitive racquetball.

Smyth recommends aerobic training such as walking, running, or cycling before stepping onto the court. "If you can maintain an aerobic activity for 20 minutes," he says, "then you're probably fit enough to play." (See "Are You Up to It?" on page 395.)

You should realize that there are two versions of squash, with slightly different methods of scoring. Canada and the rest of the world use a soft ball and a 21-foot-wide court; the United States uses a hard ball and an 18½-foot-wide court. Hard ball, because the ball doesn't bounce as much, is a tougher game. "It's very difficult to pick up hard ball without help," admits Kingsley. "Soft ball is more player-friendly."

But don't despair. If you're not up to hard ball, you can play the soft ball version on a standard U.S. court. The narrower court won't matter greatly to a recreational player.

To start, sign up for lessons: Five or six will give you a solid grounding. A racquet will run $60 to $150, and goggles are a must.

Afraid you're too old? Kingsley, who is 64, points out that there's an 80-and-over division in the U.S. Nationals.

Tussling with Tennis

Tennis has taken a bum rap in terms of its exercise potential. Granted, if it's a lazy summer day, and you're playing doubles with hubby and the Joneses from next door and hitting long, lovely lobs that your opponents lazily lob back again . . . well, it may be fun, but there's not much *exercising* going on here.

But if you play singles, or doubles of a more sprightly variety, you can get a fine workout. To maximize your workout, run hard, stretch, and lunge to reach, suggests Bill Wright, author of *Aerobic Tennis.*

How you play makes a difference not only in aerobic conditioning but also in how many calories you burn. In recreational doubles you may burn 300 calories an hour, and in recreational singles 450 an hour, but the tally rises to 600 per hour in competition.

If you've never played tennis, you'll want to take a minimum of three lessons, says Brad Patterson, executive director of the American Tennis Industry Federation. Six hours of lessons, he says, will turn you into a tennis player.

New oversized racquets make the game easier than in the past, says Patterson, and you should spend a minimum of $50. But if the bucks are burning a hole in your pocket and that $300 racquet is beckoning, go ahead—you'll end up with a racquet that's lighter, stiffer, and just that much easier to smash returns with.

Other tips: Using new balls rather than old decreases the amount of force required in each stroke, and playing on a clay court is easier on your feet and knees than playing on asphalt.

Battling at Badminton

Badminton—the word brings back fond memories of childhood summertime games on the front lawn. Remember how much *fun* it was? The indoor version is just as much fun, says Mark Hodges, executive director of the U.S. Badminton Association—and just as easy to learn.

"Within 10 minutes you can be hitting back and forth as long as you want to," says Hodges. The difference is that you're indoors, with no interference from wind or sun, and you're using a genuine feathered shuttlecock, not a plastic "birdie."

Racquets are light—modern competitive racquets run about 3 ounces—and easy to use. "Anybody who can cut bread with a knife can pick up a racquet and play," says Hodges. Because the racquet is so light, you're less prone to injuries such as tennis elbow.

Racquets average $40, while shuttlecocks run $1.25 each. Where do you play? Gyms, racquetball courts, churches, recreation halls, you name it, says Hodges.

Conditioning? Studies have found that badminton burns over 350 calories per hour.

"It's continuous," points out Hodges. "At a minimum level, playing two competition games is 20 minutes of concentrated running, jumping, and stretching." In a normal singles game, he says, a player will make 350 changes of direction.

Playing It Safe

Whatever your racquet sport, you can help lessen the chance of injury by choosing good equipment and shoes, learning proper technique, and paying careful attention to warming up and conditioning.

"Don't scrimp on shoes," advises Patterson. "If you have to save, scrimp on the racquet." Go for tennis or other court shoes or cross-trainers, all of which are designed for the stop-and-go, twist-and-turn motions of racquet sports. Cushioning is important, as is firm heel support.

And whatever your sport, warm up before you plunge into a game. Many injuries occur in those first few minutes of play while your muscles are cold. Experts advocate 5 minutes of an easy aerobic activity such as walking or slow jogging, followed by 10 minutes of stretching.

"Definitely make sure you're warmed up completely," says Dr. Hiser. "Be sure you have broken a sweat." You can also warm up by gently hitting the ball or shuttlecock.

Improving your flexibility can also help prevent injury. You should pay particular attention to stretching your Achilles tendon and posterior calf muscles, hamstrings, the muscles of the lower back and shoulders, and your adductor muscles—the ones that pull your arms and legs in toward your body. (See "Stretching" on page 440.)

That most infamous of racquet sport injuries, tennis elbow, can result from using an improper technique for the backhand or serve. Check with a club pro or instructor for techniques to keep this painful condition at bay. (And if you are contending with tennis elbow, see "Bursitis and Tendinitis" on page 92.)

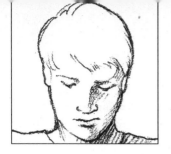

Relaxation Training

You're stretched out lazily on a blanket of soft, white Caribbean sand. The afternoon sun bathes you in a shower of golden warmth. You close your eyes and inhale deeply, relishing the feel of fresh ocean air in your lungs.

You listen to the wind whisper through a cluster of palm trees. The surf trickles its way to your feet—warm, friendly, inviting. It tickles your toes, caresses your calves. And just as gently, the sun begins massaging your body, its warmth reaching deeper and deeper inside you, rubbing out all tension, all pain, all worry.

Ten minutes later, you're back in the office eagerly poring over papers for the annual budget review.

Time to De-stress

Wait a minute! What happened to the ocean mist and swaying palms? They were a *mental* vacation, a "visualization" to accompany the practice of progressive muscle relaxation, which is one of many relaxation techniques you can use—plunk in the middle of pandemonium—to help you unload your stress. What are these techniques doing in a book on exercise? Well, learning to unwind all that tension and unclench those muscles can involve some pretty serious—although pleasurable—physical training.

If you're like most people, you think stress is inevitable. And unconquerable. You must deal with the boss, the bills, the bozo who pushes in front of you at the checkout line. So you pound your fist on the dashboard during a traffic jam. And you bellow bloody murder when the toilet overflows. Nothing else you can do, right?

Wrong. You can *learn* to relax. There's solid scientific evidence that relaxation techniques actually create physical changes that help you avoid the health fallout from stress down the road—even if that road is a bumper-to-bumper rat race.

Studies have shown that relaxation training can lower blood pressure and cholesterol levels; reduce the risk of heart attack and possibly asthma; help eliminate mouth ulcers, vertigo (dizziness), headaches, and insomnia; and alleviate symptoms related to premenstrual syndrome. It can even enhance the chances of pregnancy for previously infertile couples and reduce the pain associated with ulcerative colitis and chemotherapy. And that's just a partial list.

Untying Those Tension Knots

How do you go about relaxing your body enough to reap all those wonderful benefits? It's simple. Says stress-management expert Emmett E. Miller, M.D., "Relaxation training is a process that involves learning to operate a very sensitive, elegant instrument: the human brain."

Scientists know that we're creatures of perception. If we can vividly *imagine* we're relaxing, we guide our brain into doing it, thus creating the physiological opposite of the stress response: the relaxation response.

"Through relaxation response techniques, we can teach people to reduce the symptoms of stress by quieting the mind and increasing their awareness of the interaction between mind and body," says Eileen Stuart, R.N., director of cardiovascular programs at Harvard's New England Deaconess Hospital in Boston.

The response that relaxation therapy triggers is not unlike the actions of the body when we're sleeping, says psychologist and relaxation expert Mohammad R. Sadigh, Ph.D., director of psychology at Gateway Institute in Bethlehem, Pennsylvania.

"The body has a marvelous self-repairing mechanism, which is particularly effective at repair work during deep sleep," says Dr. Sadigh. "We can teach the body to switch from stress mode to a sleeplike repair mode, even though we're fully awake."

Getting Ready

There are many relaxation techniques—yoga, visualization, progressive muscle relaxation, meditation, self-hypnosis, focusing—but a few of the most popular are described here. Choose one that you're comfortable with. Whichever one you choose for your "exercise" regimen, there are some basic things you must do for the training to be most beneficial.

Practice the exercises at least once or twice daily for 10 to 20 minutes. "You hold the key to unlocking your brain's ability to heal pain and symptoms," says Dr. Sadigh. "Daily and consistent practice is that key."

The big bonus of regular practice is that long-term effects are cumulative, according to Herbert Benson, M.D., author of *The Relaxation Response* and one of the pioneers of relaxation training. Researchers suspect that with proper training the body becomes less reactive to noradrenalin (one of the stress hormones) over time, he says.

Make sure you're comfortable. Dress in loose-fitting clothing. Find a comfortable chair with a back and armrests, or recline in a comfortable position with a pillow under your head.

Practice in a quiet place. Pick a spot where you won't be interrupted or distracted.

Adopt an attitude of "passive concentration." If your mind wanders, don't worry about it. Just try to get back on track.

And by all means, breathe deeply. Allow your abdomen to relax outward as you inhale through your nose. Exhale slowly and completely before taking another deep breath. (For more information about the important role of deep breathing, see "Breathing Therapies" on page 333.)

All of the following relaxation response techniques involve following a set of directions. You can study the directions until you feel that you understand what you need to do. Or you can take a tip from the experts and record the directions on an audiocassette to play during your relaxation sessions. A number of excellent cassettes are available commercially as well.

Progressive Relaxation: Tension and Release

The most physical of all the therapies is progressive muscle relaxation. The purpose of this technique is to achieve total relaxation of all the basic muscle groups by concentrating on one group at a time. It's particularly effective for people so stressed out that their overtaut muscles cause back pain and headaches, says Berkeley, California, psychologist Neil Fiore, Ph.D., author of *The Now Habit: Overcoming Procrastination and Enjoying Guilt-Free Play.*

Here's Dr. Fiore's verbal prescription for folks in need of muscle relaxation. If you plan to record it, be sure to speak slowly, allowing for deep breathing and enough time to carry out the directions. If the tape seems to move you along too fast, you can always record a newer, slower version. When you're ready to begin, find a quiet, comfortable place. Sit upright in a chair and simply follow these directions.

Take a deep breath—inhale slowly, deeply. As you're doing this, press your feet together and curl your toes. Hold your breath. Study how your muscles feel, Record it in your mind. When you can't hold your breath any longer, exhale. Let it go. Just let your feet drop. Notice what it feels like. Let the blood supply and oxygen supply cleanse out the stress and tension in your legs and feet. (Repeat three times.) Uncurl your toes. Allow them to move around—really let them relax.

Now let's move to the stomach muscles.

Begin to tighten the buttocks. Pull in your stomach muscles and begin to inhale. Hold in those stomach muscles, tighten those buttocks. Push your back against the chair a bit, still holding your breath. Now exhale. Let go and let the relaxation flow through your pelvis, abdomen, and back. Just notice these relaxed feelings.

Now begin to curl your fingers as you inhale. Curl them into fists as you inhale. Allow your body from the waist down to remain relaxed. Isolate the tension in your fists as you hold your breath. Feel the tension in your hands and arms. Keep holding the muscle tension until you cannot hold your breath any longer. Then exhale completely. Feel yourself letting go of the tension. Study the feeling of relaxation. You feel like you're exhaling through your fingers. You're letting go of tension. Letting go of stress.

Now press your palms together as you take a deep breath. Include your shoulders in this movement. Raise your palms higher. Feel the tension throughout your arms. Hold and then exhale completely. Feel the sensations in your arms. Feel the tension disappearing.

Now begin to scrunch up your face, your eyes, your nose, as much of your scalp as you can, inhaling deeply as you feel the tension. Hold until you can't hold your breath any longer, then exhale completely. Allow your eyelids to float softly over your eyes. Now inhale as you begin to open your mouth wider, wider. Begin to notice any tension in your jaw. Open your mouth as wide as is comfortable for you, then slowly exhale. Slowly relax, letting your lips come together just slightly parted. Float down into the chair.

Allow your muscles to easily hold you.
Allow your feet to be supported by the
floor.

Autogenic Training:
Talking to Yourself

Autogenic training can closely approxi-
mate the sensations and physiological
changes your body experiences during
deep sleep. Here are the directions from
Dr. Sadigh. To begin, gently close your
eyes, take a deep breath, hold it for a
moment, then slowly exhale. Do this
several times. Then slowly and silently
repeat the following phrases, with pauses
in between. Do it about three times. (You
can repeat these phrases in your mind
from memory or follow along on the tape.)

> *My body is quiet (pause, repeat).*
> *My body is calm (pause, repeat).*
> *My body is beginning to relax (pause,*
> *repeat).*
> *My right arm is heavy (pause, repeat).*
> *My left arm is heavy (pause, repeat).*
> *Both arms are heavy (pause, repeat).*
> *My left leg is heavy (pause, repeat).*
> *My right leg is heavy (pause, repeat).*
> *Both legs are heavy (pause, repeat).*
> *My right foot is heavy (pause, repeat).*
> *My left foot is heavy (pause, repeat).*
> *I am relaxed (pause, repeat).*
> *My mind is quiet (pause, repeat).*
> *My whole body is relaxed (pause,*
> *repeat).*

Note: You may do the entire sequence
again, only this time say "heavy and
warm" instead of just "heavy." Then relax,
take a deep breath, and hold it. As you
exhale, stretch out your arms and legs.
Then repeat.

Visualization:
Seeing Is Believing

There are two types of visualization
technique. In *open-ended imagery* your
therapist helps you with images. For
example, says Dr. Miller, the therapist may
say, "Think of the most pleasant place you
have ever been and begin to picture
yourself there. Begin to feel it, smell it. See
its colors.

"But," he laughs, "some people complain,
'I can't think of anything!' " And so he,
like many others who use visualization,
guides his patients through the image,
suggesting many vivid details. This type
of visualization is known as *guided
imagery.* Warm beaches, deep green forests,
snow-capped mountains, quiet deserts are
included in the experts' excursions into
fantasy, along with all the physical details
you might expect.

Both kinds of visualizations are available
on audiocassette, but again, you might
also create your own. Write out the details
of your own ideal getaway, record it (with
music, if you wish), and then live it in
your mind.

Meditation: Tuning In

Meditation may seem out of place in a
chapter on relaxation therapies, but according to Dr. Benson, the practice can have a
profoundly beneficial physical effect.

The most common type of meditating
involves mentally repeating a word or
phrase. Using one that reflects your basic
belief system may help you become more
deeply involved in the relaxation response,
says Dr. Benson.

"Picking a word or phrase to focus upon

serves two purposes," says Dr. Benson. "It activates your belief systems by giving you a greater calming effect than you might have if you focused on neutral words. Second, it increases the likelihood that you'll continue using the techniques."

He cautions that the words or phrases must be short enough that they can be said silently as you exhale normally.

Sit quietly and upright in a comfortable chair. Close your eyes and focus on your breathing. After you've inhaled and exhaled several times, mentally repeat the word or phrase you've chosen over and over and over.

Here are some of Dr. Benson's suggestions.

Catholics and certain Christians might try a line from the Lord's Prayer, such as "Our father who art in heaven," or a line from the Apostles' Creed: "I believe in the Holy Spirit."

Protestants may prefer to choose a phrase from the 23rd Psalm, such as "The Lord is my shepherd," or something from the New Testament.

Jewish people might pick a passage from the Old Testament, such as "You shall love your neighbor," or single words such as "Shalom" (peace) or "Echad" (one).

Moslems might repeat words such as "Allah" (God) or a phrase from the Koran.

"Of course, you don't have to use a word reflecting a religious belief or philosophy," says Dr. Benson. A simple word like "one" will do. Other experts suggest words such as "peace," "patience," "love," or "trust." These can be equally effective for those people who do not practice a particular religion.

Tension Busters

Practicing your chosen form of relaxation training should pay off in the long run, but what if it doesn't? Or what if you just can't get the hang of those first few sessions?

While many people can learn how to relax on their own, experts say that some people need direction from a therapist. If you can't seem to unwind or relax, ask your physician to refer you to someone who can teach you. You might also contact the psychology department of your local university and ask for a reference.

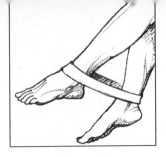

Resistance Training

Maria Fiatarone, M.D., can make invalids walk. Under her care, 90-year-old men and women, for years barely able to raise themselves from a chair—let alone walk unassisted—throw away their canes and climb stairs with relative ease. Their pace livens, they stand taller. And their strength doubles—if not triples or quadruples—giving them back a sense of power and independence they lost a long time ago.

Dr. Fiatarone is no faith healer, no religious huckster preaching salvation and mobility in exchange for a generous free-will offering. She's a physician, an assistant professor at Harvard Medical School's Division on Aging. And all she does is work the miracle of muscle, coaxing these frail, inactive nonagenarians—many of whom suffer from the debilitating drains of heart disease, osteoporosis, or high blood pressure—to lift weights with the "age-adjusted" intensity of a Hulk Hogan or an Arnold Schwarzenegger.

Powering Up

In other words, the elderly people in a training program that Dr. Fiatarone runs are working just as hard in their own way as do superathletes, even though the weights they are hoisting are far lighter.

Exercise experts are only recently coming to realize the value of an intense training routine, says Dr. Fiatarone. Even though the full range of benefits occurs only with high-intensity weight-lifting routines, Dr. Fiatarone says, most studies assessing weight lifting's benefits for the elderly and chronically ill have incorporated very easy routines with light weights. Results always were discouraging because "you realize no benefit with low stimuli," she says. But if strict resistance training enhances the health of younger, comparatively healthy folks, she says, "why not use it with the people who really need it?"

Which is exactly what she and her colleagues at Harvard did. They studied the effects of high-intensity resistance training on what she calls the "worst-case scenario"—nursing home residents in their nineties at Hebrew Rehabilitation Center for Aged in Boston. Some of the elderly people who participated in the ten-week program were so frail they barely could stand. "There was a lot of chronic disease—arthritis, high blood pressure, diabetes, heart disease, osteoporosis," she says, "but their conditions were stable."

Their exercise regimen stressed the lower body. The weight used was 80 percent of each exerciser's maximum load—only 20 percent lighter than what they could manage to lift just once. "Relatively speaking, they lifted with the same amount of difficulty as for a younger person lifting 80 percent of a higher load," Dr. Fiatarone says.

The hard-working group of nursing home residents hit the weights three times a week, doing a series of exercises for the major muscle groups of the thigh. As they became stronger, Dr. Fiatarone continually upped the load, maintaining the 80 percent lifting intensity to reflect their ever-growing strength.

Then, when Dr. Fiatarone halted the exercise program, the nursing home residents showed a marked decrease in strength. Not surprisingly, a majority wanted to continue the training, so Dr. Fiatarone inaugurated a program of continued training. "Some dropped out of the program," she says. "But most were excited and interested. Most want to continue."

Any exercise that can help 90-year-olds toss away their canes obviously has a lot going for it. Let's take a closer look at just what resistance training can do for people of all ages.

Muscle Magic

Weight lifting, weight training, bodybuilding, resistance training, pumping iron, hanging and banging, pounding plates—call it what you will, it's all the same: using muscles repetitively and forcefully against a mobile resistance, whether the resistance is a barbell, an exercise machine, a bicycle inner tube, or a sock filled with a few pounds of lentils.

Forget those images of sweaty gym giants with 500 pounds on their backs, bulging muscles, no necks, and veins like a relief map of major continental waterways.

You could try to chisel that kind of physique, but it would require a genetic predisposition to quick muscle growth and a level of exertion that most people are incapable of.

A more reasoned approach to lifting provides a panoply of benefits to men and women of any age and in varying degrees of health. It builds muscles, bones, and joints; expands flexibility; burns fat and sculpts the body with firmer, leaner lines; strengthens the heart and minimizes certain cardiovascular disease risk factors; and elevates your self-esteem.

Pumping Primer

Like your biceps or your calves, your heart is a muscle that can be trained with weights to become stronger and even larger. Lifting "increases the thickness of the heart and increases the thickness of the heart wall," enabling it to pump more blood through the body with greater force, according to Michael Yessis, Ph.D., professor emeritus of physical education at California State University, Fullerton, and author of *Kinesiology of Exercise.* Paradoxically, although pulse quickens substantially during workouts, the increase in pumping efficiency eventually lowers the resting heart rate because the stronger heart doesn't have to work as hard.

A similar paradoxical effect occurs in counteracting high blood pressure. Blood pressure increases dramatically during particularly demanding lifts. But almost immediately after training and while at rest, blood pressure drops. This effect can help people with mildly elevated blood pressure approach more healthy readings.

People with cardiovascular disease or moderate or severe high blood pressure should see their doctor before beginning a weight-lifting program—and if they do lift, they should use a lighter load—but their condition does not preclude pumping iron. (See "High Blood Pressure" on page 176.)

Bolstering Bones, Improving Image

The evidence supporting the power of weight lifting to prevent osteoporosis is as strong as the skeleton it builds. Osteoporosis causes the bones to become brittle, frail, and increasingly subject to fracture. "Resistance training may be the best way to increase bone density," says Michael Stone, Ph.D., professor of exercise science at Appalachian State University in Boone, North Carolina.

"We have not observed change in the body's *total* bone density due to lifting," says Ben F. Hurley, Ph.D., associate professor in the exercise physiology labs at the University of Maryland's Department of Kinesiology. "But we have found a significant increase of density in specific areas people with osteoporosis tend to fracture," such as the upper part of the thigh bone and the lumbar spine.

Ligaments, tendons, and joints all become stronger, Dr. Stone says. And because they're worked against resistance through their full range of motion, they also become much more flexible. The extra muscle and connective tissue built through resistance training also helps protect the joints to which it is connected. All in all, long-term training helps you become more resistant to strains and sprains when going about everyday activities.

The Promise of Body Shaping

The most visible benefit of lifting, however, is the way it can remold your body. "You can make your body look more like you want it to look," Dr. Stone says. You can create muscle in specific areas, in effect replacing amorphous flab with firm, sleek contours. "You can't spot-reduce fat by removing it only from certain areas," says Dr. Stone, "but you can spot-gain muscle."

To make your waist appear smaller, for example, you can use weight training to enlarge the width of your chest and shoulders. "You can't do that with jogging," Dr. Stone says. "In fact, because of the type of energy it demands, you may lose muscle mass with jogging if you don't also train with weights." An added benefit of building muscle is that generally speaking, the more muscle you have on your frame, the more calories and fat you'll burn when you are at rest.

Not only that, the physical changes induced by lifting can make your everyday life a whole lot easier. You can pick up that bag of garbage and carry it to the end of the driveway. You can leave the grocery cart at the store door and tote the bags to the car. You become more attractive to yourself and to others. You acquire a new inner sense of strength, independence, and self-certainty.

Hard Work, but Worth It

While "no pain, no gain" is an inaccurate and dangerous axiom, resistance training does require a little . . . well, resistance. That means you have to earn those benefits with a little sweat.

Sure, nondemanding lifting of very light weights will tone your muscles to a limited extent, preventing them from atrophying and improving flexibility. And, experts say, it's a good way to introduce yourself to resistance training and gradually work yourself into heavier loads.

But strengthening the heart, lowering blood pressure, altering the body's proportion of muscle and fat—these things *are* possible, Dr. Stone says, but they really depend on the *volume* of weight lifting performed. That's not how loud you are when you bang plates in the gym. "Volume is how much work you do," Dr. Stone says. It's how many calories you burn through the number of repetitions cranked out by the larger muscle groups, such as legs and hips, against a resistance of sufficient intensity.

To reap the full cardiovascular benefits of weight lifting, says Dr. Stone, the best volume is attained by performing each exercise for 8 to 12 repetitions and doing that at least three separate times before moving to the next body part. In lifting lingo, that's three sets of 8 to 12 "reps" (repetitions), or a total of 24 to 36 lifting motions for the same body part.

Gaining strength, larger muscles, and tempered bones is contingent on workout intensity—that is, how heavy the weights are and how much effort you make to hoist them. For each movement, intensity usually is measured by a percentage of the heaviest weight you can lift for only one repetition, explains Dr. Stone. To do high-intensity exercise, you must begin by

lifting 60 to 70 percent of your maximum repetition. (Your goal is to move up to 70 to 80 percent.) If the most you can squat once with is 100 pounds, for example, you'll do your three sets of repetitions using 60 to 70 pounds.

The optimum high-intensity, high-volume workout, then, is three sets of 8 to 12 repetitions for each body part. For each exercise you would use 60 to 80 percent of the maximum load you can lift only once for that particular exercise.

Volume and intensity are affected by how much you rest between sets. A pause of between 1½ and 3 minutes offers adequate rest to get through the next set. You need time to recover to continue your workout.

Dr. Hurley adds, "You do want to avoid overtraining and overstraining."

Heavier and Harder

As you persist through this unarguably arduous workout, your body adapts, developing a tolerance to the initial volume and intensity. Within a couple of weeks, the muscles become a little stronger, the heart a tad more durable. The exercises, amazingly enough, become easy, simple, a piece of cake, no sweat. But don't let that happen; don't let the sweat stop. Both volume and intensity, experts say, require an ever-progressing increase in the amount of weight lifted or the number of times you lift it.

You can increase the intensity of your workout in small increments, perhaps by adding just a pound or two, according to Dr. Stone. As the weight increases, the number of reps you're able to perform will naturally decrease. So you drop back to 8 reps and attempt in succeeding workouts to get your reps back up to 12.

How fast you progress will depend very much on the condition you're in to begin with and your age, explains Dr. Stone. People older than 40 "may not progress as fast," he says, because their recovery and adaptation capabilities are not as good as those of someone younger. They should proceed just a little slower and include more variety in their volume, intensity, and lifts, he says. But barring any serious and unstable joint or cardiovascular problems, for people in their fifties and sixties, "there's nothing they really can't do," he says. "Basically, they can train like anybody else."

Belly Up to the Barbell

How often should you train?

For beginners, "every other day is fine," says Dr. Hurley. You can do a total-body workout that taxes every muscle every other day or at least three times a week, says Dr. Yessis. You can also split your workout, alternating below-the-belt muscles one day with the upper body the next, Dr. Hurley suggests.

If you do want to train each specific muscle, though, here is a list of body-part-by-body-part exercises suggested by Dr. Yessis. Three sets of 8 repetitions of each exercise should be done by bending the joint slowly through its full range of motion. The exercises should not be executed so fast that momentum rather than muscle action lifts the weight. Depending on your level of fitness, you initially can use no weight or very light resistance, but remember that high intensity and high volume are necessary for peak cardiovascular and muscle conditioning.

Squats. With dumbbells in your hands or a barbell over the back of your neck and shoulders, lean your upper body forward slightly and squat, bending your knees to no more than a 90-degree angle. This one exercise works almost all lower body muscles, Dr. Yessis says, particularly the thighs and the buttocks.

Knee extensions. This exercise works the muscles on the front of the thigh—the quadriceps. You can do it with ankle weights while seated on a chair, or on a machine at the gym. Straighten your legs and hold the position for a few seconds. When lowering the weight to the resting position, never let your leg go beyond a 90-degree angle by swinging your feet under the seat of the chair. That exerts too much pressure on the knees.

Outer and inner thigh exercises. Using ankle weights, lie on your side with your legs straight, one on top of the other. Raise your upper leg as far as possible without turning your knee up toward the ceiling. Complete three sets. Then raise your lower leg for three sets. (Because this is a much more difficult movement, beginners may want to do one set only.)

Abdominal exercises. In recent years, exercise specialists have denigrated traditional bent-knee sit-ups, instead advocating crunches to isolate the abdominal muscles and avoid use of the hip muscles. To do a crunch, lie on the floor with your legs draped over a chair seat so they are bent at a 90-degree angle. Lift only your head and shoulders from the floor. (Dr. Yessis says, however, that traditional bent-knee sit-ups work both the abdominals and muscles in the hips.)

If you prefer bent-knee sit-ups, allow your back as well as your head and shoulders to rise off the floor. If you have back problems, though, stick with crunches, advises Dr. Yessis.

For the muscles of the lower abdomen you can do reverse sit-ups. Lie on your back with your knees bent. Then roll your hips up off the floor by lifting your knees toward your chest. Keep your hands at your sides, Dr. Yessis cautions, and don't tuck them under your buttocks. "That defeats the purpose, as does keeping your legs straight," he says. "It switches the work from the abdominals to the lower back, and it can be extremely dangerous."

The sides of your waist—the oblique muscles—and the muscles of your lower back can be firmed up with side bends. Hold a dumbbell in one hand by your side and bend the other arm up over your head. Without bending forward at the hips, lean sideways as far as possible, allowing the weight to hang down. Return to an erect posture, then lean to the other side. Then switch the weight to the other hand and repeat the exercise.

Chest exercises. The bench press is another multimuscle exercise, working not only the muscles of the chest (the pectorals) but also the muscles of the back of the arm (the triceps) and the front portion of the shoulder. With a dumbbell in each hand, lie back on the bench, your elbows out and the weights held slightly above your chest. Do not arch as you lift. Push the weights straight up and then lower them.

Shoulder exercises. You can either sit or stand for this next exercise. Hold the dumbbells down at your sides, one in each hand. With your arms bent just slightly at the elbows, raise the weights out and up from the sides all the way over your head. This movement works the sides of your shoulders, called the medial heads, and the trapezius—a muscle that runs from your neck down to the shoulders and upper back.

To work the rear part of the shoulder— the posterior heads—lie facedown on the bench with a dumbbell in each hand. Lift them out and up as far as possible. This also works muscles of the upper back—the trapezius and the rhomboids—both of which position the shoulders for proper posture.

Back exercises. The best way to work the muscles that wrap around your ribs and up into your back—the lattisimus dorsi—is on a pull-down machine at the gym. You sit at the machine, reach up to the bar with both hands, and simply pull it down to your shoulders. Use a wide grip with your palms facing away and pull the bar down behind your neck to strengthen the upper part of the lattisimus muscles. A narrow grip with your palms still facing away stresses the lower part of the muscle group.

Arm exercises. Curls (see the illustration on page 416) are ideal for the biceps in the front of the arms. To work the backs of the arms—the triceps—you'll need the pull-down machine again, although this time you stand in front of it and push the bar down.

Start with the bar at shoulder height. Then with your palms facing down and the upper parts of your arms again stationary, push the bar down until your elbows are almost straight. To work the triceps at a different angle, use a palms-up grip on the bar.

IRRESISTIBLE MEETS IMMOVABLE . . . AND GOES NOWHERE

Does your ski instructor tell you to press your back against the wall and crouch down as if sitting in an invisible chair? In aerobics class, does your teacher tell you to lie down, lift your shoulders from the floor, hold the position, and make those abdominal muscles burn? Do football coaches tell your young sons to hold their arms up and out to their sides to "strengthen the shoulders"?

So *are* you better on the slopes? *Is* your tummy trim and taut? Do your sons actually throw longer passes on the football field as a result of all this effort?

Probably not. Isometrics—the kind of exercises that involve working groups of muscles without actually putting them through their range of motion—have been around for a couple of decades. They were hyped, especially back in the 1950s and 1960s, for such diverse purposes as bodybuilding and bust development. The problem is, scientific studies have shown that isometrics have little value in either recreation or physical fitness. And word hasn't really gotten around to the public yet.

Use of isometrics "is still rampant. It's a real problem," says Alice Lockridge, exercise physiologist and president of Professional Fitness Instructor Training (PRO-FIT) in Renton, Washington. "They don't strengthen muscles. They only make you better at holding the position you practice."

Sitting against the wall has as much application in slaloming down a hill as it does riding in the lift to the top because "nobody really skis like that," she says. Not only is holding a sit-up dangerous, but it makes the abdominal muscles stronger "only when you're bent over. You probably don't want to be stronger in that position," she says. And holding your arms out to the sides gives you nothing more than tired arms. (Many isometric exercises are dangerous for people who have high blood pressure, because the exercises themselves cause a temporary increase in pressure.)

Lockridge says her "favorite" useless isometric—one that untold thousands may still be doing—is the fanny firmer people do while standing in a checkout line or waiting for the bus. Repeatedly tensing the buttocks (gluteal) muscles won't tone them, she says. "The only thing you get better at is squeezing your butt," she chuckles.

When irresistible force meets immovable object, it seems, you usually get nowhere fast. So why are so many people still doing isometrics?

These days little mention is made of the technique. But various types of isometric exercises were *so* popular back in the late 1950s and 1960s and were *so* highly touted that many people—including coaches and fitness instructors—are still sweating through their favorites, not to mention passing them on to the next generation.

The fact is, isometrics offer an advantage only in certain medical and therapeutic applications, according to Randall L. Braddom, M.D., a professor and chairman of the Department of Physical Medicine and Rehabilitation at Indiana University and medical director of Hook Rehabilitation Center in Indianapolis. In limited circumstances, doing isometrics will preserve some strength and will slow muscle atrophy, he says. "It's better than nothing, but we use it only in medical situations, such as in recovery after surgery on a joint."

Getting Ready for Resistance

Muster up some muscle with this beginner's weight-lifting routine. It's a good way to introduce you to the concepts and movements of resistance training.

You'll become more familiar with your body as you learn and feel where each muscle is and how it works, and you'll love the way you start to look as the muscles start to firm up.

These easy exercises call for resistance bands—large rubber-band-like loops that resemble bicycle inner tubes. They can be purchased at your local sporting goods store, or you can use bicycle inner tubes.

Repeat each movement eight to ten times to complete one set. The last movement, or "rep," should be somewhat difficult to do, and the muscle or muscles that you're working should feel tired and full. If that last rep feels easy, increase the resistance, either by doubling up the band or by buying one that offers greater resistance. Try to perform three sets of each exercise, resting for 1½ to 3 minutes between sets.

These exercises tone the hips and outer thighs. (1) Lie on your side with one leg on top of the other and the resistance band over your ankles. (2) Raise your upper leg as far as it can comfortably go, making sure your foot is flexed and your knee faces forward. You will be lifting against the resistance of the band. Switch sides and repeat. If balance is a problem, try bending your lower leg at the knee to give you a better base of support. For a greater workout, place the band just above your knees.

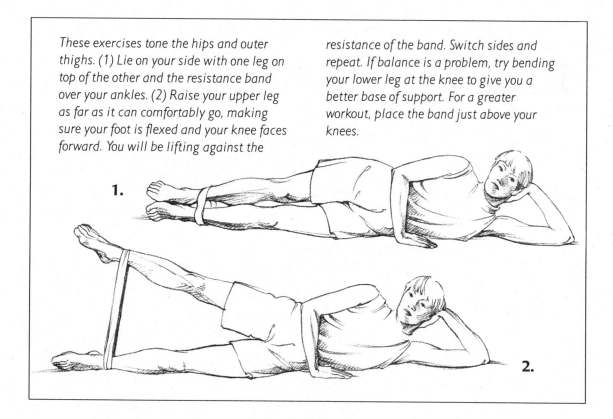

1.

2.

Getting Ready for Resistance—Continued

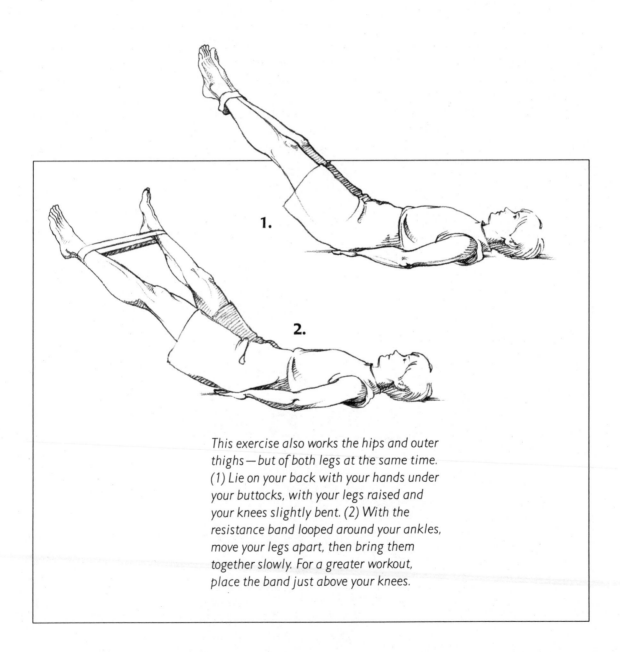

1.

2.

This exercise also works the hips and outer thighs—but of both legs at the same time. (1) Lie on your back with your hands under your buttocks, with your legs raised and your knees slightly bent. (2) With the resistance band looped around your ankles, move your legs apart, then bring them together slowly. For a greater workout, place the band just above your knees.

You can strengthen the muscles in the front of the thigh (the quadriceps) with these leg extensions. (1) Sit erect in a chair or on the edge of a sturdy table with the band around your ankles. (2) Raise one leg straight out until it's parallel to the floor, making sure to keep the other leg at a strict 90-degree angle. Repeat with the other leg. You also can try looping the resistance band over a leg of the chair or table on which you're sitting.

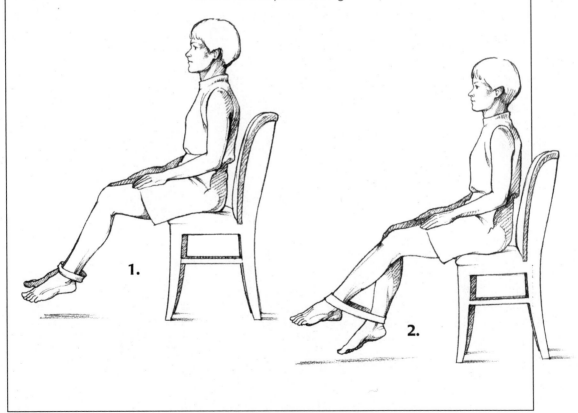

Getting Ready for Resistance—Continued

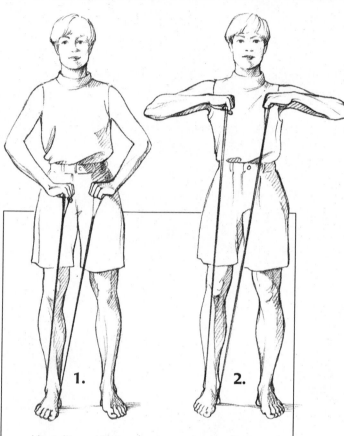

1.

2.

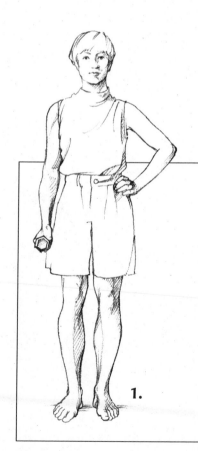

Upright rows improve posture by developing all parts of the shoulder (deltoid) muscles and the trapezius — the muscles that drape down over the sides of the neck onto the shoulders. (1) Stand on the resistance band, holding the ends in both hands at about hip level. (2) Stretch the band straight up, bringing your fists almost to your chin and your elbows as far as possible above your shoulders. The higher you go, the better the muscle is worked.

1.

Overhead triceps extensions tone the horseshoe-shaped muscle on the back of the upper arm and are good for developing strength for whenever you need to push something. (1) Hold a dumbbell in both hands behind your head. (2) Make sure your upper arms remain stationary at each side of your head as you bend at the elbows to lift the weight. You also can use weights strapped to your wrists or, if sitting, a resistance band anchored to a chair.

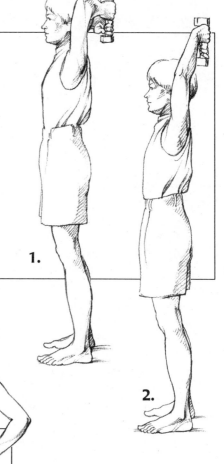

1.

2.

No need for shoulder pads—lateral dumbbell raises tone, lift, and round out the outside middle muscles (the lateral head) of the shoulder. (1) Hold a dumbbell or light hand weight at your side, then (2) raise your arm, which should be bent slightly at the elbow, out and up. The further above your shoulders your raise your arm, the more you work the shoulder and trapezius muscle. Repeat on the other side.

2.

Getting Ready for Resistance—Continued

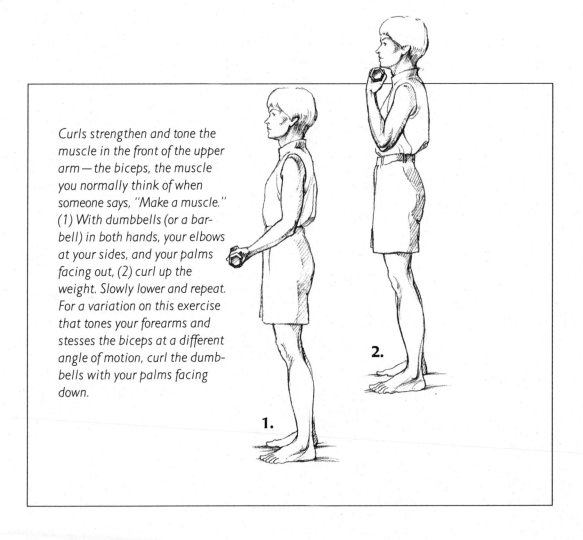

Curls strengthen and tone the muscle in the front of the upper arm—the biceps, the muscle you normally think of when someone says, "Make a muscle." (1) With dumbbells (or a barbell) in both hands, your elbows at your sides, and your palms facing out, (2) curl up the weight. Slowly lower and repeat. For a variation on this exercise that tones your forearms and stesses the biceps at a different angle of motion, curl the dumbbells with your palms facing down.

1.

2.

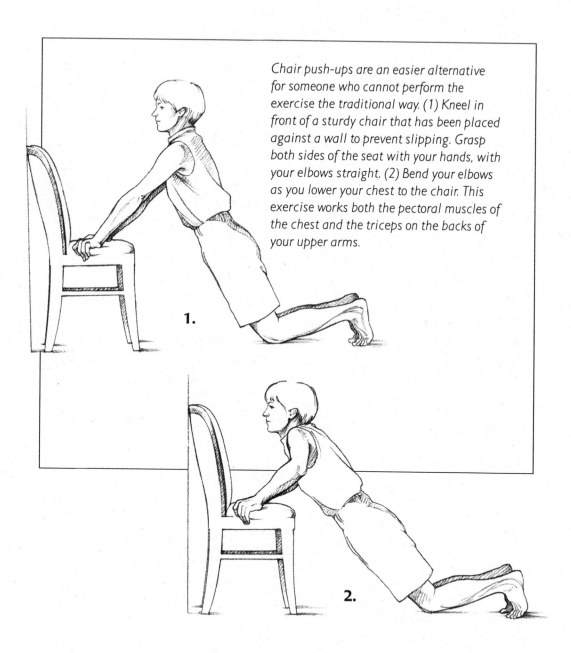

Chair push-ups are an easier alternative for someone who cannot perform the exercise the traditional way. (1) Kneel in front of a sturdy chair that has been placed against a wall to prevent slipping. Grasp both sides of the seat with your hands, with your elbows straight. (2) Bend your elbows as you lower your chest to the chair. This exercise works both the pectoral muscles of the chest and the triceps on the backs of your upper arms.

1.

2.

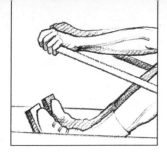

Rowing

Fredrick Hagerman doesn't mince words when he talks about rowing. And he doesn't use a lot of ifs and buts when he discusses oars.

"Rowing is a great sport. You have a tremendous feeling of power and control when you're rowing," says Dr. Hagerman, who has a Ph.D. and is a professor of zoological and biomedical science at Ohio University in Athens.

"The feeling you get when you do a good stroke is amazing," he says.

"It's like hitting a great tennis shot past your opponent. It's absolutely exhilarating."

Rowing is also one of the best aerobic exercises we can do.

"It certainly is a strong, effective cardiovascular fitness activity," says Jay T. Kearney, Ph.D., director of sports science for the U.S. Olympic Committee in Colorado Springs.

"It's rhythmic, continuous, and involves large muscle groups in the legs, back, and, to some extent, the arms. Additionally, you don't have a lot of pounding on the joints like you experience during jogging."

But before you begin, see your physician, recommends Dr. Hagerman. Rowing is a strenuous activity, comparable to jogging at 5½ miles per hour or doing 10 minutes of intense aerobic dancing.

"I don't care how old you are, even if you're a teenager, you should have a physical examination before you start a rowing program," he says.

In particular, ask your doctor to evaluate your back. If necessary, he or she can prescribe exercises to stretch and strengthen your lower back to prepare you for this intense exercise.

Stroke Those Calories Away

Rowing may burn more calories than other aerobic activities, according to a study conducted by Dr. Hagerman and his associates at Ohio University.

Sixty men and 47 women, aged 20 to 74, were asked to do four exercise tests on rowing machines and stationary bicycles. Dr. Hagerman found that workouts on the rowing machines burned more energy than exercising on the bicycles.

"It's not a mystery why rowing has a higher energy cost than cycling. When you row you're using more muscles," Dr. Hagerman says.

"Rowing is a great aerobic conditioning program. It's by far the best. It's good for the lungs, it's good for the heart, and it's good for the muscles."

In addition, it may be surprisingly good for older people. In a 14-week study of 24 men and women, aged 68 to 92, who did rowing exercises three times a week, Dr.

Hagerman found significant improvement in their exercise capacity.

"Rowing can be perfect for the elderly, especially on a rowing machine," he says. "They don't have to worry about balance, and they can pull as hard as they want to."

In some cases, rowing also might be ideal as an integral part of a cardiac rehabilitation program, says Gregory Kay, M.D., a cardiothoracic and vascular surgeon at the Hospital of the Good Samaritan in Los Angeles.

"There's absolutely no reason why someone who is 60 years old and has had coronary bypass surgery couldn't get involved in a rowing program," Dr. Kay says. (Of course, anyone who has heart disease or is recovering from a heart attack should consult a physician before doing such vigorous exercise.)

But rowing is definitely *not* an ideal workout for everyone.

"It would be ludicrous to suggest that anybody with serious arthritis or back trouble try rowing. They'd just have too much difficulty with it," Dr. Kay says. "But I think just about anybody else can get into a slow, easy program of rowing."

Take Your Paddle Indoors

After you get your physician's approval, go to a gymnasium to learn the proper rowing method, Dr. Hagerman suggests.

"Rowing isn't difficult to learn. It's not like learning how to surf or snow ski. It's much easier than those sports," he says. "But you do need to learn the proper techniques in order to avoid injury."

That's one good reason to get your initial rowing experience at a gymnasium.

Not only can you have an instructor coach you in the proper technique, but you can also find out if you like rowing well enough to stick with it. If you purchase a rower, then find out it isn't the exercise for you, it could be a costly mistake. A good rowing machine can cost more than $700, Dr. Hagerman says.

If you do purchase an indoor rower, make sure the seat rides on ball bearings, not plastic. And look for joints that are welded together, not bolted. Bolts and plastic wear out quickly.

Hydraulic cylinder rowers are the most popular at-home models. They are quiet and small enough that you can tuck them into a corner. The higher on the rowing arm you clamp the cylinder, the greater the resistance. This type can cost more than $300.

Straight-pull rowers, also called ergometers, are made with a flywheel braked by a fan belt or motor to create resistance. They cost more than hydraulic cylinder rowers but are much more effective, Dr. Hagerman says.

"An ergometer actually simulates the motion of the boat. It gives you a feeling that you're actually rowing on the water," he says. "Hydraulic rowing machines aren't like that. You're doing a rowing motion, but it's a resistance exercise. These machines don't simulate all the aerobic aspects of rowing."

The first thing you should do when you sit down on the unit is adjust the footrest to an angle that feels right for you. Otherwise, it can flex your ankles uncomfortably and prevent you from making a full stroke.

To prevent back injury, begin your

FULL SPEED AHEAD

You've seen those broad-shouldered, athletic types gliding through the water in those long, narrow boats that look as if they're about to sink. Although it may look easy, the folks pulling the oars in those sleek racing boats are getting a terrific aerobic workout.

"From a health standpoint, there's nothing like it," says Volker Nolte, Ph.D., a biomechanics expert who has been a competitive oarsman since he was 13. "It's beneficial to your whole body."

Rowing in a shell, a specialized racing boat that has a sliding seat, works out muscles throughout the body and contributes to cardiovascular fitness, says Fredrick Hagerman, Ph.D., a professor of zoological and biomedical science at Ohio University in Athens. Not only that, but a 30-minute workout in a shell burns 342 calories.

The key factor is the legs. Rowing in a shell works out more muscles in the legs than paddling a canoe, a raft, or a kayak, he says. That extra work increases demand on the heart and lungs.

Because rowing in a shell is a strenuous activity, Dr. Hagerman recommends that you see a physician before beginning.

Renting a shell from a rowing club is probably your best option, because you'd probably have to spend some big bucks to own your own.

"Rowing is a very expensive sport," Dr. Hagerman says. "You can buy a good set of golf clubs for the price of the least expensive single shell. You're not going to get one for less than $1,000."

But before you dash out to a nearby rowing club, you probably should spend some time at a gymnasium, working out on an indoor rowing machine, Dr. Hagerman says.

That's because it's much easier for beginners to learn proper rowing techniques on land than on water.

regimen with low resistance and a minimum number of strokes. Warm up by doing 12 strokes a minute for 5 minutes. Since rowing works out all of the major muscle groups, you may tire quickly. Don't feel bad if the warm-up is all you can do at first.

Gradually increase your stroke rate. Try to add 10 percent a week to the number of strokes per minute. Ultimately, aim for 22 to 24 strokes per minute. When you can row for 20 minutes, add more power to your workouts. Every 2 to 3 minutes, for example, pull harder for 10 strokes or alternate periods of hard rowing with easy rowing.

At the end of your workout, be sure to cool down with some slow stretching exercises. (See "Stretching" on page 440.)

Of course, you may find that exercising on a rowing machine doesn't pack enough challenge or excitement into a workout, or you may simply want to get outdoors. Paddling a canoe or kayak may be a good alternative for some people, says Cedric X. Bryant, Ph.D., director of geriatric research and sports medicine at Randal Sports/Medical Products in Kirkland, Washington.

Canoeing at a moderate intensity, for example, is the equivalent (in terms of calorie cost) of leisurely bicycling at about 5 miles per hour, he says.

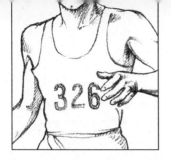

Running

You see them out there—in bone-soaking rain and howling wind, in frigid cold and blistering heat. On some mornings, they trudge past your house so early that even roosters are still asleep. Other times, they huff and puff along at night, moonlit silhouettes that make perfect targets for overprotective dogs and underattentive drivers.

No matter the weather, no matter the time, no matter how nasty their neighbor's Doberman, you can see them: taking one grueling step after another, mile after lonely mile, their feet pounding the asphalt at a force *three times* their body weight, their lungs catching the exhaust from passing cars.

And perhaps you've wondered: Are runners really *that* nuts?

After all, walking burns approximately the same number of calories per mile—roughly 100, depending on your weight—and it doesn't pummel your knees and feet nearly as much. Stair climbing also provides an excellent workout, but it doesn't subject you to the manic mood swings of Mother Nature. Ride a stationary bicycle and you'll cover even *more* miles, plus there's little chance of an up-close-and-personal encounter with a pit bull or a Buick.

Fact is, most *other* endurance exercises can give you the same cardiovascular and muscle toning as running. Like running, other exercises also help lower blood pressure, cholesterol, and your resting heart rate, improving overall health. And they burn calories and fat, helping you lose weight.

So why run?

Because running gives you benefits beyond physical exercise.

A Good Mind Workout, Too

"Sure, you can get a relatively good workout in any number of ways," says John Robinson, Ph.D., director of research for Nike, the Oregon-based maker of running and other athletic shoes. "Climbing a StairMaster or riding a stationary bicycle, for instance, will give you the same great workout as running. The question is, will you be bored out of your mind doing it? With running, you've got scenery, the sun . . . whatever you're into. It's a nice way to be out with nature."

While any exercise aids your body, few provide a better mind, body, *and* soul workout than running.

Not only does running elevate mood and reduce stress like other forms of exercise, but its high intensity helps release endorphins, the brain's natural painkillers. It's the stuff of the much-ballyhooed "runner's high."

For many—particularly stressed-out over-achievers and those on hectic schedules—this "high" can translate to a more low-key attitude, especially when it counts.

"I started running as a grief reaction when my father died 21 years ago, and it helped me tremendously," says Walter Bortz, M.D., physician, author, world-famous authority on aging, and an original member of the 50-Plus Running Association at Stanford University. (His wife, Ruth Anne, was the first woman over age 60 to cross the finish line at the 1991 Boston Marathon.) "It's a wonderful outlet for dealing with life's problems. I live a tremendously time-urgent life, but I run in the morning, and I'm mellow all day."

For your body, running does the same great stuff as other forms of aerobic exercise—only faster, and in many cases better. *Example:* Although nearly the same *number* of calories are burned per mile whether you walk or run, it takes most people *two or three times* as long to walk a mile as to run it. "People can walk for an hour and never come close to the same fitness or intensity level you can achieve by running 15 or 20 minutes," says Dr. Robinson.

Running's high intensity also releases white blood cells into your bloodstream. (White blood cells help fight disease.) It's also particularly helpful in reducing constipation—experiments show that running decreases transit time of food through the digestive system by 30 percent.

And soul? Hey, it takes plenty of that to get up—day after day—and face the open road before the rooster's crow, after work when you're dog-tired, or during weather so bad it would make a mail carrier call in sick. Sure, other forms of exercise require discipline and determination, but runners (the term *jogging* has become obsolete) seem to have that certain something—although the jury is still out on whether to call it "character" or "masochism."

Get Ready, Get Set . . . Wait a Minute

Getting scared off by our tough talk? Maybe you should be, especially if you haven't been exercising regularly.

"Running is a progression," says Stu Mittleman, director of the Fitness Evaluation Center in New York City and world record holder for the 1,000-mile run. "Most people who have been sedentary for a long time and are just starting an exercise program *shouldn't* be running. They should start off walking until they're in reasonably good shape—and then run.

"The big difference between running and walking is the intensity of the work you're doing. And the important thing in exercise is to regulate that work so it fits with *your* target heart rate zone. For some people—particularly those who are over-weight, sedentary, or otherwise out of shape—that means walking. As soon as one in three people *starts* to run, they've already *exceeded* their target zone—and you get the benefits of aerobic exercise by working *within* your target zone." (To determine your target zone and whether you are ready to start a running program, see "Are You Ready to Run?" on the opposite page.)

Getting the Right Shoes

Besides the target zone, the most important aspect of a beginner's running pro-

ARE YOU READY TO RUN?

Don't assume that all you need to start a *new* running program are a good set of legs, a good pair of shoes, and a good dose of determination. You'll also need a pencil and paper to do some math.

Here's a formula, from Stu Mittleman, a New York City–based exercise physiologist and world record holder for the 1,000-mile run, and his colleague Philip Maffetone, D.C., to help you determine whether you're in good enough shape to start a running program. It's based on the target heart rate formula that aerobic dancers use, but it will give a more precise target heart rate for activities such as running, walking, and bicycling.

First subtract your age from 180 (example: If you're 55, 180 − 55 = 125). Then you do one of the following things:

- If you are taking any kind of medication, have never exercised, or are recovering from an illness, subtract 10 from that number.
- If you have exercised but are constantly getting hurt with one injury after another, subtract 5.
- If you've been exercising but your fitness level hasn't greatly increased, don't subtract anything.
- If you've been in a regular exercise program for more than two years and are making good progress, add 5.

"Your final number is the top point of a 10-beat range that is your target zone," says Mittleman.

"You should be in that target zone at the end of about 10 minutes of exercise, whether you're doing a warm-up of walking or slow, easy running."

Mittleman suggests a 7- to 12-minute warm-up of walking to get the heart rate going at a steady and easy pace.

That means our sedentary 55-year-old starting a new exercise program has a target zone of 105 to 115 beats per minute—and shouldn't be in that zone until the end of his warm-up, or before about 10 minutes of serious exercise if no warm-up is done.

If that zone is reached *sooner* during a run, you're better off walking, or doing a run-walk combination.

This formula is especially designed for beginning runners not used to high-intensity workouts. It helps determine how fast you *get* to your target heart rate.

Note: If you're over 40 and you haven't been exercising regularly, you should get your physician's okay before beginning a running program.

gram is getting the right shoe—and the right fit—according to Joe Ellis, D.P.M., a podiatrist in private practice, consultant for the University of California, San Diego, and a biomechanical design consultant for Asics, a leading running shoe manufacturer. A good pair of running shoes will cost between $65 and $115 and should be replaced after about 500 to 750 miles, according to Dr. Ellis.

"The first thing you need to know is your foot type, and basically, types are divided into flat feet, high-arched feet, and normal feet," he says. "To determine your foot type, wet the bottom of your foot and stand on a piece of paper. Then look at the arch: Is it high and well-defined or low and flat?"

Those with high-arched feet need shoes that provide a lot of cushioning to control the "shock" of running. Meanwhile, those with feet on the flatter side need "motion control" shoes that provide stability, says Dr. Ellis.

"The best way to tell whether a shoe has what you need is to pull out the sock liner [the removable innersole, usually bearing the manufacturer's name] and look at how the shoe is stitched. If you can see the stitching that runs lengthwise down the center of the shoe, then that shoe has a lot of cushioning but will likely offer little or no stability—so it's better for high-arched people.

"If there is a board over the stitching, it doesn't have as much cushioning, but it provides stability—so it's better for those with flat feet." A tip: Heavier runners typically have flatter feet, so they're wiser buying "motion control" or "stable" shoes. (Keep in mind that *all* good running shoes provide adequate cushioning, so it's not as though you're "trading" one for the other.)

In Quest of the Right Fit

When checking for proper fit, keep in mind that running shoes should be *bigger* than other shoes. You should be able to wiggle your toes slightly.

"That's because when you run, as your foot hits the ground, your toes spread out and slide forward," says ultra-marathon man Mittleman. "Most people are wrong to buy shoes that fit like a glove. If your shoes fit that snugly, your feet won't be able to absorb the shock of running, and it'll be distributed back up to other parts of your body."

Adds Dr. Ellis: "The general rule is you should have ½ inch of space between the end of your longest toe and the shoe—and I want to emphasize *longest* toe because in 30 to 40 percent of the population, the second toe is the longest, *not* the big toe. That's about an index finger's worth."

But don't just assume you can buy a running shoe a half size larger then your regular shoe. Since many running shoes are made overseas, "size, as we know it, is thrown out the window," says Dr. Ellis. "Some manufacturers make their shoes bigger, some make them smaller. You really don't know unless you try them on."

And when you do, make sure you stand up with *both* shoes on, since your feet spread slightly while you're standing. Some people even suggest you shop for shoes in the afternoon, or after an intense workout, when your feet are more likely to swell.

You shouldn't, however, be able to wiggle the back of your foot. "One of the most important tests in proper fit is for the shoe to fit firmly around your heel," says Dr. Ellis. "If the back of your foot is slipping, *don't* buy the shoe. And by all means, don't assume you'll 'break in' the shoe. If it doesn't feel right in the store, it won't feel right when you're running."

Start Like the Tortoise

"I'd say the biggest mistake beginning runners make is they get hung up on how fast they're going and how far they're going. They try too much too soon," says Budd Coates, a corporate fitness director and nationally ranked marathoner who competed in the Goodwill Games and

THE INS AND OUTS OF RUNNING INJURIES

Among runners, "pronation" and "supination" are dirty words. But the truth of the matter is that everyone pronates and supinates somewhat. It's normal. The heel pronates—rolls outward— as the foot strikes the ground. It then has to supinate—roll back in again—to align the foot for the next step. However, *over*pronation and *over*supination lead to poor form and ultimately to running injuries. Overpronation is a leading cause of running injuries. It's caused by laxity in the joints of the foot. Overpronaters tend to be flat-footed.

Oversupination, on the other hand, is less common and causes injuries to a lesser degree. Feet that oversupinate are generally high-arched and rigid and take all the shock while pounding the pavement.

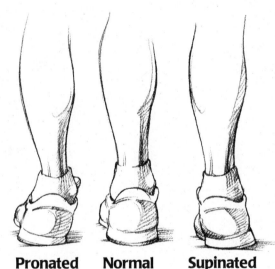

Pronated   Normal   Supinated

While a normal foot is aligned straight (center), the heel of an overpronater angles out from the leg (left). If the inside edges of your shoes are excessively worn, you may suffer from this problem. A sturdy heel counter or orthotics prescribed by a sports medicine podiatrist might be your ticket to correct foot alignment and injury-free running.

An oversupinater (right) tends to wear the outside edge of his shoe soles as his heels angle inward. A pair of soft-soled running shoes with shock-absorbing inserts or orthotics may be the answer to preventing injury for this type of runner.

U.S. Olympic Trials. "Instead of worrying about times and distance, you should mix walking with running for 30 minutes— run until you get slightly tired and then walk until you feel like running again— and work up until you can run comfortably for 30 minutes straight."

Once you get to the point of being able to run for a continuous half hour, you're already doing at least 2 miles, probably 3 to 3½.

If you want to cover more distance, great; but remember, slow and steady wins when it comes to staying injury-free.

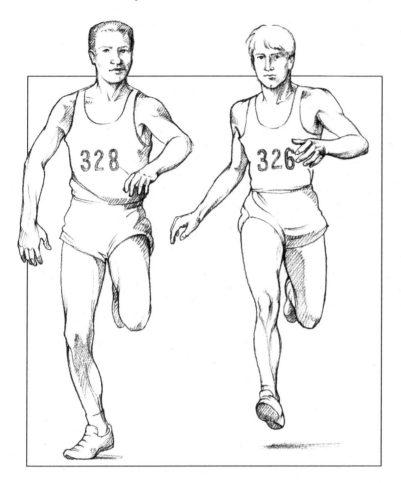

The final strides of these racers provide a contrast in form. Note the outward turn of the foot and knee, often caused by over-supination, of the third-place finisher (left) compared with the straightforward steps of the winner (right). Besides helping to prevent injuries, correcting your running form may help you turn on the speed.

"The best way to *not* get an overuse injury is to increase your mileage no more than 10 percent a week," says Jennifer Stone, head athletic trainer at the U.S. Olympic Training Center in Colorado Springs.

You'll find that whatever distance you're running, the going is easier when you let your arms take some of the work from your legs. "A big mistake a lot of people make is *not* swinging their arms; they just hold them at their sides," says Coates, who is an exercise physiologist. "The reason you

should use your arms is because arms and feet work together, like a pendulum. If you're moving your arms correctly, you're probably moving your feet correctly, too."

Avoiding Injury

Even if you follow all the rules, you may encounter some overuse injuries somewhere along the road—especially if you're new at running.

The most common injury for beginning runners—especially women—is shin splints,

NEITHER SUN, NOR RAIN, NOR SLEET, NOR . . .

If you don't want to *feel* as miserable as some runners *look* when they pant past your house, then adapt to the weather—especially in the dog days of summer, when you're likely to want to roll over and play dead instead of run.

"The key is to keep properly hydrated," says Peter Raven, Ph.D., a professor of physiology at Texas College of Osteopathic Medicine in scorching Fort Worth and past president of the American College of Sports Medicine. "That means drinking enough fluids to feel full before hitting the road. Ideally, you should drink another cup of water every 10 to 15 minutes *while* you're running. I suggest you carry a water bottle with you, so you can take frequent drinks. It's not necessary to pour it on your head; it's more important to get it in your body. After your run, weigh yourself. All of that lost weight is water loss, so drink that much back."

Dr. Raven, an expert on exercising in heat and humidity, also recommends you *not* wear a hat (unless you're bald and worried about skin cancer from sun exposure). "If you cover your head, you trap a lot of heat that should escape—so you'll feel even hotter," he says. "And also wear light-colored clothing made of natural fibers to absorb your sweat."

Warning: "Any time you feel a headache at your temples when you're running or doing any other exercise in the heat, stop *immediately*," he adds. This early warning sign of heat exhaustion tells you to immediately stop working and find someplace cool to relax.

He also suggests running in the morning rather than the evening. "Although it's more humid in the morning, temperatures tend to be cooler—and that will make you feel better. Also, there's less carbon monoxide and ozone pollution, which is bad for your heart and lungs, in the morning."

Running in the winter poses its own set of challenges, but it's no time to cut back on water. "In fact, proper hydration may be even *more* important during the cold because you're leaving a dry house (and a heated house has the same relative humidity as the Sahara)," says Jennifer Stone, head athletic trainer at the U.S. Olympic Training Center in Colorado's frigid Rocky Mountain high country. Again, drink 8 to 10 ounces of water before running and at least that much upon returning.

But don't overdress. "It's always better to wear less than more," says Stone. "In fact, if you're warm when you leave the house, you're wearing too much." In winter, wearing dark-colored clothes will help to absorb what heat the sun has to offer. If you plan on an easy pace, make sure you wear a couple of layers of clothing—that way the outer layer will trap heat.

Always cover your extremities: Use a knit ski cap for your head and socks or mittens for your hands (mittens are suggested instead of gloves because they keep the fingers together, conserving body heat). "Avoid cotton T-shirts if you can, since they absorb sweat," says Stone. "Fabrics like polypropylene are better—at least for the layer that's against your skin."

TUNE IN . . . WORK OUT . . . GO DEAF?

Although stereo headsets have become as much a part of the modern-day runner's uniform as high-priced shoes (*never* call them "sneakers"), some research suggests that listening to music during a run can destroy your hearing.

While nobody disputes that music can pump you up for a better workout, it takes only about 15 minutes of listening to a headset stereo at full volume to cause certain kinds of hearing damage, says audiologist Richard Navarro, Ph.D. The effects are *compounded* during aerobic exercise such as running.

"Noise itself triggers a release of adrenaline in your body, which causes a constriction of blood supply to your ears and diverts it to the arms, legs, and heart as a part of our 'fight-or-flight' response," he says. "On top of that, when you do aerobic exercise, it diverts blood from the ears to those extremities—the parts of the body needing the greatest amount of nutrients."

Although *either* exercise or noise can restrict blood flow to the inner ear—affecting hearing—together they cause quicker and more damaging results. This one-two punch causes some of the 17,000 hair cells in the inner ear to swell and eventually fall out.

"A Swedish study found you *double* the risk of hearing loss when you combine aerobic exercise and loud noise," says Dr. Navarro.

Another problem: Many people who exercise with stereo headsets keep the music loud. "At full volume, that's like standing next to a shotgun blast," says Dr. Navarro.

His advice: If you must have your tunes when tuning your body, don't use stereo headsets for more than one hour a day at no more than half volume (a 5 on a 10-volume control). And believe it or not, you should stick with cheaper models, which aren't as loud as the more expensive types.

---

pain in the front of the legs between the knees and ankles, says Dr. Ellis. "It usually results from wearing a too-stable running shoe, so one answer is to get different shoes, with more cushioning," he says. To prevent shin splints he suggests a little walking—but you have to do it on your heels. "Walk on your heels with your toes held upward off the ground," he explains. "I suggest taking 50 steps, with toes up and outward like a duck, and with toes up and inward *after* running." (See "Shin Splints" on page 291.)

More seasoned runners frequently get plantar fasciitis, in which the tough tissue between your heel and the base of the toes

tears. "This is marked by pain in the arch, or a pain in the heel that feels like a stone or bone bruise," adds Dr Ellis. His Rx: more support in your shoes. In the meantime, you can apply an ice pack for 15 to 20 minutes to help relieve the pain.

A good way to avoid these and other common running injuries—including cramps, side stitches, and muscle strains—is to stretch *after* running. "A common misconception is that you should stretch *before* a run," says Dr. Ellis. "Warm-ups are for getting the muscles ready to run. You stretch to make the muscles longer, and that's done best when they're full of blood—after a workout." (See "Stretching" on page 440.)

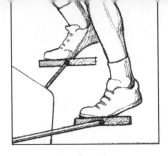

Stair Climbing

*I*f the words "stair climbing" conjure up visions of trudging up flight after flight because the elevator has broken—you're missing out on a hot new fitness trend.

The stair-climbing machine—which not only allows you to climb and climb without going anywhere but cajoles you along with flashy electronic displays—is *the* hottest trend in exercise equipment. At gyms and fitness centers, folks are lining up to use these machines.

So what's the appeal? Stair climbing gives a great workout in a short amount of time, with less jarring, bouncing, or pounding than other forms of exercise.

"It's one of the very few high-intensity, low-impact workouts around," says Craig Cisar, Ph.D., professor of exercise physiology at San Jose State University in California.

And seniors ranging in age from 70 to 89 who are using the machines in a study being conducted at the University of Florida in Gainesville report that stair climbing is, well, *fun*.

Step Up to a Fast-Paced Workout

For many folks, the allure of the stair-climber is simply that it delivers a good workout in so little time. In terms of cardiovascular conditioning, 12 minutes on a stair-climber equals a 20-minute run, according to Bob Goldman, D.O., Ph.D., president of the National Academy of Sports Medicine, director of sports medicine research at the Chicago College of Osteopathic Medicine, and director of the High Technology Fitness Research Institute in Chicago. Looked at another way, working out for 9 to 13 minutes three times a week on a climber gives you the same cardiovascular benefits as walking for 45 minutes *five times* a week.

How much energy you burn depends on the intensity level at which you set the machine—how vigorously you climb. But at a moderate setting, a 150-pound person can expect to burn about 230 calories in a 20-minute workout. That's about the same amount that you'd burn playing squash or running for the same amount of time—but with much less trauma to your joints. And the more intensely you climb, the more calories you burn.

But while you *can* get an intense workout, you don't have to. Your workout depends on how you set the machine and how long and intensely you use it. While die-hard athletes swear by the stair-climber as a conditioning tool, it has also been used to help rehabilitate people who have had reconstructive knee surgery or cardiac arrest.

A Whole-Body Tune-Up

Stair-climbers give an excellent lower-body workout, exercising large muscle groups in the back, buttocks, and lower legs—but without the pounding of jogging or walking. Combined with light upper-body work, you can tune your entire body. In a study at a YMCA in Quincy, Massachusetts, previously sedentary adults used stair-climbers three days a week for 15 minutes, followed by 5 minutes of chin-ups and other exercises for the upper body. After eight weeks, their leg and upper-body strength had greatly increased, along with their cardiovascular endurance—*plus* they lost an average of 3 pounds of fat and gained 2 pounds of muscle.

For people over 65, there can be other benefits, says Cedric X. Bryant, Ph.D., director of geriatric research and sports medicine at Randal Sports/Medical Products in Kirkland, Washington. He notes that balance problems in older adults are often related to muscle weakness in their legs. "The stair-climber can help a person regain functional strength of the lower extremity, which should improve gait, balance, and ultimately functional mobility," he says.

And because your bones must bear your weight during stair climbing, says Dr. Bryant, this low-impact activity can help build stronger bones without putting your musculoskeletal system at risk.

Meet the Stair-Climber

Before taking up climbing, you should get an all-clear from your doctor. And although most climbers are easy to use, Dr. Bryant recommends that you have some-one give you a brief orientation before you climb aboard. Tips from a pro can make a big difference when you're starting out. "The one cue we've found that makes the greatest difference is telling people to think in terms of stepping up as opposed to stepping down," says Dr. Bryant.

Your first encounter with a stair-climbing machine and what may seem like a rocket control panel may leave you in awe. But don't be intimidated—computerized climbers are easy to use, and all that information *does* have a purpose.

The StairMaster 4000 PT, a model you'll find in many health clubs, offers eight preprogrammed workouts, each with ten levels of intensity, plus a nonprogrammed workout. These machines also give you plenty of information about what's going on during your workout—including the number of calories burned, miles traveled, floors climbed, and steps per minute.

But stair-climbers, like most pieces of exercise equipment, vary greatly in design. The first climbers, back in 1983 when these things first hit the market, resembled bulky mini-escalators, with stairs that revolved on a treadmill.

Some of these machines are still around, but most modern versions are smaller, with just one step for each foot. Some climbers offer an upper-body workout, with shoulder-height handles you work as if you were climbing a ladder or levers in front of you that you push and pull.

Taking the First Step

Before you begin climbing, you'll need to adjust the machine properly. Adjustments vary from machine to machine, but you should be able to adjust both resistance and step height. On computerized climbers, this is easy. The machine will ask you to pick an exercise level, and the height of the steps is determined by how far down you push when you step.

Ready to go? Most computerized stair-climbers have built-in warm-up sessions, but it's best to warm up a bit before that. Five to 10 minutes of stretching and warming up before getting on is a good idea, says Dr. Bryant—and he also recommends a 5-minute cool-down once you're off the machine. Moderate to brisk walking can serve as both a warm-up and a cool-down.

For a beginning workout, climb only 15 minutes at a time—or less, depending on what you're comfortable with. As you build endurance and strength, slowly work up to a maximum of 30 to 40 minutes.

Finally, check your heart rate about midway into your workout to ensure that you're staying within your target heart rate zone. (See "How Good Is Your Workout?" on page 324.)

While climbing, there are two things to watch out for. First, keep your body erect, not bent. Leaning over and resting your weight on your hands can overstress both your wrists and your lower back. And make sure you don't grip and pull on the handles, says Dr. Bryant—this can cause a short-term elevation in blood pressure.

Feeling a bit stiff after a session or two? Don't worry—a bit of discomfort is normal if you're just starting an exercise program, says Willibald Nagler, M.D., physiatrist-in-chief at New York Hospital–Cornell Medical Center in New York City. "But if it continues throughout your workout or

grows progressively worse, then you should stop and try again later," he advises. Likewise, if you experience shortness of breath, dizziness, or chest pain, or if you become so tired you're losing your balance, discontinue the exercise and consult your physician.

A Climber of Your Own

So you've tried it, and you love climbing so much you want a machine of your own.

Be forewarned that climbers like the flashy models in your health club will cost you a pretty penny: $2,000 and up. While you can get workable models for less, avoid bargain-basement climbers, advises Patrick Netter, home exercise equipment expert and author of *Patrick Netter's High-Tech Fitness.* You want a machine that feels solid and doesn't wobble. You may also want enough electronic feedback, such as time, distance, and calories burned, to keep you motivated.

Before you go out shopping, realize that stair-climbers operate in one of three ways: via hydraulic pistons, air resistance, or computer. Air resistance machines will probably feel better than ones operated by hydraulics.

Computer-operated climbers, which start around $2,000, are the machines of choice—if you can afford them. One drawback of most machines that cost less is that their steps don't rotate to stay parallel to the floor as you climb. This can stress your knee by forcing it too far out over your toes, according to Michael D. Wolf, Ph.D., president of Fitness Technologies in New York City.

A big advantage of the more expensive machines is simply their high-tech flavor—

which offers a psychological advantage when it comes to motivating yourself to *use* the machine, points out David Webb, M.D., associate director of St. Francis Memorial Hospital for Sports Medicine in San Francisco.

"For a lot of people, the computerized feedback is very encouraging," says Dr. Webb. "They can see how well they've performed. They can say to themselves, 'Hey, look, I've climbed ten more flights of stairs today than last month.' "

The best way to select? Try out machines in gyms before deciding.

The Real Thing

So you don't have access to a gym or health club with a stair-climber? And you don't like the idea of planting your very own climber smack in the middle of your living room?

Yes, you *can* use the steps in your home or office building. There are, however, a few drawbacks.

First is that what goes up must come down. "Walking or running down real steps is tough on your knees," says Dr. Cisar. Studies have shown that descending stairs places significantly more force on your knees than ascending.

"Going down stairs is harder on your tendons and joints because there's a greater tension when the muscles act as brakes against gravity," says Dr. Webb. "Your knees could buckle on the way down." For these reasons, he says, a stair-climbing machine is better than your own stairs.

Descending stairs also burns off one-third fewer calories than climbing up and can cause sore legs from the force of descending.

If you want to work out on your stairs, take the same precautions as with stair-climbers—check with your doctor, and be sure to warm up and cool down. To get the most out of stair climbing, Dr. Nagler suggests that you hold your hands behind your back while climbing so you don't end up pulling yourself along by the bannister. (But if you don't have excellent balance, keep one hand lightly on the hand rail.) As you climb, be sure the balls of your feet touch the step first, and allow your heels to sink slightly. Step slowly and carefully.

To start out, climb a flight of about 12 steps three or four times. Once that routine becomes easy, then slowly increase your speed and the number of flights you climb.

An alternative that will greatly lessen the strain of going down stairs is using just one stair for your workouts, says Dr. Webb. "You're eliminating the high-impact descent," he explains. "You're descending, but you're not building up a head of steam."

Step up with your right foot, then bring your left foot up beside it. Then step down with the right foot, and then with the left. Do this slowly for 5 to 10 minutes, says Dr. Webb.

After two weeks of three to five weekly sessions, increase your time to 15 minutes, and after two more weeks, increase it to 20.

IS CLIMBING FOR YOU?

Stair climbing is a great exercise—but it's not for everybody.

If you're more than slightly overweight, for instance, you may want to approach stair climbing with caution. While you *can* use a climber safely, you should check your heart rate early into your workout—as well as midway into your session—to ensure that you're not overexerting yourself.

A study at the University of Texas found that some overweight users of a StairMaster climber—who ranged from 140 to 280 percent of their ideal body weight—reached their maximum heart rate just 5 minutes into a 20-minute session.

And while climbers are used to help rehabilitate knee injuries, they aren't for everyone with knee problems. Climbing places stresses on the knees that may aggravate certain knee problems, according to James M. Fox, M.D., author of *Save Your Knees.* He recommends strengthening thigh muscles *before* starting a stair-climbing program.

Because of those forces on your knees, certain stair-climbers can cause joint trauma in some users, says Cedric X. Bryant, Ph.D., director of geriatric research and sports medicine at Randal Sports/Medical Products in Kirkland, Washington. The potential for problems, however, can be greatly minimized by using a machine with an *independent* stepping action, with steps operating independently of one another, says Dr. Bryant. With a dependent system, the action of one step causes the opposite reaction in the other, which can be harder on your joints.

Finally, climbing can cause a rapid elevation in blood pressure—so if you have high blood pressure, this may not be a good exercise for you. If in doubt, check with your doctor.

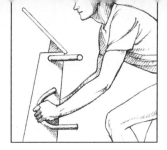

Stationary Bicycling

Stationary bikes. "Ho hum," you say to yourself. You remember trying one years ago. Your legs hurt, your seat hurt, you were soon huffing and puffing for breath, and—worst of all—you were just plain bored stiff.

Well, times have changed, and so have stationary bikes. The newest models are designed with not only fitness in mind but also comfort and *entertainment.* The latest and greatest (and most expensive) offer computer screens featuring scenery, opponents to race with, a running tally of calories burned, and individually designed workouts.

But even if you're the proud owner of a department store special—the kind that all too frequently ends up sitting unused in the corner and serving as a clothes rack—there are still ways to make your workout more comfortable and entertaining. "But why bother?" you ask.

The Beauty of Bicycling

The stationary bicycle has two enormous advantages. For one thing it's, well . . . stationary. You can sit in your living room and pedal away while the wind howls and the snow flies outside. There is no traffic to battle, no dog nipping at your heels, and no chance of

getting a flat tire far from home.

The other advantage it shares with its mobile cousin, the bicycle, is that both provide an excellent workout: They can help you lose weight, tone muscle, and improve your cardiovascular and aerobic fitness.

"The beauty of cycling is that the seat supports most of your torso weight, so there's none of the pounding on your lower joints you can get from jogging or even walking," points out Thomas C. Namey, M.D., chief of the divisions of rheumatology and sports medicine at the University of Tennessee Graduate School of Medicine in Knoxville. This makes biking particularly ideal for people who are overweight or have mild hip, knee, or ankle problems.

Studies show that people with arthritis who participate in bicycling programs experience improved muscle strength and aerobic capacity, as well as reduced joint pain and fatigue. Even people with heart disease and those recovering from knee surgery have benefited from stationary bike workouts.

"It can be better than walking or jogging," says exercise physiologist Scott Bonzheim, with St. Joseph Mercy Hospital in Pontiac, Michigan.

Okay, you're convinced, and you're ready to rush out and buy a stationary bike. Hold on a bit. You'll find a multitude of choices—a dazzling array ranging from an el cheapo model for $79 to a bells-and-whistles version that runs more than $4,000. And there are a lot of options in between.

The major difference in bikes, besides price, is the type of resistance mechanism (control of pedaling tension). Bikes under $400 usually feature either brake-pad or strap resistance. Brake-pad resistance involves brakes or pads that apply varying degrees of pressure to a moving flywheel. Strap resistance uses a nylon strap that loosens or tightens around a moving flywheel to vary resistance. Generally, the heavier the flywheel, the smoother the ride.

More expensive bikes employ either air resistance with a fan-type flywheel or computer-controlled electromagnetic resistance, which is by far the smoothest.

First things first: Decide how much to spend. If money's no object, go for whatever features really appeal to you. "You need everything motivating on your side," says Patrick Netter, home exercise equipment expert and author of *Patrick Netter's High-Tech Fitness*. But no matter what, says Netter, avoid the bottom-of-the-line specials—you don't want to end up with a bike that's cheaply made, wobbly, and noisy.

Experts agree it's best to buy your bike at a store that specializes in exercise equipment—one with knowledgeable salesclerks.

"If they don't ask you a series of questions—such as who's going to use the bike and whether you have any physical limitations—it's probably not the right shop for you," says Netter.

"I'd go to a place that has the bike in the shop and ride it before buying. There's no shortcut to trying it out," advises Morris Mellion, M.D., medical director of the Sports Medicine Center and clinical associate professor at the University of Nebraska Medical Center, both in Omaha.

In general, you want the smoothest, quietest ride on the sturdiest bike you can afford. No matter what the price, however, the bike should have an adjustment device that lets you vary resistance easily and precisely, while riding. It should also give you some feedback so you can gauge your workouts—preferably distance covered, resistance level, speed, time, and calories expended.

Test-ride the seat and handlebars for comfort and adjustability. Once adjusted, make sure they stay locked in place. Pedals should be sturdy, with a nonslip surface. Quality bikes will have at least a one-year warranty.

Taking It Lying Down

You may want to choose a recumbent or semirecumbent bicycle. These have seats that support your back and allow you to pedal with your legs stretched out in front of you. (On a recumbent, your legs are parallel to the floor, while on semi-recumbents your rear end is 6 to 12 inches higher than your outstretched legs.) Recent studies have shown many advantages to these types of bikes.

"We found that people enjoyed the bike more because of the wider seat, the more comfortable back, and the arm support," says Bonzheim, who tested 14 men with heart disease (with an average age of 60) on both upright and recumbent stationary bicycles. He found that recumbent riders had lower blood pressure than cyclists doing the same workout on upright bikes.

For older cyclists, the recumbent position offers another advantage: Because your legs are nearly horizontal, you're less likely to suffer blood pooling and swelling in your legs, says Bob Goldman, D.O., Ph.D., president of the National Academy of Sports Medicine. Cyclists are also less likely to have pain in their buttocks and lower back on a recumbent or semirecumbent, he says.

There are other advantages as well. "You can more easily relax and watch TV while you're cycling, so you can stay for an extended period of time," says Dr. Goldman. And some people prefer the recumbents because they're lower and easier to climb onto, Bonzheim points out.

Other Ways to Pedal

There are still other choices, such as dual-action bikes equipped with arm levers as well as pedals so you can work both arms and legs. A total-body workout is important for people with arthritis, says Dr. Namey. "On a dual-action bike you spread the work around—you don't let one problematic joint limit you," he says. A word of caution: On some models the action of pedals and levers isn't well coordinated, and you may bang your shins, notes Michael D. Wolf, Ph.D., president of Fitness Technologies in New York City. And dual-action bikes do tend to be noisier. (All the more reason to try the bike before you write that check.)

If you have an outdoor bicycle, consider buying a wind trainer, a device you mount your bicycle onto so you can ride it indoors. They're relatively inexpensive, and most closely simulate outdoor cycling. "This is the best choice for a low-budget person," Dr. Namey declares. You can get a decent wind trainer for $89, he says—but not a good stationary bike.

Obviously, the better the bike, the more pleasant and enticing your workout. But if you're determined, you *can* make do with a basic stationary bike, as long as it's sturdy. And these abound at garage sales and in attics. Diane Fellers, a teacher in Clinton, Tennessee, got a seldom-used 20-year-old exercise bike free from a neighbor. After investing $25 in a special saddle that supports each buttock separately, she has a functional bike she rides faithfully 30 minutes a day.

Ready to Roll

Now you've got your bike and you're rarin' to go. Not so fast! This is where you can make mistakes that could sour you on biking forever.

Think about clothing. Comfort is the key, and dressing in layers so you can shed clothes as you warm up is best, advises Lisa Sassano, director of Village Commons Health and Racquet in Cutchogue, New York. Be sure to avoid pants with heavy seams—by the end of your ride you'll be feeling every stitch.

Now for form. Many people err by setting the seat too low and by pedaling with their heels instead of the balls of their feet. Studies have shown that both make bicycling tiring and ineffective.

To find the right seat height, hop on,

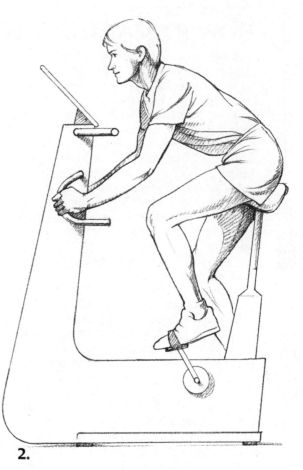

2.

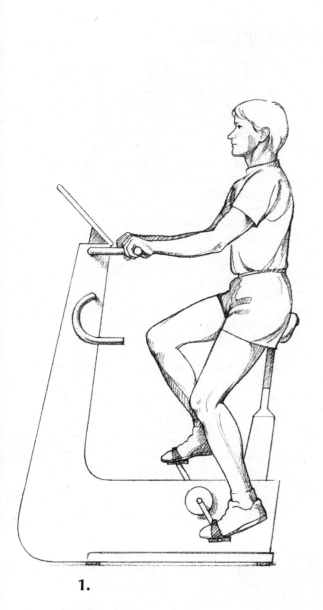

1.

Riding position is as important on a stationary bike as it is on a road bike. (1) Make sure your saddle is the right height (your knee should have only a slight bend at the bottom of the downstroke), and when you pedal, sit erect and keep your head up. (2) If your bike offers the option of double or adjustable handlebars, don't curve your back when you lean over to use the handlebars in the lower position; lean straight from the hips.

HOW TO BEAT THOSE BOREDOM BLUES

Yes, time can drag endlessly when you're sitting there churning your legs around and staring at your living room wall.

But it doesn't have to.

If you don't have a fancy computerized bike that helps entertain you, find your own entertainment—whether reading, watching TV or travel videos, knitting, or keeping track of your mileage.

"Whatever you would do sitting down, do on your stationary bike," advises Lisa Sassano, director of Village Commons Health and Racquet in Cutchogue, New York.

The creative solutions for getting through that workout are endless.

Karla Kurz, a partner in a film production company in Los Angeles, receives piles of catalogs and magazines—and saves them all for her cycling sessions. "I don't let myself look through them until I get on the bike," she says. "It makes the time go by really fast. I'll look down, and I'll already have gotten through 5 or 6 miles."

Morris Mellion, M.D., of Omaha, an avid outdoor cyclist when the weather allows, keeps his stationary bike sessions interesting by reading books for pleasure—something his busy schedule wouldn't allow him to do otherwise.

And there's always the TV. "You're going to watch a few hours of TV a day, so you might as well get something out of it," says Bob Goldman, D.O., Ph.D., of Chicago.

One woman in Brooklyn bones up on her Spanish by watching Spanish-channel soap operas on television. She also follows the calorie countdown as she pedals. "I've given up potato chips since I've seen how long it takes to ride them off," she says.

Maria Israel, a homemaker in Raleigh, North Carolina, plants herself, her wind trainer, *and* her active and demanding four-year-old in front of the television set seven days a week. Together they watch a half-hour cartoon as Maria pedals away.

Thomas C. Namey, M.D., a long-time cyclist in Knoxville, Tennessee, recommends working out with friends—with the help of a VCR and some bike touring videos.

"Pretend you're in Hawaii riding down a mountain," he suggests.

Or you can take the reward approach. A group of California women keep track of the calories they burn while cycling. At lunch afterward, they treat themselves to desserts—and the more calories they've burned, the richer and gooier the desserts they order.

---

pedal with the balls of your feet, and stop with one foot down. There should be a slight bend in your knee (about 10 to 15 degrees), says Dr. Mellion. If you aren't sure the seat's high enough, raise it another notch. You'll know when you've gone too far, he says: "Your knees will get really straight, and you'll have to rock from side to side to pedal."

The seat should be level or nearly so (some people prefer it tilted a bit up or down). You should be able to reach the handlebars comfortably by leaning forward slightly—with your back straight, not curved.

Don't jump on and start hammering away. A common mistake is to start off with the resistance too high, which can wreak havoc with your knees—not to mention your resolve. Beginners should ride 10 to 15 minutes, three times a week, with very little resistance, suggests Dr. Mellion. Begin by trying to pedal 40 to 45 revolutions per minute for the first few minutes, increase to 60 to 80 rpm, and then finish off with several minutes of cool-down at 45 rpm.

Make sure, however, that you don't pass 70 percent of your maximum heart rate during the warm-up phase. (To calculate your target heart rate, see "How Good Is Your Workout?" on page 324.) When you're just starting out, check your pulse after just 1 minute of warm-up, says Dr. Namey. "You may be surprised to see that it's already too fast," he says, "or conversely, it may not have budged."

Your goal should be to ride a minimum of 20 minutes three times a week, always with warm-up and cool-down periods of 2 to 5 minutes. As you become fitter, you may want to increase your workouts to 30 to 60 minutes by adding 5 minutes to each workout every week. If you're within your heart rate guidelines and still want a tougher workout, advises Dr. Mellion, increase your rpm or increase the resistance.

Finally, you can find all kinds of special goodies for you and your bike—book rack, seat cover with gel inserts, padded cycling shorts and gloves, and more. (Why should the outdoor bicyclists keep all those wonderful accessories for themselves?) The general rule is: Treat yourself to whatever it takes to make your workouts interesting and comfortable.

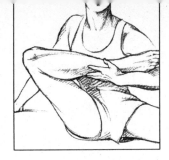

Stretching

Although it sometimes seems as if the gap between inactivity and fitness is wider than the Mississippi River, you *can* cross over to a more vigorous life. You just have to build a bridge.

"Stretching is the bridge from a sedentary to an active life. If you're sedentary and you want to start an exercise program, stretching is the way to do it," says Bob Anderson, author of the now-classic book *Stretching*. Anderson has taught his techniques to thousands of athletes, including Olympic competitors and National Football League players.

Despite what you might think, stretching isn't a torture invented by an evil physical education teacher. Instead, it's an easy way of preventing injuries, improving your physical performance, and maintaining range of motion in your joints. That, in turn, probably will encourage you to try more strenuous exercises.

"There's absolutely no doubt that stretching can improve your physical performance," says Chuck Corbin, Ph.D., a professor of exercise science and physical education at Arizona State University in Tempe. "If you don't have flexibility, you can't do any sport that demands a significant range of motion. But no matter who you are, you're probably better off if you stretch than if you don't."

Even if you're not doing it to prepare yourself for exercise or sports, just doing a few stretches every day can help keep your body limber throughout your life, says Anderson.

"Some people have what I call creeping rigor mortis," he says. "They get stiffer and stiffer throughout their life. I don't think you necessarily have to get stiff as you age. As long as you challenge yourself by stretching daily, you can maintain the flexibility that you have today for a very long time."

Stretching also can relieve stress and have a profound effect on your mood, says Dean Ornish, M.D., director of the Preventive Medicine Research Institute in Sausalito, California.

"Stretching can help you feel more peaceful and relaxed," he says. "Just as your mind affects your body, so can your body affect the mind."

Reach for the Sky

The beauty of stretching is that it can be done almost anywhere.

"I try to make stretching accessible to people even at their most sedentary times, like watching television or sitting in an airport," Anderson says.

"Sometimes people will tell me that they wake up and their muscles feel very tight. I'll tell them that they should do a few stretches before they get out of bed."

Two stretches that Anderson believes are particularly useful are the knee-to-chest stretch and the upward reach side stretch (see the illustrations on pages 446 amd 447.)

"I think those two stretches complement each other very nicely," he says. "The knee-to-chest is good for hip and knee flexion. The other stretch will elongate parts of your body—such as the back, legs, and feet—that tend to get cramped up and lose flexibility."

Other experts say stretching the lower back is important because most Americans have weak, tension-ridden muscles in that area of their body.

One good exercise to strengthen that area is called the lotus, says William Cornelius, Ph.D., an associate professor of physical education at the University of North Texas in Denton. (This easy stretch should not be confused with yoga's famous pretzel-legged meditation posture of the same name.) To perform the lotus, lie on your stomach. Then without straining, prop up your upper body on your elbows and forearms for support. You should feel your lower back arch a bit. Hold that position for 10 to 20 seconds. Repeat two or three times, says Dr. Cornelius.

Out of Bounds

There are numerous safe and healthy stretches for the lower back, and for every other part of the body as well. (See the illustrations on page 443.)

When stretching, however, you do need to take some precautions. You should only do "static" stretches that require you to reach out and hold a position for several seconds. Bouncing stretches—such as reaching down and touching the floor several times in rapid succession—can trigger a reflex mechanism that will actually tighten the muscles you're trying to stretch.

"'A person who doesn't have good muscle tone is more likely to tear a muscle by sudden bouncing movements," says Peter Francis, Ph.D., a professor of biomechanics at San Diego State University and coauthor of *If It Hurts, Don't Do It.*

Don't stretch in ways that force the joints beyond their normal range of motion, Dr. Francis says. Pressing a joint too far actually weakens the ligaments around it.

In the traditional hurdler's stretch, for example, one leg is extended while the lower portion of the opposite leg is bent outward, away from the body, with the sole of the foot pointing away. That kind of stretch puts an unnatural strain on the knee, Dr. Cornelius says.

"You're stretching the inside of the knee, and there's no reason to do that," he says. "It just makes the knee less stable. If you're doing an exercise like that, you're doing something wrong."

A safer stretch, which is also designed to reach the large muscles of the thighs, can be substituted for the hurdler's stretch. (See the illustration on page 444.) Hold for about 10 seconds, then switch legs.

Stretching Your Goals

Once you've made stretching a part of your daily routine, you might want to use it as a foundation for more vigorous exercise.

But remember, while you may not need to do any elaborate warm-up if you're just going to stretch, you probably should include 5 minutes or so of an activity such as walking or slow jogging to warm the muscles before you stretch. And a brief warm-up followed by a stretch is excellent preparation for strenuous exercise such as running.

"For the average inactive person, a good warm-up is essential before stretching and vigorous activity," Dr. Francis says. "Warming up lubricates the muscles and prepares them for a good workout." To get the best results, Dr. Francis suggests stretching before *and* after your workout.

"If you stretch beforehand, you're better prepared to achieve the range of motion that the activity requires," he says. "If you stretch afterward, when the muscles have been worked out, you will make a good contribution to maintaining the long-term elasticity of those muscles."

Every Day and in Every Way

Whether you're preparing to exercise or just trying to improve your mobility, remember to do a variety of stretches. You also should stretch as often as possible, preferably every day, Dr. Cornelius says.

"You have to do stretching exercise for all the joints in your body," he says. "One stretch doesn't stretch your whole body. If you only do one stretch, that doesn't mean you're a flexible person. It only means that you're flexible in that one joint."

"It's important to do general types of stretching for any activity," Anderson agrees. "For cycling, for example, you need to stretch your lower back and quadriceps [the large muscles in the front of the thighs]. But if you think about it, you'd realize that you should stretch your neck, shoulders, and hip flexors, too. You don't want to have a stiff neck in any sport. If I have a stiff neck, I'm not going to run or cycle very well, am I?"

Finally, be patient and don't overdo it. It took months, possibly years, for your muscles to become as tight as they are, so it will take some time for them to become more flexible, Dr. Francis says.

In other words, you shouldn't try to do too much too soon. "Some people have the attitude that the farther you go, the better; if it hurts, it must be good," Anderson says. "We'd be much better off if we treated ourselves like racehorses. Horse trainers warm those horses up, cool them down, and generally treat them very well. But we don't do that for ourselves because we're not taught the value of stretching.

"Animals like cats and dogs stretch naturally, and it's natural to us, too. We just don't think of it that way," he says. (Also see "Yoga" on page 480.)

Get the Lead Out

Whether you're sitting at your desk or preparing for a long morning run, stretching should be an important part of your daily routine.

Here are a few stretches to get you started. They are easy to do, they require no special clothing or equipment, and they can be done almost anywhere.

Many experts suggest that you do 3 to 5 minutes of walking or slow jogging to warm up your muscles before you stretch. Be gentle with your body, and don't try to stretch your muscles more than feels comfortable for you.

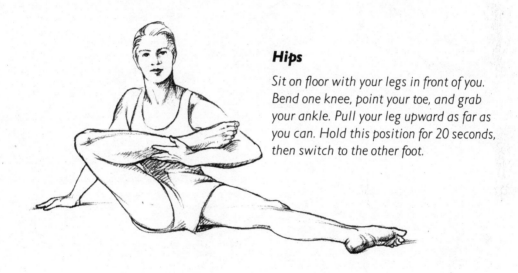

Hips

Sit on floor with your legs in front of you. Bend one knee, point your toe, and grab your ankle. Pull your leg upward as far as you can. Hold this position for 20 seconds, then switch to the other foot.

Lie on your back, bend your knees, and place the soles of your feet together. Use your hip muscles to slowly push your knees to the floor. Hold for 30 seconds.

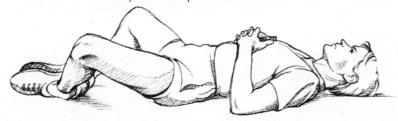

Get the Lead Out—Continued

Legs and Hips

Sit on the floor with your legs spread as far as feels comfortable. Keep your knees straight. With your back straight, lean over one leg, reaching your hands out toward your toes. Hold this position for 10 to 20 seconds. Repeat to the other side.

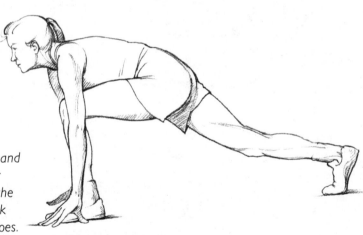

Step forward with one foot and bend that knee. Place your hands on the floor next to the front foot. Extend your back foot until you are on your toes. Gradually lower your body until you feel a stretching sensation along the back of your thigh and in the groin area. Hold for 10 to 20 seconds, then switch feet. Hint: Keep your forward knee directly above your forward foot.

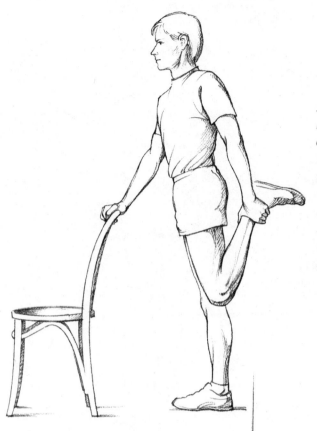

Stand on your right foot (if you need additional support, hold on to a wall or chair). Bend your left leg and grab your left ankle with your left hand. Hold for 10 to 20 seconds. Then repeat on right side. Warning: Your foot should never be pulled all the way up to your buttocks but should be held at least 12 inches away. Don't let your knee sway outward in back. Instead, try to keep it straight in line with your body.

Calves

Stand about 3 feet away from a wall with your feet pointing straight. Step forward with one foot, keeping the other foot back. Allow the knee of the front leg to bend. Lean forward as far as comfortable, keeping your heel on the floor, and feel the stretch in your calf and Achilles tendon. Hold for 10 to 20 seconds. When you become more flexible, try standing farther away from the wall.

Get the Lead Out—Continued

Back

For this upper-body stretch, stand with your back to a wall and 1 to 2 feet away. Your feet should be shoulder-width apart and your toes pointed straight. Slowly turn your upper body around until you can touch the wall with your hands at about shoulder height. Turn in one direction, hold for 10 to 20 seconds, then turn in the other direction. Do this stretch slowly and cautiously if you have knee or back problems.

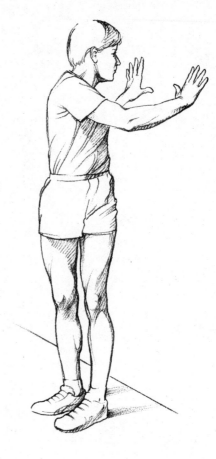

To do this stretch, which affects the lower back and hip muscles, lie on your back and bring one knee up to your chest. Hold for 5 to 10 seconds. Repeat four or five times with each leg.

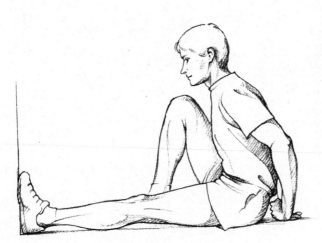

Back and Legs

Sit with one leg extended and your foot flat against a wall. Bend the other leg so that the sole of that foot is close to your buttocks. Clasp your hands behind your back and bend forward. Keep your lower back as straight as possible. Allow the bent knee to move up so your upper body can bend forward to a stretched but comfortable position. Hold for 10 to 20 seconds, then switch legs.

Arms

Get down on the floor on all fours. With your palms flat and your fingers pointed toward your knees, slowly lean backward so that your forearms and wrists are stretched. Hold for about 20 seconds. Be sure to keep your palms flat and don't overstretch.

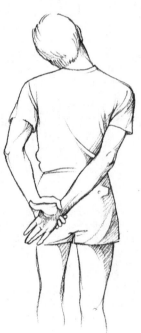

Neck and Shoulders

Hold your right arm behind your back with your left hand. As you lean your head sideways toward your left shoulder, pull your right arm down and across your back. Hold for 10 seconds, then switch and repeat on the opposite side.

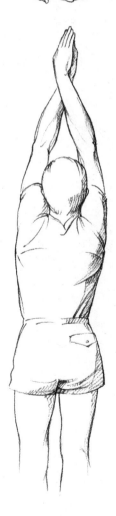

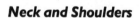

Sides

With your arms extended over your head, place your palms together. Breathe in and stretch your arms upward and slightly backward. Hold for 5 to 8 seconds.

Get the Lead Out—Continued

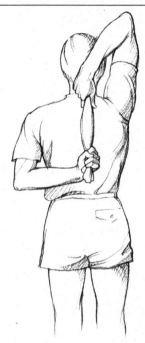

Shoulders

Grasp a towel with your right hand and hold your arm, with your elbow bent, over your head. Dangle the towel behind your back. Grab the other end of the towel with your left hand and pull it taut. Hold for 10 seconds, then switch arms.

Chest

Stand in a doorway with your arms raised to shoulder height and your elbows bent. Grab the door frame with your hands, palms facing away from you. Place one foot in front of the other. Slowly lean forward through the doorway, bending your forward knee. Hold for 10 seconds.

Put your hands shoulder-width apart on a file cabinet, refrigerator, or other ledge. Let your upper body drop as you keep your knees slightly bent. Place your hands at different heights until you find a position you can hold for 30 seconds.

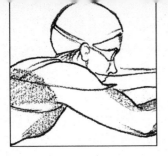

Swimming

Get up at 5:00 A.M. so you can hop in the pool and swim for an hour before work? It may not *sound* enticing, but Scott Petrequin, 60, finds his daily swim gives him more energy, increases his sense of well-being—and even gives him a chance to plan the day's activities as he does his laps.

"After a morning workout I'm particularly productive and energized," says Scott, a vice president at a paper mill in Cohoes, New York. "When I'm traveling I miss it; it throws my rhythm off."

Swimming is not only invigorating, it also gives your muscles, heart, and lungs a great workout. A study of previously inactive, middle-aged adults who participated in 12 weeks of intense swim training showed their oxygen uptake increased an average of 20 percent and their heart pumped more blood with each beat without elevating their blood pressure.

When you're swimming, the buoyancy of the water essentially carries your body weight, supporting your joints and providing a cushion of safety against injury. Not only that, your heart rate is lower when you're swimming than it is during other sports.

For these reasons, medical experts see swimming as a good exercise even for people with arthritis and joint problems as well as for those recovering from heart disease.

If you're looking for an exercise just for weight loss, however, this may not be the best choice. Swimming may stimulate your appetite so that you find yourself *gaining* weight. If you're aiming for weight control, you'll have to watch your portions and possibly increase the intensity of your workouts. (See "In the Swim" on page 255.)

Taking the Plunge

In many respects swimming is an ideal exercise. The problem is that most of us can't just leap into the pool and start churning out laps. You can march down to the local Y with the best of intentions— but if you find yourself gasping for breath after one lap while lithe bodies glide effortlessly past, you probably aren't going to be eager to go back.

The trick is to do some toning up *before* you get into the water, says Jerome Ciullo, M.D., medical director of the Sports Medicine Center of Metro Detroit and clinical assistant professor at Wayne State University Medical School in Detroit. "Don't use swimming to get into shape," he says. "You want to be *capable* of doing the activity you want to participate in."

He recommends walking or riding a stationary bicycle to tone the heart and muscles—that way you'll be fit enough to stay in the water longer when you do get in. "If you can ride a bicycle for 10 or 20 minutes and you feel comfortable doing that, then you're capable of starting swimming and not getting frustrated," he says.

If you're out of shape, you should also have a complete physical before starting swimming, advises Allen B. Richardson, M.D., an orthopedic surgeon, assistant professor of surgery at the University of Hawaii in Honolulu, and chief medical officer for the U.S. Olympic swimming team.

Once you're ready, the rest is easy. All you need to start is a swimsuit (the sleeker and more streamlined, the better), a pair of goggles, and a swim cap.

What Comes Next

Experts recommend stretching before swimming, either in or out of the pool. This warms up muscles to increase blood flow and also increases flexibility.

Good stretches are shoulder rolls, head turns, trunk turns, triceps stretches, and runner's hamstring stretches, says Jane Katz, Ed.D., world masters swimming champion, professor of physical education at the City University of New York, and author of many fitness books. (See "Stretching" on page 440.) She also recommends running in water and doing an arm and leg stretch in the pool. To do this stretch, stand in waist-deep water and grasp the pool edge with your right hand. Raise your right foot to rest on the edge right next to your hand. Now reach with your left arm in an arc toward that foot. Hold, and repeat for the other side. (This particular

stretch requires a fair degree of flexibility. If you can't quite get your foot up there, place your foot at a lower point on the wall.)

Next comes light swimming or easy drills to warm up. "The muscles have to be warmed up gradually," warns Dr. Ciullo. "To exert them suddenly leads to sprain and strain injuries."

You can also use your warm-up period to inventory how you're feeling and see what muscles may be a bit sore, says Terry Laughlin, director of Total Immersion adult swimming camps and publisher of *SwimSmarts,* a newsletter for fitness swimmers.

If all you can do is stretch, warm up, paddle for only a single lap, and then cool down, then that's what you do. "You have to remember you're not competing against anybody else," says Dr. Ciullo. "You're trying to better yourself."

Don't force yourself through a painful or exhausting workout, he advises: If you're too tired, you're going to get hurt. "You do have to exert yourself to make progress, but the old idea of 'no pain, no gain' is ridiculous," he says.

As in other sports, you eventually want to aim at your target heart zone. (See "How Good Is Your Workout?" on page 324.) In swimming, your target heart rate is 10 to 15 percent lower than in other sports. (This means that to calculate your maximum heart rate you should add 13 to your age and then subtract that total from 220. Take 60 to 85 percent of that number to get your target heart rate.)

Good times to check your pulse are after your warm-up, about midway into your

THE WELL-EQUIPPED SWIMMER

Find your workout getting dull? You can enliven your pool time—*and* get a better workout—by using various swim "toys."

First on your list might be a set of fins. These can not only give you extra kick to help you along but also improve the workout your legs get. University of Texas swim coach Mark Schubert has used fins in his team's workouts for years to help build leg strength and endurance.

Many swimmers tend to drag their legs, letting their upper body do all the work. Fins force your legs to work in both directions, working your thigh, calf, and abdominal muscles in the process. They can also make your feet and ankles more flexible and are helpful when you're recovering from knee injuries.

Another handy workout item is the pull-buoy. It consists of two Styrofoam cylinders held together with cords. You place it between your upper legs, and it holds your lower body up in the water—letting you work on your arm stroke without worrying about what your legs are doing. A kickboard is the counterpart of the pull-buoy: a flat piece of Styrofoam you hang on to, to work on your kick.

Hand paddles or webbed gloves increase resistance against the water and are designed to help strengthen your arms. They can also increase the incidence of shoulder problems, however, and in most cases should be avoided, says Allen B. Richardson, M.D., orthopedic surgeon and assistant professor of surgery at the University of Hawaii in Honolulu.

You can purchase any of these items at your local sporting goods store or pool center.

workout, and after your cool-down, says Dr. Katz.

To make your pool time more interesting, you may want to learn different strokes. "Many people think of swimming as the crawl, period," says Dr. Katz. In her book *Swim 30 Laps in 30 Days,* she describes a progressive water exercise and swim program that begins with a 1-lap workout and progresses to 30 laps. It includes learning five strokes: crawl, backstroke, breaststroke, sidestroke, and butterfly, in five progressive levels. Another advantage of knowing other strokes is that each stroke works the muscles in a different way. You can also adapt your workout to rest sore or weary muscles.

Okay, you've got the all-clear from your doctor, and you've walked around the neighborhood briskly every evening to increase your fitness level. What if you *still* find yourself thrashing through the water and gasping for breath?

The problem may not be your fitness level but *how* you're swimming. "I'd say 95 percent of the people who swim are swimming at a novice level," says Laughlin.

Thrashing and Splashing

A common mistake, he says, is an unstreamlined body position, often caused by swinging or jerking the head too much.

Thrashing the arms wildly in the crawl is also common. You can solve this problem by imagining a line down the center of your body and keeping each arm on its side of the line.

Breathing is the most common problem area, says Dr. Katz. Some swimmers hold their breath and haven't gotten the hang of exhaling underwater and forming bubbles so the air exchange is continuous.

If you can't iron out your problems on your own, sign up for lessons. "Some skills are almost impossible to obtain on your own," says Laughlin, who videotapes swimmers underwater to show them stroke problems. Swimming's not like running or biking, he says, where you can improve your skills just by doing the activity. When you swim poorly you just *continue* swimming poorly.

You can also get coaching in masters swim groups, which participate in organized competitive swimming events specifically for those ages 19 and up but exclude current college or senior national-level competitors. An added benefit of masters groups and swim clubs is the social aspect of meeting people and swimming with friends.

Swimmer's Woes

As comfortable a sport as swimming is, things can still go wrong. A classic problem is swimmer's shoulder. This is an overuse injury that's not surprising when you consider that a dedicated swimmer's shoulder may churn through 10,000 revolutions a week.

Improving stroke mechanics may be the key. If you're an experienced, top-notch swimmer, you may be overusing your shoulder muscles rather than rolling enough in the water. If you have inflexible muscles, however, you may well be rolling *too much*—and cheating yourself by not calling more of your muscles into play.

Too much body roll in the crawl is often caused by breathing on the same side all the time, says Dr. Ciullo. "If you use one side, it means you dip down too far, and the other shoulder has to go over a wider arc to hit the water," he says. The solution is simple: Breathe on alternate sides.

Swimmer's ear—a bacterial or fungal infection—is often caused by prolonged immersion in water that washes away protective earwax in your ear canal. The most common symptom of infection is ear pain, but there may also be itching, hearing loss, or discharge from the ear.

If you have an infection, a visit to the doctor is in order. But a few precautions can help prevent the problem. After swimming, tilt your head to either side and jump vigorously to let water run out. You can also gently swab your ears with rubbing alcohol after swimming, or use an over-the-counter preparation of alcohol or glycerin drops.

Ear plugs can help keep the ear dry, notes Dr. Richardson, although standard, commercially available wax-type ones can push ear debris into the ear canal. Silicone plugs are a better choice, according to some doctors. You may want to try cotton wool coated with petroleum jelly, which swimmers in a London study reported to be most efficient, comfortable, and easy to use.

WISE PRECAUTIONS

Even skilled swimmers should always take certain precautions:

- Never swim alone.
- Check water depth.
- Make sure a lifeguard is on duty.
- Listen to your body and stop when you're fatigued.

For outdoor swimming, you must also:

- Check water temperature and roughness.
- Check for obstacles.
- Watch out for undertow and weedy areas.
- Swim parallel to the shore.

Water temperature should also be considered. Swimming in water that's too cold causes you to lose too much heat and stresses your cardiovascular system, according to Dr. Richardson. Water that's too warm, on the other hand, *inhibits* normal loss of body heat and also stresses your system.

Many pools are kept at 80° to 83°F, which requires you to move briskly to stay warm. Most of us can swim comfortably in temperatures of 82° to 86°, but the 92° to 98° temperature of therapeutic pools is designed for limited movement only and is too warm for vigorous swimming.

Protecting Your Body

Pool and ocean water can take their toll on hair, skin, and eyes.

Goggles are a must, says Dr. Richardson. Take the effort to find a pair that fits properly. If you're allergic to rubber goggle rims, there are other versions available.

Wearing either hard or soft contact lenses in water without goggles is a mistake, doctors agree. Hard lenses can easily wash away, while soft lenses can get contaminated, and pool or lake water can actually suck moisture out of them so they stick to the eye.

Leave lenses off, or protect them with goggles. Or you can buy prescription goggles.

Copper in pool water can bond with light-colored hair to turn it a shade of green. Head to the store for special shampoos, or better yet, avoid the problem by using swim caps and hair conditioners. Dr. Katz recommends applying conditioner to your hair tips *before* your swim for extra protection. Always rinse pool or salt water from your hair after swimming.

Both chlorine from pools and salt from the ocean dry out the skin, so shower afterward, and add moisturizer as needed.

Stroking Your Swim

Year after year, in poll after national poll, millions of Americans cite swimming as their favorite exercise. If you want to get the most out of this leisure-time activity, you need to pay attention to some basics.

The best strokes to give you an all-around workout are the crawl (or freestyle), backstroke, breaststroke, and sidestroke. The crawl and backstroke use essentially the same shoulder motion and move you through the water mainly by the action of your arms and forearms. They primarily work your shoulder muscles, as well as those of your chest, upper back, and arms. Your legs don't work as hard, and they take on a secondary role.

The breaststroke uses many of the same muscles, although instead of working the top and back of your upper arm, it hits the front, or biceps. The kick uses the inside of your legs as well as the front and back of the thighs. Your legs will get a good workout, because the stroke uses your arms and legs with about equal intensity.

When you're looking for an easy way to warm up, slow down, or cool down, the sidestroke can't be beat. It won't give you quite the aerobic workout the crawl and backstroke provide, but its gentle movements and long glide periods provide a nice change of pace.

The shaded areas in the illustrations indicate which muscle groups are used during each swim stroke.

Crawl

A common mistake in the crawl is to allow your arms to wallow around underwater. You want to use a clean S-shaped stroke for maximum efficiency.

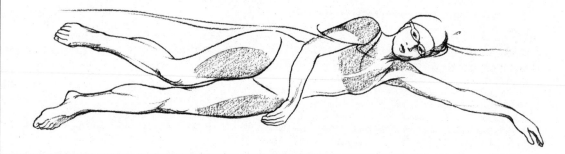

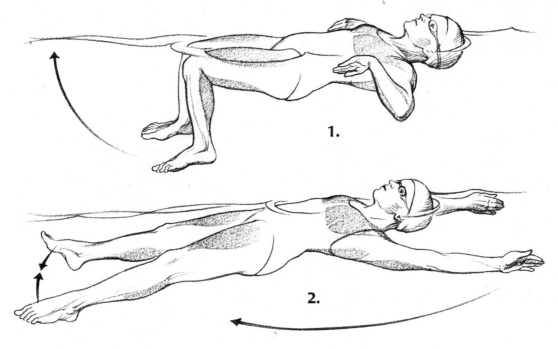

1.

2.

Elementary Backstroke with Whip Kick

There are several varieties of backstroke, depending on how you move your arms and legs. (1) In the elementary backstroke, you pull your arms along the side of your body and use a whip kick. (2) The kick is performed by dropping your heels, spreading your knees apart, and then snapping your ankles and legs together. In another version, you use a flutter kick, like that in the crawl, and windmill your arms through the water.

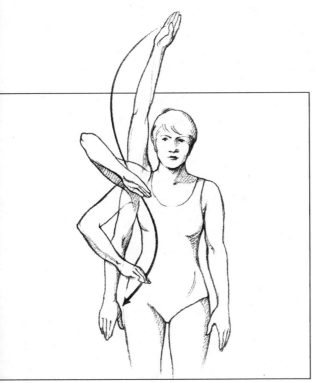

Stroking Your Swim—Continued

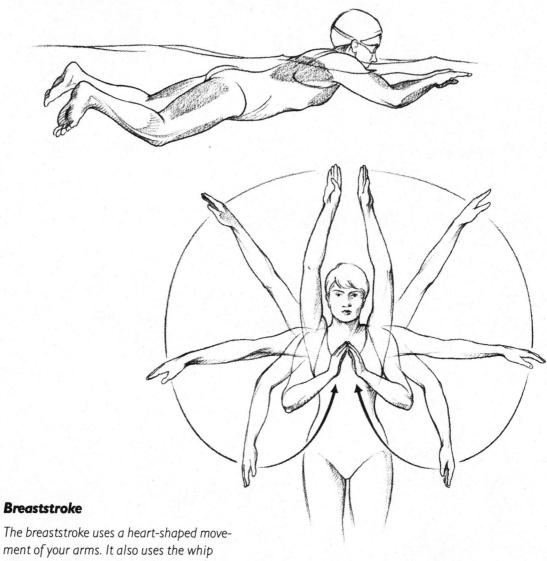

Breaststroke

The breaststroke uses a heart-shaped movement of your arms. It also uses the whip kick, except your knees will drop and separate before you snap your ankles together.

Sidestroke

The sidestroke is especially comfortable, as
your head stays out of the water. (1) This
stroke features a scissor kick, in which your
legs move just like a pair of scissors,
(2) followed by a long, relaxing glide.

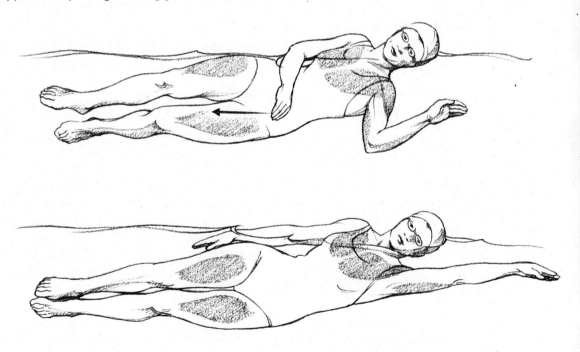

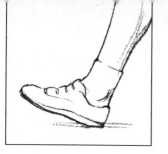

Walking

If a carnival barker at a county fair was promoting walking, you might scoff at his claims.

"Step right up, friends," he would say. "I'm gonna tell you about a miracle of the modern age that is actually a forgotten part of our ancient wisdom. A discovery that will change your life. This potent elixir is more powerful than most prescription drugs. It will help prevent heart disease, control diabetes, lower your blood pressure, relieve depression and anxiety, prevent osteoporosis, and spark creativity.

"It will help you live longer, relieve back pain, combat asthma, increase your immunity, improve your memory, and enhance your self-esteem and your social life. It can make you more energetic, reduce stress, control your weight, relieve PMS, prevent insomnia, and best of all, my friends, improve your sex life.

"It doesn't come in a bottle, and it's not a pill I can sell you . . ."

That's a tall order for something as simple and natural as walking. But you know what? Every single word is true.

"There's absolutely no doubt whatsoever that walking is one of the world's best exercises," says Peter Francis, Ph.D., a professor of biomechanics at San Diego State University. "If you want most of the health benefits of exercise and the least chance of injury, then walking is it."

That's something that ordinary folks all over the country are discovering.

Join the Parade

"I find walking is a joy. I know it's keeping me in extremely good condition for my age," says Fred Pattle, a 70-year-old retired television weatherman in Newport, Oregon.

"If I don't walk, my day is a disaster," says Fred, who walks about 3 miles a day. "I just feel rotten. I need to get out and get my circulatory system going every morning. Walking also relieves stress and depression. When I do it, all that stress and depression just melts away."

And in Palm Desert, California, Dale Warner, a 51-year-old salesman, lost 124 pounds in 18 months, thanks to walking and a low-fat diet. But more important, he dramatically improved his fitness level.

"My [total] cholesterol is now 142, well within the safe range, and my 'good' HDL cholesterol is high," he says. "My blood pressure is much better, too: 130/72. And my resting pulse rate is 50: that of a fit man. At my last visit, my doctor said, 'Walking has changed your life. In fact, I'm sure walking has saved your life, or at least extended it by 20 years.' "

Doctors aren't just delivering that message to their patients. Many of them are living it, too. For example, Neil Block, M.D., who has practiced family medicine in Orangeburg, New York, for more than ten years, not only encourages his patients to walk, he also does it himself.

His walks take him around the neighborhood, a nearby lake, or a local mall. His favorite walking times are before lunch or dinner, but sometimes he heads out the door just before bedtime.

"I not only sleep very well after I've walked, but I'm also able to fall asleep faster. As a result, I feel more energetic the next day," says Dr. Block, who began walking to relieve moderate back pain.

"Walking is a part of a healthy lifestyle," he says. "My card says 'Family Practice— Lifestyle Changes.' Correct habits create health. Walking creates health."

Science Marches On

Based on the findings of medical science, the enthusiasm that many people have for walking is certainly warranted. In fact, a number of scientific studies have confirmed the amazing preventive and healing power of regular activity such as brisk walking.

"The evidence is overwhelming that doing regular exercise and other physical activities you enjoy is one of the very best health decisions you can make," says James Rippe, M.D., director of the Exercise Physiology and Nutrition Laboratory at the University of Massachusetts Medical School in Worcester.

In fact, researchers at the University of North Carolina at Chapel Hill point out that an inactive person's risk of heart disease is the same as that of someone who smokes a pack of cigarettes a day.

Studies have shown that walking really can slash your total cholesterol levels, help control high pressure, reduce your risk of heart attack and stroke, and help relieve the pain of angina and intermittent claudication.

Walking is a terrific way to build strong bones and help prevent osteoporosis. And if you have diabetes, then walking should be an important part of your daily routine, doctors say.

In addition, walking may offer protection against certain types of cancers, including those of the colon, thyroid, and bladder.

Evidence suggests that walking helps relieve premenstrual syndrome (PMS) symptoms, such as anxiety, breast tenderness, and mood swings. In fact, doctors say that walking is one of the best mood-enhancing things we can do. Research has shown that regular walking for as little as 10 minutes a day can reduce stress and anxiety.

Walking also may improve your relationships, says Cynthia Strowbridge, a New York psychotherapist who encourages clients to walk together, especially if they've been experiencing tension in their relationship.

"The tension can be dispersed through the exercise, rather than channeled into an outburst of emotion. Being in step together in the out-of-doors can be amazingly healing to the body and spirit," Strowbridge says.

Walk This Way

"For most people, walking is the easiest way to get more physical activity into their

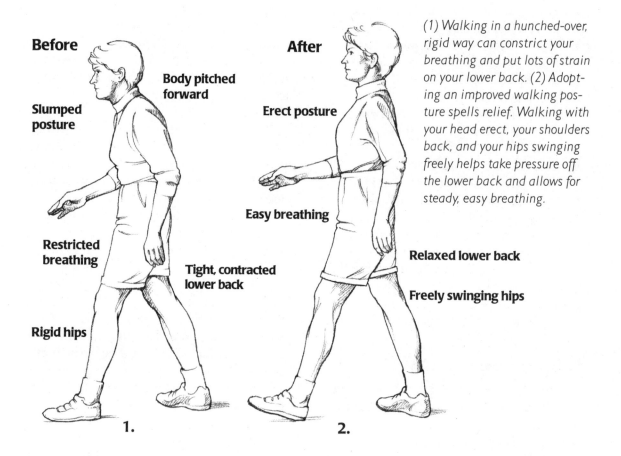

Before

Slumped posture

Body pitched forward

Restricted breathing

Tight, contracted lower back

Rigid hips

1.

After

Erect posture

Easy breathing

Relaxed lower back

Freely swinging hips

2.

(1) Walking in a hunched-over, rigid way can constrict your breathing and put lots of strain on your lower back. (2) Adopting an improved walking posture spells relief. Walking with your head erect, your shoulders back, and your hips swinging freely helps take pressure off the lower back and allows for steady, easy breathing.

day," says Dr. Rippe, coauthor of *Dr. James Rippe's Complete Book of Fitness Walking.* "It's a very beneficial thing to do.

"People have the misconception that they have to walk 5 miles a day or train for a marathon in order to be fit," he says. "Walking ½ to 1 mile a day at a pace you enjoy is certainly enough to decrease your risk of heart disease, as long as you stick with it."

Before you can enjoy walking, you need to learn how to do it properly. We know that sounds odd, but many of us have

forgotten a few basics in the years since we took our first steps, says David Balboa, a sports psychotherapist and co-director of The Walking Center of New York City.

"People are told to go out there and walk, but nobody bothers to tell them how to do it properly. So a lot of people go out there and walk in a distorted manner, and it doesn't feel right, or they hurt themselves, so they drop out," says Balboa, coauthor of *Walk for Life.*

When you start your walk, your shoulders should be relaxed, and your arms

KEEPING IN STRIDE

It's too hot, it's too cold, it's too wet, it's too dry, it's 2:00 in the morning! . . . My feet hurt, I'm tired, I'm depressed, I ate too much chocolate . . . I don't have time, I'd rather spend time with my family . . . No, *you* go, I'll do it next time . . .

Sometimes it seems like there are more excuses for not walking than there are hamburgers at a fast-food restaurant.

"When you're in the excuse mode, almost anything can become an excuse," says James Rippe, M.D., director of the Exercise Physiology and Nutrition Laboratory at the University of Massachusetts Medical School in Worcester.

"In my experience, most of the barriers that stop people from exercising are simple barriers. They're not complex at all."

The good news is that most of these excuses can be solved with planning and fine-tuning your attitude toward exercise.

"Say to yourself that your health and well-being are as important as any meeting, 'So I'm going to walk,'" Dr. Rippe says. "After that, set a time to walk and make it a priority."

Yet the number one excuse that Dr. Rippe hears is "I don't have time."

"People who don't exercise have the same amount of time as everyone else," he says. "Of all the activities you can do, walking should pose the least time problem, because all you have to do is step out your front door."

To overcome this obstacle, plan your day carefully and recognize that there are lots of ways to incorporate a walk into your daily schedule, including walking to work, he says.

Make a checklist of all the things you need for walking comfortably, such as shoes, clothing, and a portable radio, then get them, Dr. Rippe suggests.

"Spend a little money on boots, gloves, and walking clothes so on the days you don't feel like going out there, you can feel good about putting on the clothes. Then once you have those clothes on, you'll probably be motivated to do your walk," says Howard Dananberg, D.P.M., a podiatrist in New Bedford, New Hampshire.

To stay cool in the summer, try walking at an indoor mall. Many malls across the country are opening their doors to walkers before the stores open. If you're walking outside, wear light, loose-fitting clothing and a hat to keep the sun off your face. Drink lots of water and walk in the early morning or early evening when the sun is less intense and temperatures are cooler.

In the winter, schedule your walks during the lunch hour when the sun is high in the sky. Cover your face and lips with petroleum jelly and wear a scarf on your face to warm the air that you breathe. Wear a warm hat and layers of clothing that will give greater insulation and can be removed as you walk.

Encourage your spouse or family to walk with you, Dr. Rippe suggests. "Far from taking time away from your family, your walks can enhance communication and closeness within your family," he says.

If you think you're too tired to walk or are just in a bad mood, remember that walking may invigorate you and change your disposition.

Finally, remember that your first step out the door, no matter how short, is a step in the right direction.

should be slightly bent at the elbow, he says. Allow your arms to swing naturally to counterbalance the action of your legs. Imagine a center line going down the path. Walk with your usual stride and plant your feet parallel to the line, Balboa says. Allow your hips to be freer and to turn forward toward the line with the movement of each leg.

Walk as smoothly as possible. Try to develop a gliding motion. Be aware of the sensation of your foot rolling from the heel up to the toes. But don't pound your heel hard on the ground, Balboa warns. Eventually that pounding can hurt your body.

And don't lean forward from the waist in an effort to go faster. Don't worry—as your muscles get stronger and you build up your endurance, you'll be able to zip down the road more quickly.

Breathe deeply when you walk, Balboa advises. If you draw air deeply into your lungs, you'll walk better and keep your abdominal muscles strong.

Finally, set realistic goals that are attainable and will keep you motivated.

Taking Those First Steps

But how do you do that when you haven't been on a serious walk in years?

Start gradually, experts say. Remember that you don't have to walk the equivalent of the distance between Walla Walla, Washington, and Wausau, Wisconsin, during your first month of training.

"If you take someone who has been completely sedentary and tell them to walk a mile, they can't do it," says Howard Dananberg, D.P.M., a podiatrist in New Bedford, New Hampshire. "What I usually suggest to sedentary people is they begin by walking 5 minutes away from their home, then come back. Do that five times the first week. Then add 5 minutes to your walk each week until you're walking at least 25 minutes a day."

Eventually you should be able to walk about 1½ miles in those 25 minutes, he says. But in the beginning, walking duration is more important than distance or speed.

"I think time is the crucial thing," says Sharon Bruce, an exercise physiologist who specializes in cardiac rehabilitation at the Hospital of the Good Samaritan in Los Angeles.

"If you go and walk really fast for 10 minutes, you're not going to get the same benefits that you would if you go out and walk for 30 minutes.

"Thirty to 40 minutes is definitely the recommended amount of walking time for you, because you're going to get an aerobic effect, and you'll burn a sufficient number of calories," she says.

In fact, walking for 30 minutes at a moderate pace of 3½ miles per hour burns about 175 calories. That might not seem like much, but think of it this way. If you do it five days a week, that burns 875 calories a week, 3,500 a month, and 42,000 a year. Since a pound of fat equals 3,500 calories, that modest amount of walking translates to a weight loss of 12 pounds a year.

Even better, the calories burned during those walks take you almost halfway to the threshold of 2,000 calories that some researchers say you need to burn through physical activity each week in order to lengthen your life.

Of course, it may take time for you to

FULL SPEED AHEAD

One nice thing about walking is there's no speed limit.

"Somebody has estimated that there are about 200 terms for walking fast—speedwalking, powerwalking, striding, fitness walking," says James Rippe, M.D., director of the Exercise Physiology and Nutrition Laboratory at the University of Massachusetts in Worcester. "There are a lot of different words for it, but the idea is basically the same. You're trying to walk at a pace that will improve your cardiovascular fitness."

And walking fast certainly has the potential to do that. In one small study, for example, Dr. Rippe had ten marathon runners do brisk walking.

"All ten were able to keep their heart rate elevated up to their training levels," Dr. Rippe says. "They had to walk at 5 miles per hour, which is pretty fast, but it shows that virtually anyone can train by walking if they do it fast enough."

Walking fast also burns more calories. Many fitness walkers cover 1 mile in about 15 minutes (a speed of 4 miles per hour), burning 365 calories an hour. But if you push your speed up to 5 miles per hour, you increase your calorie burn to 585 an hour. Those extra 220 calories you burn each day translate to a weight loss of about 15 pounds in a year.

"I'm all for speedwalking, because it really helps you burn calories, and you challenge your cardiovascular system to work harder, especially if you use light, 1-pound hand weights," says Sharon Bruce, an exercise physiologist at the Hospital of the Good Samaritan in Los Angeles.

So how do you get started? Ease into your speedwalking program. Don't assume that just because you're a veteran walker, you can go from 4 to 5 miles per hour in one day.

Begin your walk at your normal pace; then near the midpoint of your workout—when your muscles are warm—pick up the pace. Maintain the faster pace for no more than 1 minute. Do the same on the next two days.

On day four, extend your time to 2 minutes. Hold at 2 minutes for a few days, then add another minute of speedwalking. The progress may seem slow, but eventually you should be able to speedwalk for 10, 15, or even 30 minutes.

You should be able to speedwalk for at least 10 minutes before you consider increasing your pace again.

Just because you're walking fast doesn't mean you should overstride. Your stride should be a natural one. If you take an exaggerated step, your posture will be thrown off. A huge stride also can lead to groin strain.

If you are more than 15 to 20 pounds over your ideal weight, experts say that you shouldn't speedwalk. Instead, maintain your regular walking program until you approach your ideal weight. Then try speedwalking to knock off those last 10 pounds.

---

notice changes in your body shape and fitness level, but be patient. It's worth waiting for.

For instance, it took three years for Suzanne Levine, D.P.M., a New York City podiatrist, to lose 52 pounds after she modified her diet and began walking. She now weighs about 128 pounds and walks an average of 4½ miles four to five times a week.

"Gradually, I increased the number of walks I took each week, the distance, and the pace. . . . For the first time in my life I felt comfortable with my body," says Dr. Levine, author of *Walk It Off: 20 Minutes a Day to Fitness and Health.*

Stepping Lively

Once you get through the initial weeks of walking, try picking up the pace.

"You want to walk at a pace that we call a comfortable push," Bruce says. "You want to be able to carry on a conversation, so you really don't want to be out of breath. At the same time, you want to feel as if you're pushing yourself a bit."

So what's an easy way to gauge if you're walking at a good pace? Try singing. If you can belt out the National Anthem as if you were in front of 40,000 baseball fans, you're probably not working hard enough to benefit your heart and lungs. But if you're so winded you can't gasp a note, you're walking too fast. Something between a songfest and speechlessness should do nicely.

When you get into shape, you should be able to walk 1 mile in about 15 minutes or about 4 miles per hour, three to five days a week, experts say.

Dr. Levine suggests walking Monday through Friday, particularly if you are a beginner. Doing it on weekdays will make walking part of your daily routine and free you to do other activities on the weekends.

Adding distance and choosing more challenging routes are good ideas, too. Find a course that has more hills, for example, Bruce says. Take a 3-mile walk to the mall rather than fight your way through a tangle of aggravating traffic.

Stepping Lightly

Don't attempt to do too much too soon, Dr. Dananberg warns. Just because you can walk a mile to the grocery store doesn't mean you're ready to tackle the Appalachian Trail next week.

"The general rule of thumb is you don't want to increase your exercise level more than 10 percent in any one week," he says. "If you start a walking program because a friend wants you to go on a 20-mile hike, you need a lot of time to prepare for that. You just can't do it in two months. You need to train for it."

But whether you're walking around the block or hiking in the Rockies, you need to take care of your feet. Blisters are likely to be your prime nemesis. If you do get one, try to keep it intact, says Philip Sanfilippo, D.P.M., a podiatrist in private practice in San Francisco.

"Popping a blister is not recommended," he says. "By not popping it, you're leaving a natural biological dressing over the top of it. It actually keeps it cleaner, and you don't have to worry about putting antibiotics on top of it." If your blister pops, you may want to cover it with an over-the-counter antibiotic cream and a plastic bandage. But see your doctor if it becomes inflamed, suggests Dr. Sanfilippo.

If the blister is in an awkward place and is likely to burst on its own, place a nonadhesive padding, such as a plastic bandage or taped-on cotton ball, over it.

But the best "cure" for blisters is prevention, Dr. Dananberg says. Pay careful attention to purchasing appropriate shoes and socks. (See "If the Shoe Fits, Wear It" on the opposite page.) Put talc or cornstarch on your feet before you put on

IF THE SHOE FITS, WEAR IT

You think it's going to be a simple task when you stroll into the local shoe store to buy a pair of walking shoes and good socks.

Then the clerk asks a fateful question— "What kind do you want?"—and points to a sea of socks and a wall of walking shoes.

Wading through the confusion of purchasing the right shoes and socks can give even the most patient pedestrian a migraine. In fact, some of the leading manufacturers make more than 300 models of athletic shoes.

Fortunately, there are few hints that will save you money and aching feet.

First, remember that fit, not style, should be your prime consideration. In other words, use some common sense.

"No matter how many technical features a shoe has, it has to fit. If it doesn't fit, it's not right," says Howard Dananberg, D.P.M., a podiatrist in New Bedford, New Hampshire.

Make sure the shoe bends easily across the ball of your foot. "The most important aspect of a shoe is how flexible it is across the forefoot," Dr. Dananberg says. "If the shoe is stiff, don't buy it. It's going to hurt you, and you're going to develop real foot problems."

You should be able to wiggle and stretch your toes inside the shoe, says Philip Sanfilippo, D.P.M., a podiatrist in San Francisco.

The shoe should be lightweight, padded at the heel and tongue, have an absorbent, smooth lining, and be elevated at least ½ inch above the sole at the heel, says Dr. Sanfilippo. And the sole should be tilted upward at the toe in order to enhance your natural walking motion, he says.

Shop for shoes in the late afternoon, because that's when your feet are the biggest.

To prevent foot injuries, follow this rule: If you walk 25 miles a week or more, buy new shoes every six months. If you walk less than 25 miles a week, you'll need a new pair about once a year.

The fit of your walking sock is just as important as the fit of your shoe. Too tight and you'll constrict the toes. Too big and the extra fabric will bunch up, causing discomfort, friction, and blisters. The sock should slip on comfortably but fit smoothly over your entire foot, with room for the toes to move and stretch. Remember sock sizes are usually a size or two larger than shoe sizes. One sock size accommodates two shoe sizes.

Synthetic fibers such as Orlon retain their shape and texture longer, and they wick away sweat. But natural fibers such as cotton may be a matter of personal preference. They tend to absorb moisture and perspiration.

Some sock packages have the American Podiatric Medical Association seal. This means the manufacturer has submitted the socks for review by a committee of doctors of podiatry who have examined the product, worn it, and reviewed its advertising claims.

---

your socks. That will create a slippery surface that is less abrasive.

"Taking breaks, especially on long walks, to cool down your feet is very helpful," Dr. Dananberg says. "Stopping every hour or so, washing off your feet, then reapplying talc or cornstarch is just about the best thing you can do."

If you do feel pain, don't try to walk through it. Stop and try to solve the problem. It may be as simple as a pebble in your shoe.

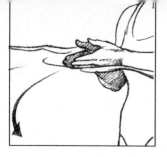

Water Exercise

*E*ver watch a baby kicking and splashing in her bath? Or kids jumping, running, and shrieking in a backyard pool? They are having a great time—and are completely unaware they're also getting a great workout.

Adult water exercise may be a little more structured—and perhaps less noisy—than the exercise that kids get playing "sharks and minnows," but the idea's the same. You're working out in water—and having a great time doing it.

Do you have trouble associating the word *exercise* with having a good time? Rest assured: Water exercise *is* a kinder, gentler form of exercise.

"Let's face it—when it comes to land-based exercise, most people don't enjoy all the sweating, straining, and pounding," says Jane Katz, Ed.D., world masters swimming champion, professor of physical education at the City University of New York, and author of *The W.E.T. Workout.* "The magic of water is that it leaves you refreshed, not fatigued; exhilarated, not exhausted."

And no special skills are required. You don't need to know how to swim; you don't have to be in good shape. All you need is a swimsuit and a pool.

Water exercise covers a wide range of activities—just about everything *except* swimming. It can be water aerobics with your Y class, supervised sessions prescribed by a physical therapist, or running or doing jumping jacks in your backyard pool. It can be done with your head completely above water or can include bobbing underwater. It can be done in deep water or shallow, in a regular pool or a heated therapeutic facility. The common ingredients are movement and water.

What's Special about Water

Water is a superb workout medium, says Dr. Katz. The natural buoyancy of water aids movement, letting you do exercises that might be too painful or stressful on land.

Unconvinced? Think about it. Water effectively reduces your body weight by 90 percent. So if you weigh 150 pounds, in water your limbs only have to support 10 percent of that, or 15 pounds. Stress on your joints, bones, and muscles is kept to a minimum.

But water has other advantages. It helps cool you off as you exercise, and in many cases any stiffness or pain you may be feeling will decrease in water. In heated or therapeutic pools there's little or no cooling effect, but the warm water helps relieve the pain of stiff joints or injured limbs.

And because water provides resistance

to movement, pushing to move through it can tone and strengthen muscles and improve your range of motion.

Who's Suited

All this means that water exercise is great for people who are pregnant, obese, or recovering from injuries and for those with arthritis, musculoskeletal problems, or multiple sclerosis. Plus, of course, anybody who just wants to get fitter.

Athletes at the University of Texas in Austin regularly work out in the pool, both to help rehabilitate injuries and to improve fitness levels.

"We use it for just about every injury you can think of," says Spanky Stevens, head athletic trainer. "There are guys who think exercising in the water is for wimps. It's not. But it *is* one of the best ways for anybody to keep fit and healthy."

Perhaps you're overweight or out of shape and uncomfortable exercising around others in a gym or on a track. In a pool you don't have to be as conscious of how your body looks. "Water is a very forgiving medium," says Dr. Katz. "I've seen women climb into the pool wearing layers upon layers of clothing so that no one can see their shape. But once they're in shoulder-deep water, they're thrilled. They feel light as a feather."

For older people who fear painful falls on land, exercising in water can be the perfect solution. And for people with painful rheumatic diseases such as arthritis, moving in water may be the *only* way they can exercise, notes physical therapist Roxane McNeal, president of Aquatic Therapy Services in Abingdon, Maryland.

How much exercise do you get in water? That depends, of course, on your level of activity. If you're putting in an intense workout, you're burning about the same number of calories as you would in an intense workout on land—and getting similar benefits—but without the jarring and pounding. Studies have shown, for example, that running in either deep or shallow water makes similar metabolic demands on the body as running on land.

Doing gentle, slow exercises in water, on the other hand, may not burn off lots of calories or produce an aerobic training effect, but it *will* improve your muscle tone and range of motion—which may be just what you're looking for when you climb into the pool.

Off and Splashing

Ready to start? Check with your doctor first, advises Dr. Katz, particularly if you have any health problems or haven't been exercising for a while.

Once you've got the go-ahead, you can sign up for a class at the community pool or create your own workout. (If you're under the care of a physical therapist, your therapist will design your program for you.)

Whatever your program, start out slowly and listen to your body. Spend 5 minutes warming up in the pool to get your body ready. Some good warm-up exercises:

- Sit on the edge of the pool with your feet in the water and your hands next to your hips for support. Move your feet in circles. Then move your legs up and down in a flutter kick.
- Stand in chest-deep water. Inhale, then

HOT ENOUGH FOR YOU?

Pause before you plunge into that pool: Water temperature is an important consideration. You don't want to vigorously exercise in a pool that's toasty warm, nor do you want to be shivering as you do gentle movements in a frigid pool.

Many pools are kept at 80° to 83°F, which requires that you keep moving to stay warm. In pools less than 84°, you may begin to feel like a polar bear if you can't exercise vigorously. For most pool exercises, a good range is 82° to 86°.

Therapeutic pools are kept warmer—from 92° to 98°. Pools this warm are for pain relief and gentle range-of-motion exercises, however, and aren't safe for exercise programs. Because the water is so hot, you won't be able to lose the heat you generate from exercise. You could overstress your heart or even pass out.

Water temperature affects your heart rate as well. As with other sports, for aerobic benefits your exercise goal should be to reach a target heart rate zone. But when you're in cool water—in the 70° to 80° range—your heart rate is 10 to 15 percent *lower* than while doing a workout of the same intensity on land. This means you figure things a bit differently when gauging the intensity of your workout. To calculate your maximum heart rate, follow the directions in "How Good Is Your Workout?" on page 324, but subtract your age *plus 13* from 220.

If you're exercising in warm water (86° to 88°), however, you can figure your heart rate range the same as if you were on dry land.

bend your knees slightly until your chin is at water level. Exhale, then bob underwater and continue exhaling. Repeat this movement several times.

- In water that comes to your shoulders, stand with your back against the pool wall. Press your back, head, shoulders, buttocks, and heels against the wall. Step away from the wall, retaining your posture, then step back to the wall and check your position.
- Stand in chest-deep water with your side to the pool wall. Place one hand on the wall; push your shoulder against the wall for 30 seconds. Change sides and repeat.

For other warm-ups, you can jog in place or in circles, or pretend you're jumping rope. You can also do shoulder shrugs.

A good beginning workout, says Dr. Katz, might include a 5-minute warm-up, a 15- to 30-minute main set, and a 5-minute cool-down, three times a week. (See the illustrations on page 470 for activities you can include in your workout.)

Another workout you can do on your own is pool walking or jogging. After a warm-up, spend 10 to 20 minutes traveling back and forth across the pool. To introduce variety, try walking sideways or backward. If the slippery pool bottom makes you uneasy, try a pair of rubber-soled water socks (you can find them at sporting goods stores).

Extra Equipment

Although you can complete most water aerobics classes with nary a bit of paraphernalia except your suit (and a swim cap if you want to protect your hair), you may enjoy using some equipment to vary your workout.

A flotation vest can help ease your mind about being in the water if you're a nonswimmer and also is a safety device for deep-water exercises. If you're pool-running, for example, it will keep you upright with your head above water as you run so you don't have to struggle to keep your balance. Or you can use it while "running" in deeper water to keep an injured foot or ankle completely off the pool floor.

Other devices that may be useful:

- A waterproof watch with a second hand: You can time yourself to make sure you do each exercise for the specified time.
- A swim cap: This will help keep your hair dry and protect it from the ravages of chlorine.
- A pull-buoy and kickboard: These are Styrofoam floats you can use for drills or to push through the water for added resistance.
- Fins: You can use these to vary lower-leg exercises and kicks.
- Hand paddles: While these aren't recommended for swimming because you can strain shoulder muscles, it's okay to use them to increase resistance for arm exercises.
- Floats: These inflatable vinyl pouches that can be worn on your arms or legs make it easy to stay afloat.

A Splashing Good Routine

Looking for a no-sweat exercise routine? Then try this one, originally designed for senior citizens. Don't be fooled, though. Part of the "Top of the Hills" program put together by the YMCA, these water exercises are challenging enough to give people of all ages a good workout. The exercises don't require a lot of fancy equipment—a bathing suit and a kickboard are all it takes. (Goggles and bathing cap are optional.) If you can't find a kickboard at your local sporting goods store, you can use the lid of a large Styrofoam cooler. It should be about 12 by 18 inches.

As with any exercise program, it's important to warm up before you start the exercises and cool down afterward. Stand in chest-deep water with your feet comfortably apart for all the exercises. To start the warm-up series, do a few simple neck and shoulder stretches. Turn your head from side to side, then tilt it from shoulder to shoulder. Then roll your shoulders forward and backward.

Once you've completed the routine, let yourself cool down gradually. Rest your elbows on the edge of the pool and stretch your legs out in front of you. Do 2 minutes of simple kicks, scissor kicks, the bicycle, and rocking your bent knees from side to side. Finish up with head turns and tilts and shoulder rolls as before.

Get your doctor's okay before you dive in—and be prepared for a refreshing workout!

Warm-Up

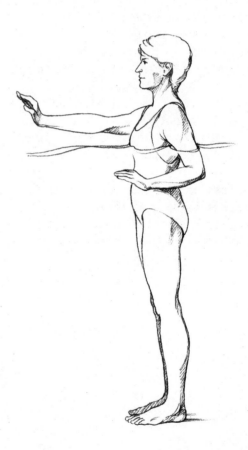

Hold your arms at shoulder height. Alternately reach them out to the front. Reach out 20 times with each arm.

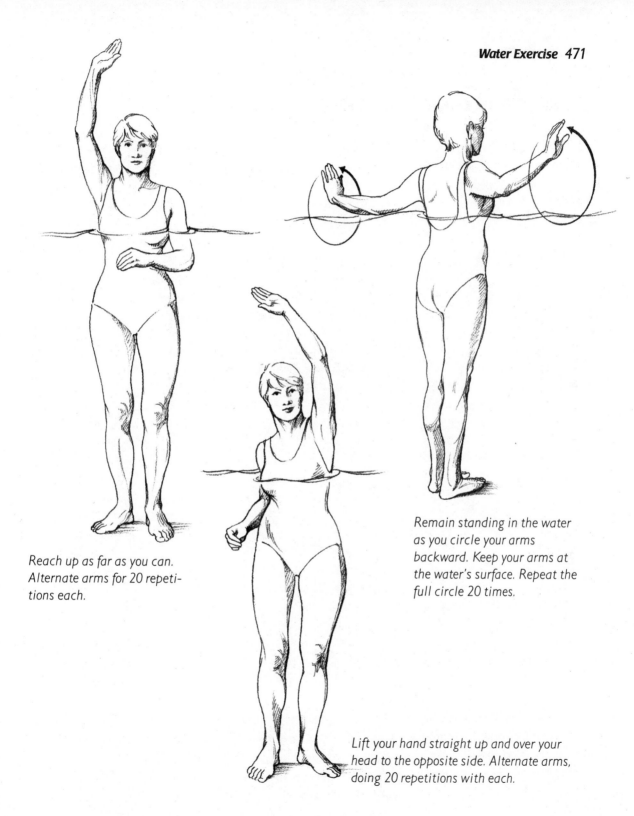

Reach up as far as you can. Alternate arms for 20 repetitions each.

Remain standing in the water as you circle your arms backward. Keep your arms at the water's surface. Repeat the full circle 20 times.

Lift your hand straight up and over your head to the opposite side. Alternate arms, doing 20 repetitions with each.

A Splashing Good Routine—Continued

Finish up your warm-up with the breaststroke. (1) Start with your palms together and your elbows at your sides, then push your hands out at shoulder height. (2) Swing your arms out to the sides, then bring your hands together once again before pushing them forward. Repeat the stroke 20 times.

1.

2.

Now move your arms as if you were doing the crawl or freestyle stroke. Move each arm alternately through 20 repetitions.

Kickboard Exercises

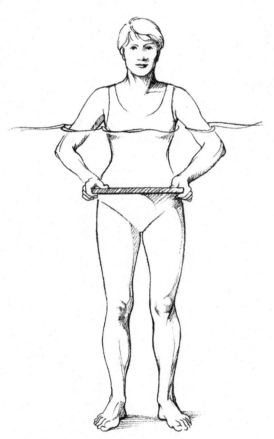

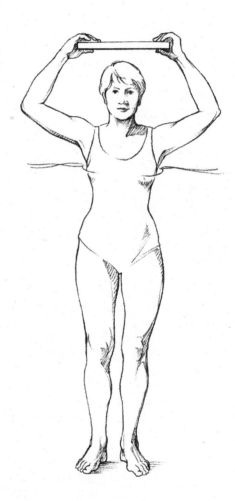

Hold the ends of the kickboard. Keeping it flat, push it straight down into the water until your arms are fully extended. Control the movement as you bring the board back up to the surface. Repeat 20 times.

Press the board down into the water as in the previous exercise. When you bring the board up, however, lift it out of the water and over your head. Repeat 20 times.

A Splashing Good Routine—Continued

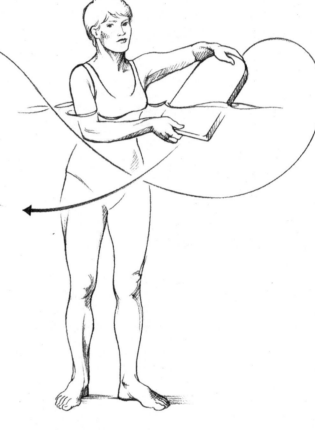

Hold the kickboard vertically. Keep the bottom half in the water as you swish it from side to side. Swish the board 15 times to each side. Switch hands and repeat.

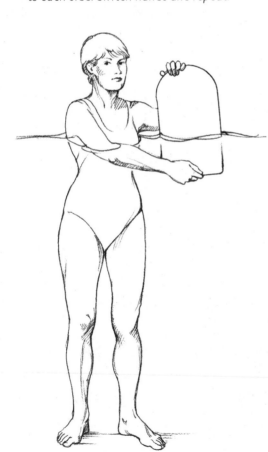

Scoop the board through the water in a complete figure eight. Repeat 15 times.

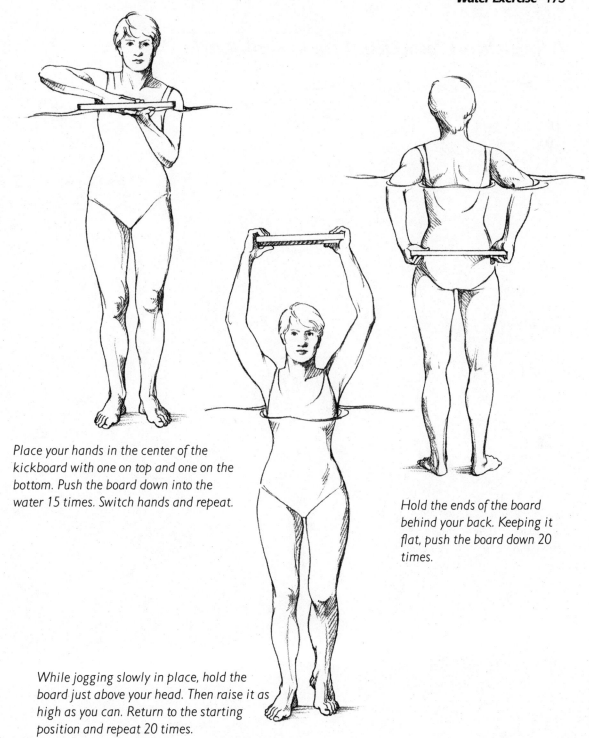

Place your hands in the center of the
kickboard with one on top and one on the
bottom. Push the board down into the
water 15 times. Switch hands and repeat.

Hold the ends of the board
behind your back. Keeping it
flat, push the board down 20
times.

While jogging slowly in place, hold the
board just above your head. Then raise it as
high as you can. Return to the starting
position and repeat 20 times.

A Splashing Good Routine—Continued

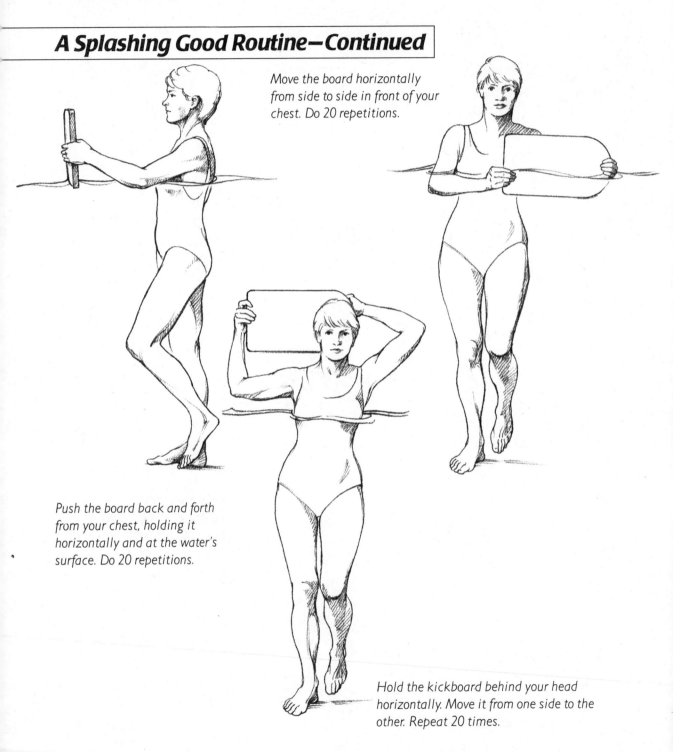

Move the board horizontally from side to side in front of your chest. Do 20 repetitions.

Push the board back and forth from your chest, holding it horizontally and at the water's surface. Do 20 repetitions.

Hold the kickboard behind your head horizontally. Move it from one side to the other. Repeat 20 times.

Arm and Leg Routine

Hold your arms out from your sides at shoulder height. Make small circles with your hands, first with your palms up, then with them down. Do 15 repetitions each. Then reverse the direction of the circles and do them with palms up, then down. Do 15 repetitions in each direction.

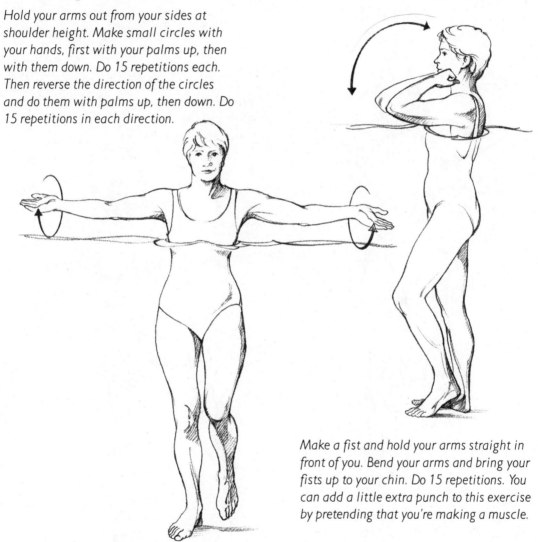

Make a fist and hold your arms straight in front of you. Bend your arms and bring your fists up to your chin. Do 15 repetitions. You can add a little extra punch to this exercise by pretending that you're making a muscle.

A Splashing Good Routine—Continued

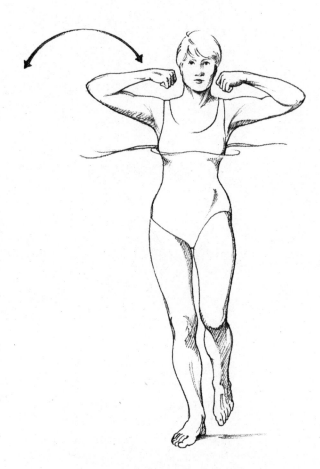

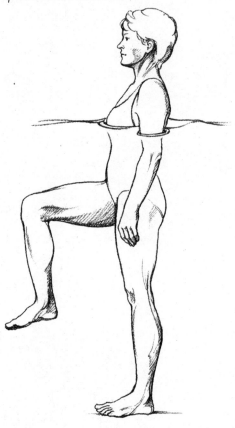

March in place, picking up each knee as high as you can. Alternate knees, picking up each knee 20 times.

Flex your arms as in the previous exercise, except this time hold your arms out to the sides. Be sure to keep them at shoulder height. Flex your arms 15 times.

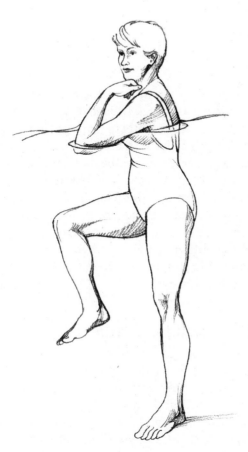

Bring your left foot up behind you and try to touch that foot with your left hand. Make your effort lively by swinging your right arm up in the air. Then switch sides in a quick, smooth motion. Alternate from side to side 15 times.

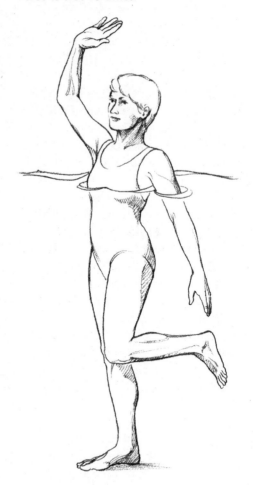

Pick up your right knee and swing it toward your left elbow. Don't worry if it doesn't touch. Alternating knees and elbows, do 15 repetitions on each side.

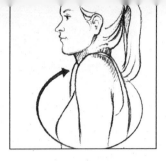

Yoga

Does the word *yoga* conjure up images of phenomenally flexible Eastern yogis sitting around in poses only a pretzel could manage? Not for you, you say? Not interested in being able to put your feet behind your head or balance yourself in a handstand while you do a split?

Yoga does seem to have a bit of a public relations problem. But before you decide it's not for you, make sure you're not already doing yoga! This 5,000-year-old discipline is the mother of many forms of exercise: Just about every stretch mirrors a yoga pose that does the same thing. Many relaxation exercises—both breathing therapies and progressive muscle relaxation, for example—are taken from yoga techniques. So are range-of-motion exercises for stiff arthritic joints and some commonly prescribed back-pain-relieving exercises. Even the famed Kegel squeeze, prescribed to tone muscles around the bladder and vagina, has its counterpart in sexually energizing yoga.

Another commonly held impression—that yoga is only slow and relaxing—is a half-truth. While yoga can provide the ultimate in relaxation and flexibility, forms of it can be quite vigorous, building muscle strength and endurance as effectively as most fitness programs.

And it's plain untrue that only limber people can do yoga. (It is true, though, that yoga inevitably limbers you up.) Yoga can be done in a chair, in a wheelchair, or even in bed. Yoga poses can be modified, sometimes with pillows or benches, to accommodate people with arthritis, multiple sclerosis, heart disease, or even partial paralysis. A good yoga instructor can teach just about any willing person, selecting and modifying poses based on a student's physical limitations.

Designed for Fitness

Even though they often provide fitness as a bonus, many forms of exercise were developed primarily for fun (like tennis), transportation (like walking), or proof of one's competitive prowess (like football). The type of yoga that concentrates on the body, however, was designed strictly for fitness, says Patricia Hammond, a yoga instructor in Sarasota, Florida, and a spokesperson for the American Yoga Association.

"In yoga philosophy, these exercises were done to make the body perfectly healthy so you could sit perfectly still to meditate," she says. "That's because it's hard to concentrate on anything that's going on in your mind if your body is ill, tired, stiff, or in pain, because the body has such strong pull on our attention."

Each yoga pose supposedly has particular health-restoring effects. One pose may stimulate the thyroid gland in the neck, for instance. Another may improve breathing or give the heart a bit of a rest. And many affect the whole body.

But are these claims true? *Can* yoga make your body perfectly healthy—or at the very least heal whatever's ailing it?

Yoga masters over the centuries have contended that a yoga program, faithfully followed, can cure just about any health problem: asthma, diabetes, heart disease, arthritis, back pain, and mental disorders such as nervousness or depression, to name just a few. And certainly more than one student of yoga has experienced its curative potential. But there's not much in the way of what Western medical practitioners call "scientific proof" to back up those claims. (There's no study, for instance, that compares the insulin requirements of diabetics who do yoga with those of diabetics who do not practice yoga.)

On the other hand, there's little doubt that yoga's blend of stress-management techniques and flexibility training, along with dietary advice that sounds like it's straight out of the Pritikin Program (veggies and more veggies) and a spiritual orientation that reduces hostility and nurtures acceptance, incorporates most of the lifestyle strategies thought to help prevent every disease from atherosclerosis to cancer. That's one reason doctors like Dean Ornish, M.D., author of *Dr. Dean Ornish's Program for Reversing Heart Disease* and director of the Preventive Medicine Research Institute in Sausalito, California, include the practice of yoga in their research programs.

"Everyone does at least 1 hour and 15 minutes of yoga a day, but some do it twice a day," says Barbara Musser, a yoga instructor helping in Dr. Ornish's research. "Although the study was not designed to determine this, it seems that those who are getting the most heart disease reversal are those doing the most yoga."

Some studies, mostly from India, have examined the physical aspects of yoga—the poses, or *asanas*—separate from yoga's dietary and spiritual aspects. These studies show that yoga poses can change the way the body functions, at least temporarily.

The Pose That Refreshes

Take blood pressure, for instance. One study showed, not too surprisingly, that the so-called corpse pose—which calls for lying flat on the floor, relaxing all the muscles, and breathing slowly and deeply—leads to a temporary drop in blood pressure. Other exercises, such as the bellows breath—which calls for rapidly pumping the diaphragm, taking in quick, short breaths—have been found to lead to a temporary increase in blood pressure. And some, such as the headstand or shoulder stand, can cause regional variations in blood pressure in the body. (Blood pressure drops in the feet and rises in the head or neck.)

"Those findings are not surprising, since blood pressure is affected by the body's position and by breathing rate," Hammond says. "They support the theory that yoga can be used to redirect or increase blood flow to particular organs or parts of the body."

The heart disease patients in Dr. Ornish's

program practice a shoulder stand, according to Musser. "We have found it very beneficial," she says. "It allows blood to flow freely to the heart and brain." People in the program who have back problems must do a modified version of the shoulder stand—they lie with their legs up against a wall, or with their feet up on a chair.

Several studies also show that people with high blood pressure who do a general yoga program that includes quiet, meditative poses experience a drop in pressure. One U.S. study looked at people aged 55 and older with mild to moderate high blood pressure. These people participated in the "Easy Does It Fitness" program, sponsored by the American Yoga Association. (Some of the exercises for this program are included in this chapter.) Every single one of the participants had a decrease in blood pressure (average drop, about 5 points) that held constant throughout the 12-week program and during a 12-week follow-up period, reports Hammond, who coordinated the program.

"We think it worked mostly by relaxing people," she says. "If you can relax your body, mind, and breath, the muscles that control the diameter of blood vessels are also relaxed, so dilation occurs, and blood pressure drops. Relaxation also means less stress hormones are being produced in the body. Your overall ability to return more quickly to a steady-state level is improved."

And some studies have found that certain yoga poses change the amount of pressure within body cavities such as the colon. Poses that put a squeeze on the abdomen were found to raise colon pressure. Some forms of advanced breathing exercises, called locks, may increase or decrease pressure in the colon and even change its position slightly.

Even less vigorous poses can provide beneficial stimulation to organs and glands, Hammond says. "The shoulder stand, for instance, is said to stimulate the thyroid gland by increasing pressure on the gland," she says.

Newcomers to her yoga classes report an immediate improvement in intestinal problems, she says. "Exercises that put pressure on the lower abdomen, both pressing forward and stretching back, or twisting, get the intestines moving," Hammond explains. "Most people get gas, constipation, or bloating simply because they are not moving. The knee-to-chest press is the best, but any pose that motivates the intestines to move gets the system going again."

Studies also show that yoga increases flexibility, a benefit that becomes apparent to most yoga students after only a few weeks of practice. One researcher found that only three weeks of regular yoga practice produced significant increases in strength, coordination, and stamina.

Back Basics

Yoga's impact on flexibility and muscle strength makes it useful in the treatment of back pain, says Hammond. "Yoga addresses both the stiffness and weakness associated with most back pain." Yoga exercises work on back and stomach muscles, both important for back support. And yoga helps you maintain good posture throughout the day, with both poses and body awareness, she says. "Once posture improves, many aches just disappear." (See "Posture Training" on page 387.)

Yoga stretches differ from many kinds of stretching because they are so gentle and held so long, sometimes for minutes, Hammond says. "Because there is no forcing or bouncing," she says, "you're less likely to injure muscles." Her "Easy Does It" students especially enjoy the back-soothing knee-to-chest squeeze, done in a chair or on the floor. (See the illustrations on page 496.) "We do several of those, alternating one leg and both legs, and we even suggest that people who wake up in the morning with a backache do that stretch in bed before they get up," she says.

Gentle yoga exercise—such as the sacral rock and yoga sit-ups—are beneficial because they help your back relax and they strengthen the abdominal muscles to provide back support from the front, says Mary P. Schatz, M.D., a certified yoga instructor and author of *Back Care Basics: A Doctor's Gentle Yoga Program for Back and Neck Pain Relief.*

Here are two yoga poses adapted from Dr. Schatz's book. To do the sacral rock, lie on your back on a firm surface with a folded towel or blanket under your head and neck, with your knees bent and your feet on the floor a few inches from your buttocks. Keeping your knees together and your feet on the floor, move your knees slowly to the right about 6 to 8 inches, then back to the starting position, then slowly to the left. After you've done that a few times, you can clasp your knees toward your chest and rock slowly from side to side for a few minutes, massaging your back muscles against the floor. Get up carefully, Dr. Schatz warns. Roll to the side and push yourself up to a sitting position with your arms and hands.

To do the yoga sit-up, lie on your back with your calves resting on a chair seat. Cross your arms in front of your chest and place your hands on your shoulders. As you exhale, flatten your lower back against the floor and raise your shoulders only 6 to 10 inches off the floor. (Do not come all the way up into a sitting position.) Continue exhaling and lower your shoulders back to the floor. Inhale deeply once again. Then as you begin a long, slow exhalation, flatten your lower back against the floor, raise both shoulders off the floor, lower your right shoulder to touch the floor, raise it back up, and, still exhaling, lower both shoulders to the floor. Repeat the exercise, this time dropping your left shoulder. Continue the sequence until your abdominal muscles feel warmed up. Then do one or two more and stop, Dr. Schatz directs.

For those who have had back surgery or an injury, even scar tissue in and around the back muscles and spinal ligaments can be stretched if a yoga pose is held from 90 to 120 seconds, Dr. Schatz says. "This promotes a return to more normal mobility in areas where movement is restricted by scarring," she explains. If you have had surgery on your back, or if you have a back injury, you should work only with a yoga instructor who has had training in therapeutic work, advices Dr. Schatz.

Yoga poses done while standing help strengthen the muscles of the legs, buttocks, abdomen, back, and shoulders for improved support of the lower back, says Dr. Schatz. "These poses provide the foundation for better flexibility of the hips, shoulders, and middle spine and thus decrease the excessive demands placed on the lower back when these areas are stiff.

HOW TO FIND A GOOD YOGA CLASS

If you feel ready for a limber body and more peace of mind and would like to give yoga a try, keep the following tips in mind when looking for a class.

Ask others for their opinions. "Ask the people who have experienced a certain technique, 'What are the results of your practice?' 'Are you happy with the class?' " says Steven Brena, M.D., chairman of the board at the Pain Control and Rehabilitation Institute of Georgia.

Inquire about the style before signing up. There are numerous different "styles" of yoga, not all of which emphasize relaxation. While most styles do incorporate relaxation techniques, some are downright strenuous. Check up front with the instructor before making assumptions.

For suggestions about what to look for in a yoga teacher, write to the American Yoga Association, 513 South Orange Avenue, Sarasota, FL 34236.

The heart program created by Dean Ornish, M.D., director of the Preventive Medicine Research Institute in Sausalito, California, uses a style called Integral Yoga. For a referral to a certified teacher of Integral Yoga in your area, write to Satchidananda Ashram—Yogaville, Route 1, Box 1720, Buckingham, VA 23921.

Look for a teacher who individualizes instruction. Everyone's different, and instructors should adapt exercises to accommodate your arthritis, low back pain problem, or other physical concerns.

Take a trial class if you can before you invest long-term. An instructor who's concerned with meeting your needs will allow you to get a taste before you slap down payment for a whole series of classes.

Be suspicious of any institute that asks for a lot of money. Yoga classes are offered by many YMCAs and independent teachers. Average prices range from $5 to $15 for a group session to up to $20 to $30 for private lessons. Some yoga institutes hold weekend and week-long retreats that may include meals and lectures on health and nutrition, and they are, of course, more expensive.

"Properly aligned rotation of the spine—such as passive, relaxed spinal twists—allow the small muscles that rotate the spine to be stretched to achieve greater flexibility, increased spinal rotation, and improved disk nutrition." (She adds that in order for a muscle to lengthen in response to a stretch, the stretch must be maintained for at least 20 seconds.)

Yoga poses that help increase flexibility and strength can do wonders for some people with arthritis, yoga instructors say. Yoga also benefits those with arthritis by lubricating shoulder, knee, and hip joints and the joints of the back. Certain poses can help prevent the muscle shortening that can lead to painful arthritic contractures in hands or hips, Dr. Schatz says.

Overall Tension Easer

Even if you're not battling some specific bodily ill, yoga may have something to offer. One thing just about every student of yoga comments on is the growing sense of calmness and well-being that comes with regular practice, Hammond says.

Gentle Yoga: The Aaahhhh *Routine*

Yoga is wonderfully relaxing and energizing and, along with medical care, can ease back pain, stiff joints, anxiety, and a host of other physical and emotional upsets.

The following yoga routine is a series of exercises designed for the novice. The series is provided by the American Yoga Association, whose founder, Alice Christensen, developed programs and manuals for beginners of all ages, including the "Easy Does It Fitness" program for older adults.

You'll note that the routine includes a warm-up and cool-down. For maximum relaxation, do both! Stretch only as far as you comfortably can, then hold the pose. Relax and breathe normally. With time, you'll be able to stretch farther. If you enjoy the routine, consider taking a yoga class. Detailed verbal guidance during these poses can help you master them.

Warm-Up

The Complete Breath

The complete breath is considered a relaxing breath. Do three sets, both before and after a yoga session. (1) In a comfortable seated position, place your hands on the lower part of your rib cage, with your fingers just touching. Exhale fully, contracting your abdominal muscles. Now relax your belly and inhale, pushing forward with your abdominal muscles and slightly arching your back. (2) Continue to inhale, trying to expand your rib cage not just forward but also to the side. Your fingers should naturally come apart. While still inhaling, straighten your shoulders and stretch your spine a little and feel the breath pushing into the very top of your lungs. Then exhale, reversing the process. Repeat several times.

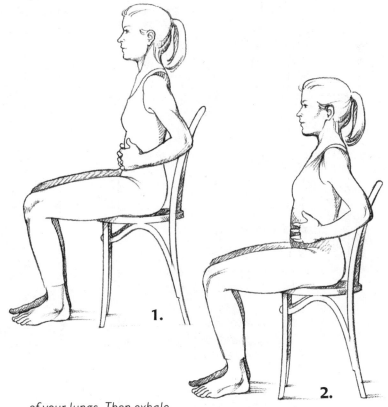

1.

2.

Gentle Yoga: The Aaahhhh Routine—Continued

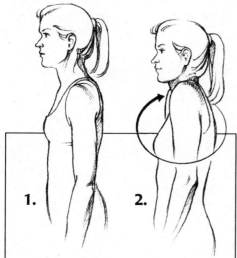

1.   **2.**

Shoulder Rolls

(1) Stand with your arms at
your sides. Let them hang loose
just like wet spaghetti. (2) Lift
both shoulders up toward your
ears, then roll them in a circle—
back, down, forward, and then
up toward your ears again. Do
three to five repetitions in each
direction. Shake out your arms
and relax them.

Neck Stretch

(1) Raise your arms parallel to
floor, palms up. (If this is tiring,
put your hands on your hips or
let them hang at your sides.
You want your shoudlers relaxed.)
Start by lowering your chin to
your chest, (2) then lift your
chin. Do three repetitions,
breathing normally. (3) Next,
starting with your head straight,
tilt your head to the right side,
with your ear over your shoulder,
(4) then lift your head up and
gently tilt it toward the opposite shoulder. Try not to lift your
shoulder up toward your ear;
move only your head. Breathe
normally.

1.

2.

3.

4.

Gentle Yoga: The Aaahhhh Routine—Continued

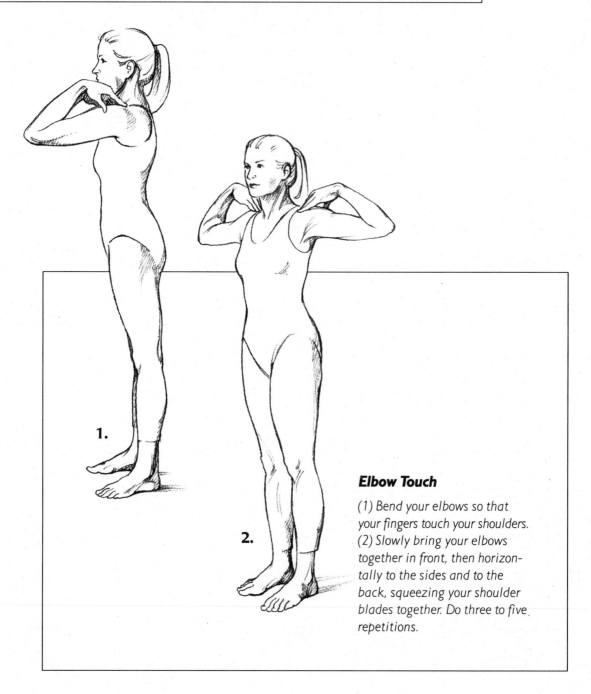

1.

2.

Elbow Touch

(1) Bend your elbows so that your fingers touch your shoulders. (2) Slowly bring your elbows together in front, then horizontally to the sides and to the back, squeezing your shoulder blades together. Do three to five repetitions.

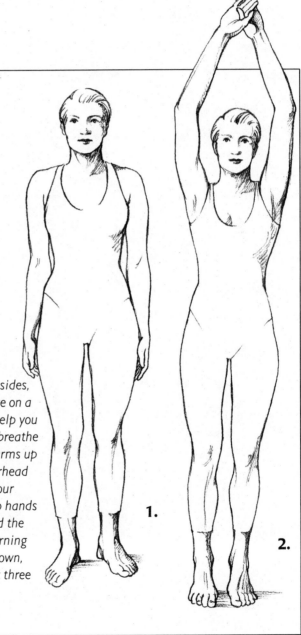

Standing Reach

(1) Standing with your arms at your sides, breathe out completely. Fix your gaze on a spot on the floor or wall—this will help you keep your balance. (2) Now start to breathe in, at the same time bringing your arms up in a wide circle to the sides and overhead while rising up on your toes. Hold your breath for just a second as you clasp hands and stretch a little farther up toward the ceiling. Then breathe out while returning your straight arms to the side and down, and lower your heels to floor. Repeat three times.

1.

2.

Gentle Yoga: The Aaahhhh Routine—Continued

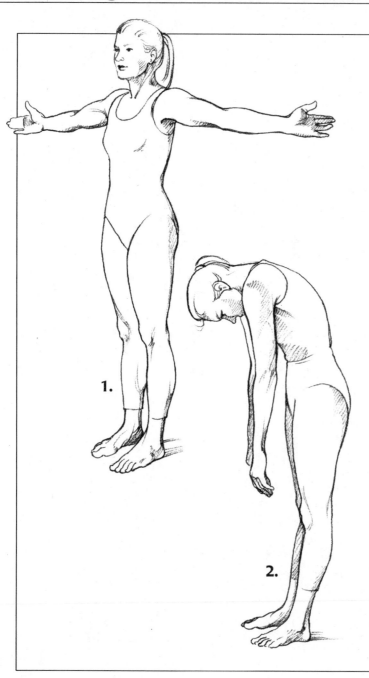

Easy Bend

Stand straight with your feet together and your arms at your sides. Breathe out. (1) Breathe in and raise your arms at the same time until they are outstretched parallel to the floor. Your chest should be fully expanded. (2) Start to breathe out and slowly drop forward into a slouch, letting your head and arms relax completely. Bend only halfway (even if you can easily bend much farther) so that your hands hang down at about the level of your knees. Then start to breathe in as you slowly rise to a standing position, bringing your arms up and out to the sides again and rolling your spine up one vertebra at a time. Do three repetitions, in a kind of pumping motion. After the last inhalation, just breathe out and relax, slowly lowering your arms to your sides. (If you have back pain, don't do this pose.)

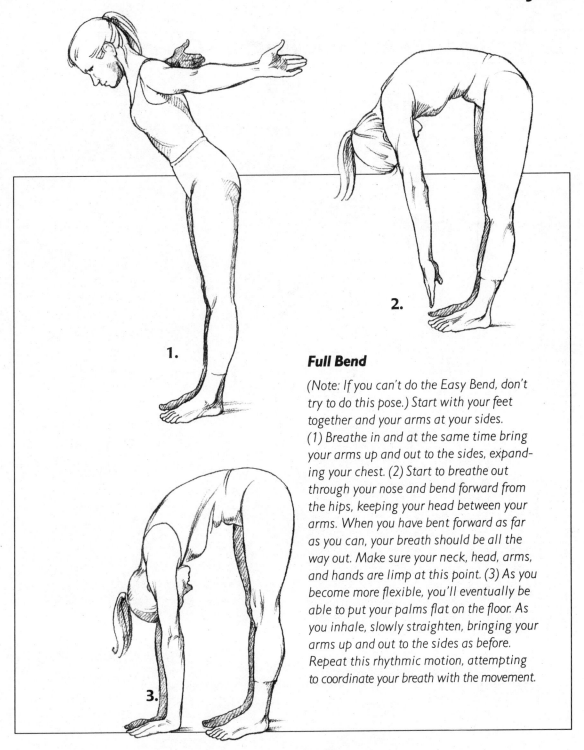

1.

2.

3.

Full Bend

(Note: If you can't do the Easy Bend, don't try to do this pose.) Start with your feet together and your arms at your sides. (1) Breathe in and at the same time bring your arms up and out to the sides, expanding your chest. (2) Start to breathe out through your nose and bend forward from the hips, keeping your head between your arms. When you have bent forward as far as you can, your breath should be all the way out. Make sure your neck, head, arms, and hands are limp at this point. (3) As you become more flexible, you'll eventually be able to put your palms flat on the floor. As you inhale, slowly straighten, bringing your arms up and out to the sides as before. Repeat this rhythmic motion, attempting to coordinate your breath with the movement.

Gentle Yoga: The Aaahhh Routine—Continued

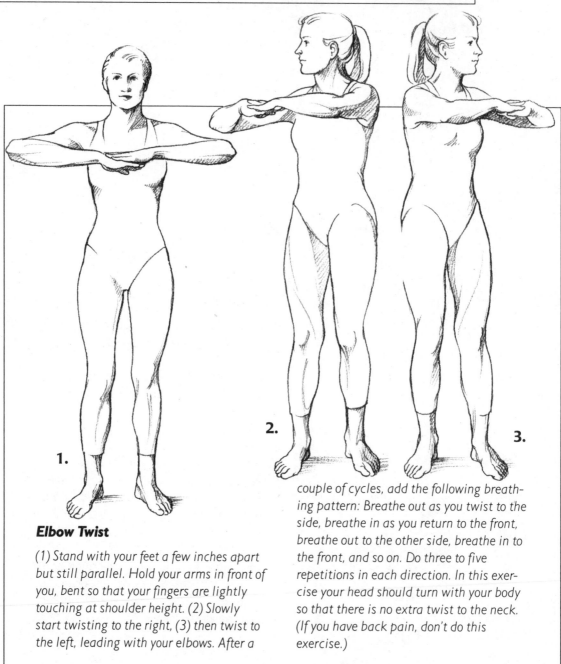

1.

2.

3.

Elbow Twist

(1) Stand with your feet a few inches apart but still parallel. Hold your arms in front of you, bent so that your fingers are lightly touching at shoulder height. (2) Slowly start twisting to the right, (3) then twist to the left, leading with your elbows. After a couple of cycles, add the following breathing pattern: Breathe out as you twist to the side, breathe in as you return to the front, breathe out to the other side, breathe in to the front, and so on. Do three to five repetitions in each direction. In this exercise your head should turn with your body so that there is no extra twist to the neck. (If you have back pain, don't do this exercise.)

Exercises and Poses

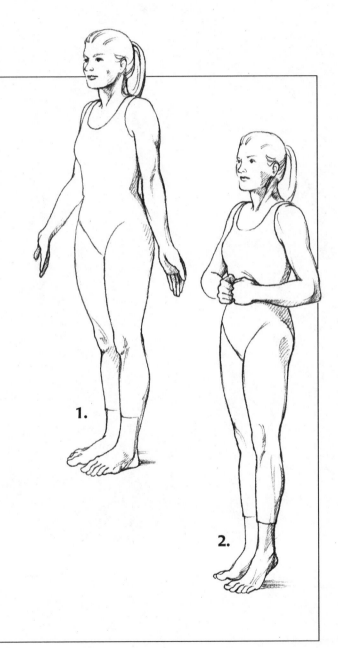

Easy Balance

Stand with your arms at your sides and exhale. (1) Start to inhale, bringing your arms out slightly and rising up on your toes. Fix your gaze on one spot to help you balance. (2) After you've completed your inhalation, make your hands into fists and press them into your diaphragm — just below your rib cage — while holding your breath in. Hold for just a second. Then relax, breathe out, and come back down on your heels, with your arms relaxed at your sides. Concentrate on a fluidity of movement as you do three to five repetitions.

1.

2.

Gentle Yoga: The Aaahhh Routine—Continued

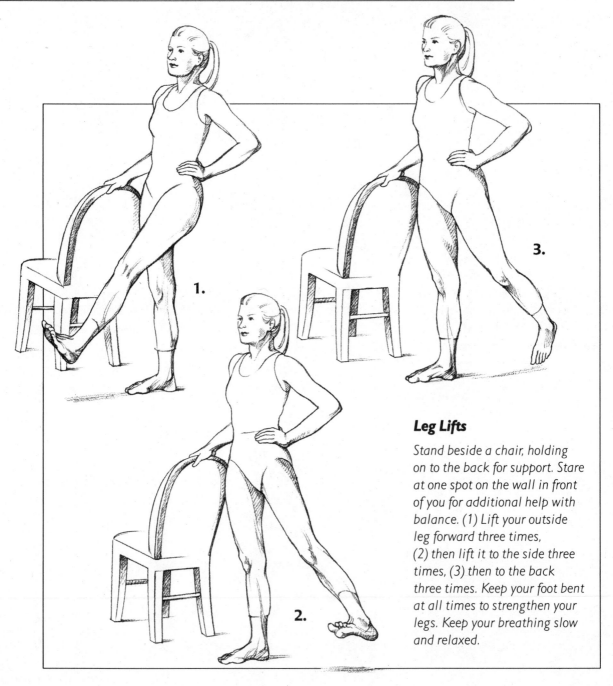

1.

3.

2.

Leg Lifts

Stand beside a chair, holding on to the back for support. Stare at one spot on the wall in front of you for additional help with balance. (1) Lift your outside leg forward three times, (2) then lift it to the side three times, (3) then to the back three times. Keep your foot bent at all times to strengthen your legs. Keep your breathing slow and relaxed.

Tree Pose

Stand with your feet together. To get the feeling of balancing on one leg, first shift your weight to your right foot and rest your left foot on top of the right. Steady yourself by fixing your gaze on a spot on the wall or floor in front of you. (At first you can hold on to the back of a chair or the wall for support.) Pick up your left foot and place it against the inside of your right leg as high as possible, with the toes pointed toward the floor. You may find it easier to hold your foot in place if you are barefoot. If your foot will not go high enough to rest on your inner thigh, just brace it against your knee. Try to breathe steadily. Consciously relax your breath by relaxing your abdominal muscles. When you feel that your balance is steady enough to let go of your chair support, slowly raise your arms straight up overhead with your palms together. Keep breathing normally. Hold for about 10 seconds at first; work up to 30 seconds or more. Repeat once on each side.

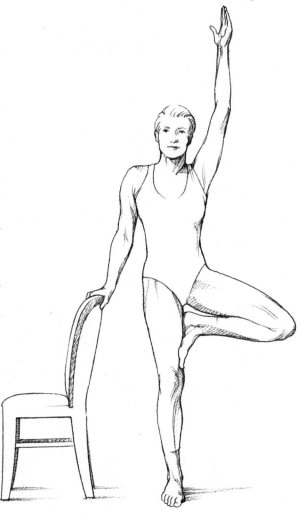

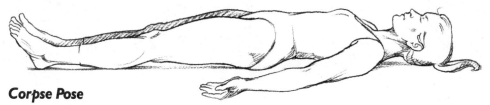

Corpse Pose

Lie down with your arms at your sides or slightly out from your body with the palms facing up. With your eyes closed, relax your face, your shoulders, your abdomen, and *any other areas of your body that hold tension. Just lie there for a couple of minutes and enjoy the deep relaxation that this pose engenders.*

Gentle Yoga: The Aaahhhh Routine—Continued

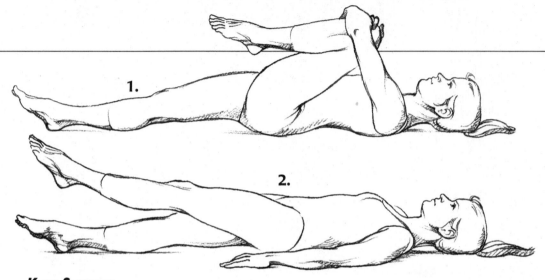

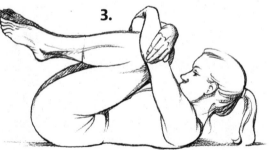

Knee Squeeze

Lie flat on your back with your arms at your sides. (1) Inhale as you raise your left knee to your chest. Wrap your arms around your knee and hold your breath as you squeeze your knee to your chest. (2) Exhale and slowly relax, straightening your leg. Repeat with your right leg. Do three repetitions on each side, alternating sides, then rest a moment, breathing gently. Then try the same exercise, but lift both legs. In this variation it is helpful to breathe in first, then hold your breath while you squeeze. After a week or so of doing the double knee squeeze, you may add the following step: (3) After you squeeze your knees to your chest, lift your forehead as far as possible between your knees; then relax and breathe out. (If you have knee pain while doing this exercise, grasp your thighs behind your knees.)

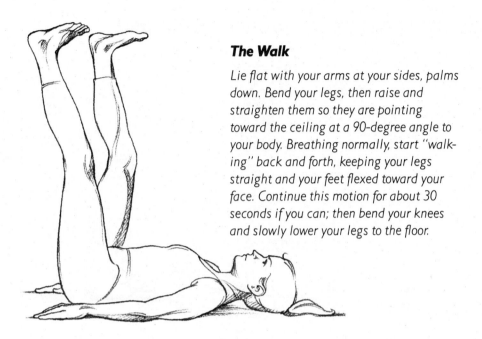

The Walk

Lie flat with your arms at your sides, palms down. Bend your legs, then raise and straighten them so they are pointing toward the ceiling at a 90-degree angle to your body. Breathing normally, start "walking" back and forth, keeping your legs straight and your feet flexed toward your face. Continue this motion for about 30 seconds if you can; then bend your knees and slowly lower your legs to the floor.

Foot Flaps

Sit with your legs straight in front of you. (1) Rest your hands on your thighs and make them into fists, simultaneously flexing your toes back toward you as far as you can without strain. (2) Then open your hands and push your feet forward. Repeat several times.

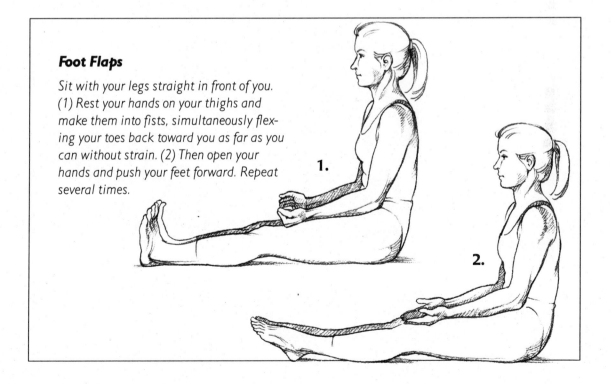

Gentle Yoga: The Aaahhhh *Routine—Continued*

Baby Pose

(1) Sit on your heels with the tops of your feet flat on the floor. Bend forward until your head touches the floor. (2) If that is comfortable, bend your arms back with your elbows out to the sides, so that your neck and shoulders can relax. Your elbows and head should be resting on the floor. Don't turn your head to the side. Breathe normally and relax as much as possible. If putting your head on the floor creates too much abdominal discomfort, try separating your knees or crossing your arms in front of you and resting your head on your arms. (If you have knee pain, don't do this pose.)

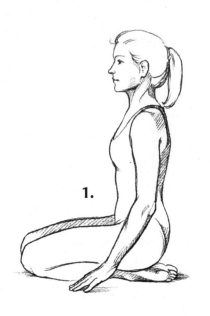

1.

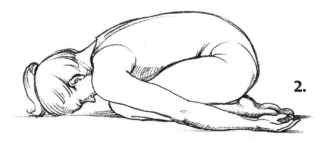

2.

The Complete Breath

To close the routine, do the complete breath again, this time lying down. (1) Put your hands on your rib cage with the fingers just touching. (2) Relaxing your abdominal muscles, breathe deeply into the bottom portion of your lungs. Then continue to inhale, trying to expand your rib cage not just forward but also to the sides. Your fingers should come apart slightly. Finally, fill the upper portion of your lungs. This slow, deep inhalation should be done in one continuous motion. Then exhale slowly. Both the inhalation and the exhalation should be through the nose. Do several complete breaths before you get up and go about your business.

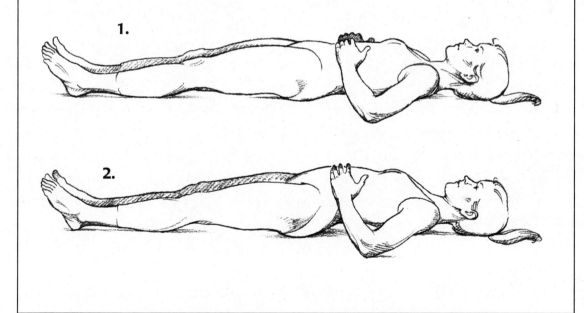

1.

2.

Index

Note: Page references in *italic* indicate illustrations.

A

Abdominal breathing. *See* Breathing, deep
Abdominal exercise
    for constipation, 126
    for fatigue, 149–50
    in resistance training program, 408–9
Abdominal muscles, back pain and, 77, 78
Achilles tendon, stretching of, 95
Addiction, alcohol and drug, 130–33
Aerobic exercise
    aging and, 7–9
    for arthritis, 23
    for back pain, 77
    cancer and, 108–9, 110–12
    for chemical dependencies, 130, 131–32,
      132–33
    cholesterol reduced by, 8, 118, 119–20
    for depression, 134, 135, 137
    for diabetes, 138–42, 144
    for enhancing creativity, 128–29
    for enhancing sexuality, 8, 286–87
    for fatigue, 147–48
    for glaucoma, 160
    for heart disease, 165–75
    for high blood pressure, 176, 178–80
    infection and, 122–24
    for insomnia, 183–85
    for low self-esteem, 206–8
    for lung disease, 210–12
    for memory improvement, 220–22
    for muscle pain, 237
    noise and, 428
    for PMS, 224–25
    in pregnancy, 272
    TMD and, 313, 315
    for varicose veins, 316–17
    for weight loss, 252–53, 254–56
Aerobics, 321–26
    benefits of, 321–22
    breathing during, 323
    cross-training for, 324–25
    injury from, 322
    instructor for, 326
    intensity vs. impact of, 322–23
    low-impact, 323
    music and shoes for, 325
    workout effectiveness, 324
Aging, 3–11
    aerobic exercise and, 7–9
    exercise benefits and, 3–6, 308
    orchestra conduction exercise and, 11
    physical signs of, 6–7
    stair climbing and, 430
    weight lifting and, 9–10, 404–5
Airplane, exercises on, 192–93, *193–94*
Alcohol dependency, 130–33
Alexander Technique, 391
Allergies, 12–13
Americans, older, exercise by, 4
Anaphylaxis, exercise-induced, 13
Angina, 14–15
Ankle exercise
    for arthritis
        flexibility, *50–51*
        range-of-motion, *36–37*
        in water, *67*
    for shin splints prevention, *294–96*
Ankle sprains, 299–305
    balance exercises for, 301, *305*
    range-of-motion exercise for, *301*